Clinical Health Psychology in Military and Veteran Settings

Larry C. James • William O'Donohue
Jeanne Wendel
Editors

Clinical Health Psychology in Military and Veteran Settings

Innovations for the Future

Springer

Editors
Larry C. James
Chief, Behavioral Medicine Service,
Department of Behavioral Health
Tripler Army Medical Center
Honolulu, HI, USA

William O'Donohue
Department of Psychology
The University of Nevada
Reno, NV, USA

Jeanne Wendel
Department of Economics
The University of Nevada
Reno, NV, USA

ISBN 978-3-031-12062-6   ISBN 978-3-031-12063-3 (eBook)
https://doi.org/10.1007/978-3-031-12063-3

This Springer imprint is published by the registered company Springer Nature Switzerland AG
The registered company address is: Gewerbestrasse 11, 6330 Cham, Switzerland

Contents

About the Editors

Larry C. James, PhD, is the chief of behavioral medicine service at the Tripler Army Medical Center, Hawaii, and is the former dean and professor in the School of Professional Psychology at Wright State University. Dr. James is also a retired army colonel and the former chair of the Department of Psychology at Walter Reed Army Medical Center directing weight loss programs and conducting bariatric surgery psychological evaluation since 1994. Dr. James is a fellow of the Academy of Clinical Health Psychologists, and he has been seen as a national leader in the development of innovative obesity treatment programs. He is board certified by the American Board of Professional Psychology (ABPP) in both clinical and clinical health psychology.

William O'Donohue, PhD, is Professor of Psychology at the University of Nevada, Reno. He has published over 80 books and 300 journal articles and book chapters. His interests include quality improvement, evidence-based care, integrated care, and the assessment and treatment of crime victims.

Jeanne Wendel, PhD, is Professor Emeritus of Economics at the University of Nevada, Reno. Dr. Wendel earned her PhD from Southern Methodist University and joined the faculty at the University of Nevada, Reno in 1985. She has published journal articles on health economics and the economics of regulatory issues. She also has experience implementing and supporting a hospital quality improvement program.

Chapter 1
Introduction

Larry C. James, William O' Donohue, and Jeanne Wendel

In the mid-1990s, the first author of this book was practicing as a Clinical Health Psychologist at Tripler Army Medical Center in Honolulu, Hawaii. At that time, not only was he the Director of the Army's Fellowship in Clinical Health Psychology, he was also the Director of an innovative Behavioral Medicine inpatient plus outpatient program. The patients who were enrolled in the program had several comorbid disorders such as obesity, type II diabetes, hypertension, and chronic pain. The patients would be admitted to this healthy lifestyle inpatient program for 3 weeks as a cohort of 8–15 patients and then required to participate with their cohort in weekly group cognitive behavioral therapy (CBT) follow-up for 12 months. The program was very successful, and the author published his work widely (1997a, b, 1998).

On one afternoon, the medical director of the hospital "just showed up" at Dr. James' office unannounced. He posited the question to Dr. James, "Major James, do you have any data to show that your program is not only clinically effective but does it save my hospital money… Son, we've got to make some hard budget decision and if you cannot produce a draft of a peer reviewed paper ready for submission in one year, I will shut your program down." Dr. James, in his review of his program, told an audience that "the medical director lied! He actually only gave me 6 months to demonstrate that my program was not only clinically effective but also that we saved the hospital money. This question, or direct order as it were, to show that the program "saved the hospital money," was a daunting task!"

L. C. James (✉)
Department of Behavioral Health, Tripler Army Medical Center, Honolulu, HI, USA

W. O' Donohue (✉)
Department of Psychology, The University of Nevada, Reno, NV, USA

J. Wendel
Department of Economics, The University of Nevada, Reno, NV, USA
e-mail: wendel@unr.edu

L. C. James et al. (eds.), *Clinical Health Psychology in Military and Veteran Settings*, https://doi.org/10.1007/978-3-031-12063-3_1

Very few if any clinical health psychologists - and psychologists working in today's hospital settings - are prepared to apply medical cost offset as a dependent variable to determine if their program is "effective."

This book fills an important gap: there are no comprehensive psychology books on the market that cover this important topic. The US population includes more than one million veterans who served in Iraq. The long-term healthcare expenditures for these veterans are expected to require billions of dollars of expenditures by the Department of Defense, the Department of Veterans Affairs and private sector payers. The authors bring a wealth of experience in treatment of service members and veterans, implementation of innovative research programs within military settings, and analysis of health economics issues.

The book *Clinical Health Psychology in Military and Veteran Settings: Innovations for the Future* will offer the reader two parts.

Part I will examine key economic challenges facing civilian, military, and veteran healthcare providers.

The economics section of this book provides a broad overview of issues and trends in the US healthcare system. These issues and trends are relevant for clinicians, innovators, managers, and administrators working with military/VA patients because of the following:

- Public sector and private sector healthcare providers and payers face similar issues and pressures.
- Budget systems and payment systems create incentives for individuals working in care delivery organizations, and these incentive systems shape decisions made within those organizations. A conceptual framework can help clinicians and managers analyze incentive design options and understand constraints imposed by existing incentive systems.
- Clinicians recommending care strategies may need to understand enough about Medicaid and Medicare payment systems to design care strategies that are financially feasible for patients who are eligible for multiple types of insurance.
- Psychologists who plan to implement innovative care strategies in primary care settings may need to demonstrate that the innovation is cost-effective. Innovators designing program evaluation studies will need to consider a series of study planning issues.
- Many healthcare payers and providers, including the VA system, are designing strategies to address the "social determinants of health." Familiarity with the evidence demonstrating the importance of social determinants of health and with programs deployed by some private sector organizations can help clinicians and managers identify and analyze strategic options.
- Health information technology (HIT) offers substantial potential benefits and ongoing implementation challenges. Understanding these issues can help clinicians and managers work with electronic health records systems.
- The US healthcare system is continually evolving. Clinicians will need to understand, assess, and adapt to ongoing changes. Understanding current issues and trends will provide a foundation for developing insights about these changes.

For example, Drs. Patterson and Wendel will offer the reader a review of the US healthcare system and discuss in detail its critical components. Dr. Mary Paterson will discuss critical information that should be required reading for all clinical health psychologists entitled "Clinical Practice & Financial Management." As COVID-19 continues to rage upon our healthcare system, Alan Yang and Steve Lebedoff offer the reader a "deeper dive" into advances in healthcare communication and Dr. Jeanne Wendel will offer a chapter entitled "How Will You Know Whether Your Efforts To Strehgthen Patient Health Are Effective and Efficient" which is simply outstanding.

Part II will discuss innovative clinical health psychology applications in military and VA hospitals and clinics from around the country. Each chapter will have a comprehensive literature review and a presentation of exciting and novel clinical applications in the military hospitals. Case reports will also be a part of each chapter as well as easy-to-use "apps" to offer military and veteran patients. In Chap. 9, Dr. Justin Matsuura et al. will discuss innovations in pain management for service members and veterans. In addition, Dr. Matsuura and his team provide a discussion of innovative and future trends in military-related pain treatment strategies for the future. In Chap. 10, Dr. Schumm and his colleges push the envelope and draw the association between chronic pain and post-traumatic stress disorder which is rarely discussed in the current literature.

COVID-19 has had devastating consequences not only on our patients in DOD medical centers around the world but also on the clinical health psychology providers. Drs. Prictchard and James offer the reader a new perspective on the role of clinical health psychologists in the COVID-19 response. Larry James and Aina Katsikas continue the important and innovative discussion on the health psychologists' telehealth applications for the COVID-19 response. These authors discuss, as a result of COVID-19, telehealth applications as well as practical and ethical considerations when providing services via telehealth.

In Chaps. 13 and 14, Dr. Susan George and her colleagues have offered chapters on areas that have never been discussed in a health psychology book. The authors respectively discuss clinical health psychology applications related to transgendered veterans and the health psychologist's role in family domestic violence. Just one example of importance of these two chapters is the work of clinical health psychologists at Tripler Army Medical Center in Honolulu. The health psychology service at this hospital has responsibility for the assessment and treatment of transgendered service member, and there is a paucity of research or treatment manuals for the delivery of behavioral health services to this population. Thus, Dr. George et al.'s work can be seen as critical and a landmark discussion of these issues. Finally, in our last chapter, we recognize that many military health psychologists in the Department of Defense are credentialed to prescribe, order medical labs, and conduct physicals. Thus, Chap. 15 is a very innovative discussion on how to apply medical labs and tests as assessment tools for health psychologists. Chapter 15 will serve as **the** clinical guide for military and veteran health psychologists around the country in doing health assessments for many years to come.

References

James, L., Folen, R., Garland, F., & Davis, M. (1997a). New Frontiers for clinical health psychology: Our leadership role in inpatient weight management programs. *Professional Psychology: Research and Practice, 28*(2), 146–152.

James, L., Folen, R., Garland, F., Noce, M., Edwards, C., Gohdes, D., Bowles, S., & Kellar, M. (1997b). The Tripler LEAN PROGRAM: A healthy lifestyle model for the treatment of obesity. *Military Medicine, 162*, 328–332.

James, L. C., Folen, R. A., & Noce, M. A. (1998). A healthy lifestyle program for the treatment of obesity in minority men. *Journal of Clinical Psychology in Medical Settings, 5*(3), 259–273.

Part I
Health Economic Challenges Facing the Civilian Healthcare Industry

Chapter 2
The US Healthcare System: Components and Functional Areas

Mary Paterson and Jeanne Wendel

1 Introduction

Psychologists delivering integrated care to VA patients may work in Veterans Administration (VA) facilities, or they may work in private sector provider organizations under the Community Care Program. In either situation, these clinicians may provide care to patients who receive some types of care covered by the VA and other types of care covered by Medicare, Medicaid, or private sector insurance. In this situation, clinicians may need to coordinate care funded through multiple sources that is delivered by multiple provider entities. A broad system perspective can support these coordination efforts, by helping individuals working in diverse organizations develop a shared understanding of the constraints imposed by payment system incentives, budget realities, and service delivery strategies. This shared understanding is essential for clinicians working to strengthen the coordination needed to achieve the triple aim (Berwick et al., 2008).

In addition, these providers and payers are working in a system that is continually evolving and creating opportunities and challenges for healthcare providers and entrepreneurs. Clinicians and managers working in the VA face uncertainty about the strategy that will be used to adjust to ongoing changes in numbers and locations

M. Paterson
Conway School of Nursing, Catholic University of America, Washington, DC, USA
e-mail: paterson@cua.edu

J. Wendel (✉)
Department of Economics, The University of Nevada Reno, NV, USA
e-mail: wendel@unr.edu

L. C. James et al. (eds.), *Clinical Health Psychology in Military and Veteran Settings*, https://doi.org/10.1007/978-3-031-12063-3_2

of veterans. Private sector provider organizations face decisions about whether to sign new types of insurance contracts, whether to accept (or make) merger or buy-out offers, and whether to expand the practice or reduce its scope. Clinicians and managers working in both environments face questions about whether to implement new programs and strategies such as integrated care or programs designed to address issues raised by social determinants of health. Continued adjustments in Medicare payment systems are likely. General revenues currently provide a larger source of funds for the Medicare program than Medicare payroll taxes, which were initially intended to be the primary source of funds for this program (Medicare Payment Advisory Commission [MedPAC], 2021a). In this dynamic environment, it is useful to conceptualize the US healthcare system as a "system" comprised of interlocking components that evolve in response to new technologies and new political and social pressures.

This system perspective will be increasingly useful for VA clinicians, if Congress and the VA decide to expand the VA Community Care Program. One source of pressure for change in the VA system stems from the fact that the Veterans Health Administration (VHA) owns facilities in fixed locations while veterans increasingly live in the south and in the west. This is leading to a mismatch between the locations of VA facilities and the locations of veterans. David Roe (Ranking Member of the 2019 US House of Representatives Committee on Veterans' Affairs) summarized the problem facing the VA in 2019: "the VA and the demographics of the country are shifting where, as we said before, veterans are moving south and west. … And the VA needs to be more nimble, I think, in how it is able to move … we can't keep a thousand buildings under-utilized or not utilized at all" (Roe, 2019). At the same committee hearing, Dr. Richard Stone (Executive in Charge, Veterans Health Administration) described the magnitude of the problem facing the VA: "As we sit here today, about 63 percent of our beds are filled; that is not an efficient running system at 63 percent" (Stone, 2019). As of 2021, the GAO rates VA Health Care as a "high-risk" program (Dodaro, 2021). Authorizing veterans to obtain care from private sector providers is one possible strategy for adjusting to shifts in veterans' demographic and geographic characteristics.

This chapter provides an overview of components of the US healthcare system, relationships among those components, and impacts of payment systems on healthcare provider strategies. While we frequently hear complaints about the system, and we might have opinions about strategies to improve the system, this chapter focuses on the task of understanding the existing public/private blended system that has evolved over several centuries. This perspective is useful for clinicians and managers working to build collaborative relationships and systems for coordinating patient care that span public sector and private sector provider organizations.

This chapter includes four sections. The next section discusses components of the US healthcare system. This includes discussions of roles of public sector and private sector entities working at three functional levels in the system and relationships among these entities. It also provides an overview of the historical evolution of the current system, to provide a context for considering ongoing forces for change. Section 3 focuses on payment system structures and the impacts of these structures on provider incentives and risk. The fourth section provides concluding remarks. Each subsection of Sects. 2 and 3 begins by providing descriptions and explanations of the health system components and forces creating pressures for change and then discusses implications for providers.

2 The US Healthcare System Includes Public Sector and Private Sector Entities Working in Three Functional Areas: Funding, Administering, and Providing Care

2.1 Funding Healthcare

We will consider the three public health insurance programs administered by the Centers for Medicare & Medicaid Services (CMS): Medicare which provides health insurance for qualifying individuals who are at least age 65 or those who have a qualifying disability, Medicaid which provides health insurance for low-income individuals, and CHIP which provides health insurance for qualifying children and adolescents who do not qualify for Medicaid and do not have other insurance. This section will also note the integrated systems of health insurance and healthcare provided by the Department of Defense and the Department of Veterans Affairs. Smaller public programs that provide care for Native Americans and federal prisoners are not considered in this chapter.

This section will also describe two types of private sector programs defined by their payment and incentive structure: payments made by private sector insurance companies and out-of-pocket payments made by individuals. Private sector insurance companies include those offering employer-sponsored insurance (ESI) and insurance purchased by individuals.

We examine the relative roles of public and private funding sources from two perspectives: (i) percentages of expenditures funded by public and private sources and (ii) percentages of individuals insured through public and private programs.

2.1.1 Percentages of Personal Healthcare Expenditures Insured by Public and Private Sources

Major Private Sector Sources of Funds Services covered by private health insurance accounted for one-third of the nation's personal healthcare expenditures in 2019.[1] In addition, individuals pay for 13% of personal healthcare expenditures out-of-pocket (see Fig. 2.1). Thus, private sector sources provide 46% of the funds for personal healthcare expenditures (Centers for Medicare & Medicaid Services [CMS], 2020).

Major Public Sector Sources of Funds Services covered by the major federal programs (Medicare, Medicaid, and CHIP) account for 41% of personal healthcare expenditures. Services provided by the Department of Defense and the Department of Veterans Affairs account for 4% of personal healthcare expenditures, with services provided by the Department of Veterans Affairs accounting for two-thirds of these expenditures (CMS, 2020).

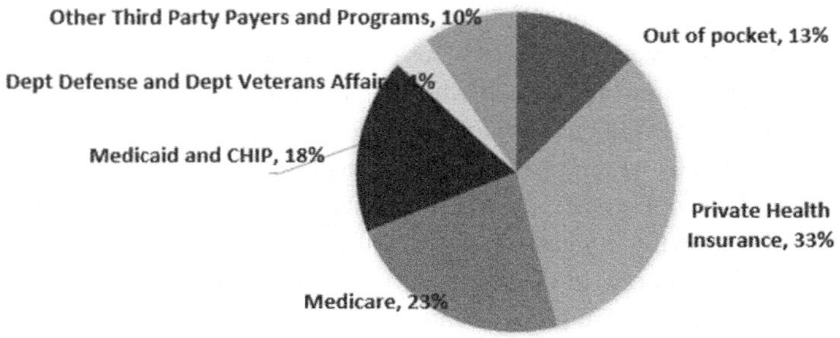

Fig. 2.1 Personal health care expenditures by funding source

Note: Personal healthcare expenditures include expenditures for personal healthcare. It excludes administrative expenditures and health insurance company's operating costs. The category "out of pocket" includes expenditures made by insured individuals, to meet deductibles, make required copayments, and pay for healthcare services not covered by insurance. It also includes expenditures made by uninsured individuals, which accounted for 9% of the US population in early 2020. (Cohen et al., 2021).
Source: CMS, (2020)

[1] These percentages are computed from the National Health Expenditure Data, which are maintained by the Centers for Medicare & Medicaid Services (CMS). In these data, personal healthcare expenditures are defined to include "the total amount spent to treat individuals with specific medical conditions." These expenditures do not include expenditures for public health programs, federal research programs, or expenditures to fund administrative costs of running government programs or health insurance company operating expenses. Source: National Health Expenditure Accounts: Methodology Paper, 2019 Definitions, Sources, and Methods. P 6. https://www.cms.gov/files/document/definitions-sources-and-methods.pdf

Other Sources of Funds The public sector and private sector sources of funds noted above account for 88% of personal healthcare expenditures. The remaining expenditures are funded by relatively small public and private programs categorized as "other third-party payers and programs" (CMS, 2020).

2.1.2 Percentages of Individuals Covered by Public Sector and Private Sector Funders

While private insurance pays for one-third of personal healthcare expenditures, individuals for whom private insurance is the primary source of coverage constitute 56% of the US population (see Fig. 2.2). This includes individuals covered by employer-sponsored insurance and individuals who purchase insurance directly. The difference between the percentage of expenditures and the percentage of individuals covered by private insurance highlights the importance of the specialized roles assigned to private sector insurance and the major public sector programs such as Medicaid and Medicare. Individuals covered by employer-based insurance use relatively few healthcare resources because they are relatively young and healthy. In contrast, Medicare accounts for 23% of personal healthcare expenditures, but Medicare is the primary source of insurance for only 14% of individuals residing in the United States (CMS, 2020).

Each major funder finances care for a specific patient population. Because the characteristics of the covered individuals vary across the major sources of funds, and the covered services vary across the funding sources, the types of care financed also vary across the funding sources. For example, hospital expenditures account for 41% of personal healthcare expenditures for individuals covered by private

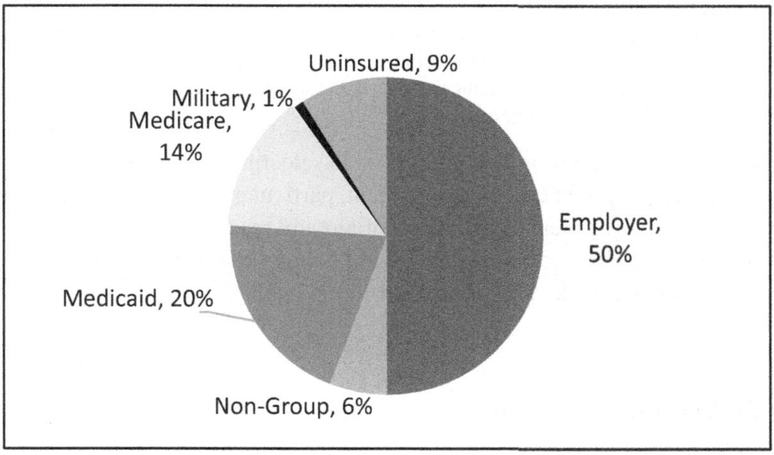

Fig. 2.2 Percent of population by insurance type. Source: KFF, (n.d.)

insurance, 43% of these expenditures for individuals enrolled in Medicare, and 65% of these expenditures for care funded by the Department of Veterans Affairs (VA). Home Health Care accounts for 1% of VA expenditures, while it accounts for 6% of Medicare expenditures. Traditional Medicare does not pay for routine dental care (CMS, n.d.-a), and the Department of Veterans Affairs only pays for dental care for veterans who specifically qualify for this coverage (US Department of Veterans Affairs [VA], 2020). In contrast, these expenditures account for 6% of personal healthcare expenditures funded by private insurance (CMS, 2020).

Because public programs and private sector programs were developed to cover individuals with specific characteristics, some individuals are eligible for coverage from more than one funder. For example, half of individuals enrolled in the VA health system are enrolled in Medicare, 7% of individuals enrolled in the VA health system are enrolled in Medicaid, 28% are also enrolled in a private sector plan, and 8% are enrolled in a long-term care plan (Huang et al., 2018).

The challenge posed by individuals who have more than one health insurance plan is known as the dual entitlement problem. Insurers develop policies to guide the coordination of health insurance benefits. This approach specifies which payer will be considered the primary payer and which will be considered a secondary payer. The secondary payer will pay for items on the healthcare account that are not covered by the primary payer but which are insured by the secondary payer. This "coordination of benefits" is guided by policies written by the insurers that define exactly how the healthcare account for an individual will be submitted and managed.

Clinicians working in healthcare systems are seldom aware of the details of these policies; however, patients frequently engage with this issue. For example, veterans who are entitled to both VA benefits and Medicare must choose which payer they will select for an episode of care as explained in the guidance contained in the Medicare coordination of benefits publication for Medicare recipients:

> If you have or can get both Medicare and Veterans' benefits, you can get treatment under either program. When you get health care, you must choose which benefits to use each time you see a doctor or get health care. Medicare can't pay for the same service that was covered by Veterans' benefits, and your Veterans' benefits can't pay for the same service that was covered by Medicare. Also, Medicare is never the secondary payer after the Department of Veterans Affairs (VA). (CMS, n.d.-b)

Assisting VA beneficiaries or their caregivers in selecting the coverage for a particular health event has a clear clinical component, particularly when the episode of care may overlap with other services the patient already receives or has received in the past from the VA. These are areas which clinicians skilled in communication and patient education may play an important role.

2.2 *Delivering Healthcare*

While public programs fund approximately half of the care delivered in the United States, most of this healthcare is delivered by private sector providers. The Veterans Health Administration (VA) system has traditionally been an outlier, because it operated as a largely self-contained program that funded care, performed necessary administrative functions, and also delivered care in publicly funded VA facilities. However, this situation has been changing. The 2014 Veteran's Choice Act[2] and the 2018 Mission Act[3] expanded the criteria under which individuals eligible for VA-funded care may obtain this care from private sector providers. Individuals are now eligible to seek private sector care if they are not able to access care in VA facilities due to excessive distance or lengthy waits for appointments. Private sector care purchased by the VA accounted for 9% of the VA healthcare budget in 2014, and it served 21% of VA patients in that year (Farmer et al., 2016). The Farmer et al. study projected continued growth of this demand for purchased care due to (1) shifts in the location of veterans from the east and mid-west to the south and west and (2) increasing complexity in the care required due to aging of the veteran population and the associated need for specialty care. In this situation, cooperation and contracting between VA and private providers may increase in parts of the country that do not have sufficient VA care facilities to adequately serve the qualified population seeking care.

Private sector healthcare was traditionally provided by small independent physician practices and free-standing hospitals. However, it is increasingly being provided by physicians and hospitals that are members of larger integrated systems (Furukawa et al., 2020). This trend reflects the results of three related forces:

- Horizontal mergers between physician practices (or acquisitions of small practices by larger practices) are producing a smaller number of practices, while a larger percentage of practices would count as larger practices. Similarly, horizontal agreements between previously free-standing hospitals (or acquisitions of hospitals by existing hospital systems) are producing a smaller number of hospitals with most of these counting as larger hospital systems.
- Vertical acquisitions occur when hospitals acquire physician practices. These acquisitions are producing integrated systems that offer a broad range of care from primary care to specialized hospital-based treatments.
- Competitive interactions may contribute to these trends. If larger entities enjoy lower costs than smaller entities due to economies of scale, the larger entities will grow over time, and some smaller entities will shrink or disappear. For example, larger physician practices might enjoy a cost advantage over smaller practices if larger practices have greater ability to spread the fixed cost of Health Information Technology (HIT; including electronic health records systems) over more patient encounters than smaller practices. In addition, larger practices might be better positioned to analyze patient data and use the results to support quality improvement efforts, and managed care companies may streamline their contracting efforts by focusing on large practices. Finally, practice size is correlated with ability to bear financial risk if the practice signs reimbursement con-

[2] Veterans Access, Choice, and Accountability. Act of 2014. 38 USC 101 note. Aug. 7, 2014. [H.R. 3230].

[3] S.2372—115th Congress (2017–2018). Public Law No: 115–182 (06/06/2018).

tracts that include cost control incentives.[4] Larger practices are also better positioned to handle the financial risk of having an unusually large proportion of patients with high healthcare expenditures. In 2016, only 1% of US families accounted for 20% of US healthcare expenditures, and the most expensive 5% of families accounted for 46% of healthcare expenditures (Sawyer & Claxton, 2019). If a practice has its "fair share" of expensive people, average expenditures will be consistent with actuarial estimates. However, if an unlucky practice has an unusually high proportion of patients who are expensive, average expenditures per patient could be substantially higher than actuarial estimates. The financial risk of having, for example, double the expected number of expensive patients is higher in a small practice than in a large practice (Paterson & Wendel, 1996).

As a result of these consolidation trends, 49% of primary care physicians were affiliated with systems in 2018. More than two-thirds of hospitals and 91% of hospital beds were affiliated with vertically integrated health systems in that year (Furukawa et al., 2020). While there is broad consensus that these trends are ongoing, there is also uncertainty about the long-term impacts of these trends on quality of care, rates paid to provider organizations, and total healthcare expenditures. Some analysts conclude that consolidation among hospitals leads to price increases and hospital acquisition of physician practices leads to increased utilization of hospital-owned diagnostic equipment (Miller et al., 2021; Tollen & Keating, 2020). In contrast, others conclude that increases in physician practice size lead to statistically significant reductions in healthcare expenditures (Zhang et al., 2021).

Private sector funding and provider trends impact VA clinicians in a variety of ways. For example, the VA Community Care Program will clearly require meaningful coordination between VA providers and private sector providers. Ongoing consolation among private sector providers will pose challenges for VA clinicians as shifting alignments of provider care organizations may require adjustments in care coordination plans. Consolidation can also affect care coordination strategies if it leads to changes in payment system structures or risk management strategies used by the VA's private sector partners.

In this environment, private sector provider organizations face difficult questions about the optimal organizational structure for providing care. Individual providers and provider organizations work in a shifting landscape. Fixed costs are increasing for many practices due to acquisition and maintenance of electronic health records systems, reporting activities required by managed care companies and publicly funded programs, and activities required to support contract negotiations. Compared with small practices, larger practices can spread these overhead expenses over larger numbers of patient visits; hence, larger practices have a competitive advantage that is not enjoyed by smaller practices. In this situation, providers must decide whether to merge with other providers, acquire other providers or be acquired by them, or

[4] The CMS payment incentive system for providers with patients enrolled in traditional Medicare, MACRA, includes cost control incentives.

sell to a national firm specializing in practice management. Other industries have gone through this type of consolidation process. This process offers challenges and opportunities to providers, but it is not always easy to distinguish between the two.

Finally, many private sector provider organizations use activity-based costing strategies[5] that constrain excess capacity and tightly allocate and monitor the use of expensive resources such as physician time and expensive diagnostic technology. This is less true in budget-driven systems that have more flexibility in allocating resources within the larger budget envelope. These differences in organizational flexibility can impose strains on coordination strategies. Similarly, DeVore (2021) notes that hospitals with substantial fee-for-service revenue experienced greater adverse financial impacts from COVID-19 than hospitals that derived larger portions of their revenues from capitated payments.

2.3 Administering Healthcare

Private insurance companies and government healthcare funding programs such as Medicare can either conduct the rate setting and administrative functions in-house (DIY approach), or they can subcontract the tasks to a private sector entity. Many funders use a combination strategy in which they use the DIY strategy for some covered individuals, while they use the subcontracting strategy for others. If the VA Community Care Program is continued and expanded, the VA could consider the diverse array of administrative contracting strategies used by CMS and by private sector employers (MedPAC, 2021a, b). The major categories of strategies used by public and private funders are illustrated in Table 2.1.

When an employer sponsors health insurance plans for employees, the process of administering payments is typically conducted by an insurance company or a third-party administrator. The decisions to contract with an administrative entity and the type of entity selected to perform the administrative tasks are typically shaped by the type of payment structure used by the employer. Employers typically contract with third-party administrators to perform administrative tasks when they utilize a fee-for-service (FFS) payment system, and they contract with managed care companies to perform these tasks when they prefer to make a fixed monthly payment for each individual enrolled in the plan.

Some large self-insured employers use the DIY strategy of contracting directly with selected provider organizations. These large employers have sufficient resources to organize, manage, and pay for healthcare administrative functions and assume the associated financial risks. They must also comply with regulations such as confidentiality protections for sensitive health information (HIPAA) and antitrust

[5] Activity-based costing is a direct costing approach that traces all actual costs required to produce a defined service or product. When true activity-based costing is used as the basis for cost reimbursement, reimbursements are for documented costs of production only. Unallocated funds and reserve costs cannot be expensed to the service.

Table 2.1 Administrative strategies for purchasing healthcare by funding source and type of healthcare provider

Ownership of healthcare provider	Funding source			
	Public		Private	
	Entity conducting the administrative tasks		Entity conducting the administrative tasks	
	Entity providing the funds	Private sector contractor	Entity providing the funds	Private sector contractor
Public	Care delivered by VA personnel and facilities			
Private	Medicaid or Medicare with in-house administration VA Community care	Medicaid or Medicare contractor administers payments	Employer uses direct contracting (approximately 10% of private insurance market)	Employer contracts with insurance company or third-party administrator to administer payment process

laws. This approach, which is known as direct contracting, has been adopted by 11% of large US employers (Gaal & Gusland, 2019). The federal Center for Medicare and Medicaid Innovation is testing a strategy for using direct contracting in the Medicare program (MedPAC, 2021a).

2.4 *Strategies for Performing the Tasks in the Three Functional Areas*

Figure 2.3 illustrates the array of strategies used by public programs and employers to perform the tasks in the three functional areas of funding healthcare, administering health care (including contracting, payment, and auditing), and delivering health care. As shown in Row A, the VA was traditionally a vertically integrated organization that performed all three functions. (To illustrate the fact that all three functions are performed by the same entity, the three segments of the bar in the row A are all the same color.) Faced with a growing demand for care, however, the VA had to choose between expanding and realigning their own service delivery capacity or purchasing services from the private sector. Economists refer to this decision as a "make vs buy" decision. The passage of the Veterans Choice Act in 2014 opened access to private providers for veterans who were not able to access care in VA facilities due to excessive distance or lengthy waits for appointments. For patients receiving community care, the VA is the funder and the administrator, but it does not deliver the care. This situation is illustrated in row B.

When Medicare utilizes the FFS payment structure, the federal Centers for Medicare & Medicaid Services (CMS), which administers this program, also administers the FFS payment process, as illustrated in row C of Fig. 2.3. This

		Fund	Administer Payments	Deliver Care
Veterans Health Administration (VA)				
A	VA			
B	Community Care			
Medicare				
C	FFS (traditional Medicare)			
D	managed care (Medicare Advantage Plan)			
E	Accountable Care Organization (ACO)			
Employer Sponsored Insurance				
F	FFS with third-party payer or managed care			
G	managed care plan integrated with providers or ACO			
H	Direct Contracting			

Fig. 2.3 Relationships among entities that fund, administer, and deliver healthcare

includes setting rates, verifying provider credentials, receiving and processing claims, making payments, and conducting activities to prevent and detect fraud. When Medicare utilizes the managed care payment structure, CMS contracts with private sector managed care companies to perform these tasks, as illustrated in row D of Fig. 2.3.

If care is provided by a large integrated provider organization, such as an Accountable Care Organization,[6] this organization may perform many of the administrative tasks as illustrated in row E. In this situation, however, Medicare would retain some oversight and audit tasks.

When employers provide employer-sponsored insurance (ESI), the employer provides funds but usually does not administer payments or directly deliver care. If the employer uses a third-party administrator (TPA) or a managed care company, these administrative entities process the claims and pay providers according to the policy agreements between the insurer or TPA and the employer. Each of the three functions is conducted by a separate entity, as illustrated in row F. Alternately, the two functions of administering payments and delivering care could be conducted by an integrated entity such as Kaiser Permanente or an Accountable Care Organization, as illustrated in row G. If the employer uses the direct contracting strategy, the employer contracts directly with providers. This type of employer performs the administrative functions in-house, typically locating those functions in a unit that

[6]The 2010 ACA defined Accountable Care Organizations (ACOs) for patients enrolled in traditional Medicare. An Accountable Care Organization is an organization of providers, typically led by a hospital or a physician organization. Medicare assigns a panel of patients to an ACO and makes capitated payments to the ACO. The ACO is responsible for providing care as specified in the contract while demonstrating strong performance on quality metrics. Because ACO members include hospitals, physicians, and other healthcare providers, the capitated payment gives the ACO members a strong incentive to collaborate, communicate, and coordinate.

does not share information with other components of the organization. This situation is illustrated in row H.

The possible situations illustrated in rows C–E of Fig. 2.3 indicate that the terms "single payer" and "Medicare for all" are not well defined. Each of these concepts has several potential interpretations; hence, the task of forecasting impacts of these policies is not straightforward. Consider the possibility that Medicare could be designated as the single entity that would fund healthcare for all US residents. The Medicare program could discharge that responsibility by either undertaking the administrative contracting or purchasing tasks itself, or it could subcontract these tasks (Terry & Muhlestein, 2021). The proportion of Medicare beneficiaries enrolled in managed care advantage plans has been increasing, so expanded use of the subcontracting strategy is likely (Freed et al., 2021a). In this scenario, healthcare providers would continue to bill multiple entities, they would continue to deal with incentive systems and healthcare payment policies specified by multiple entities, and they would continue to engage in rate negotiations with multiple entities.

If Congress and the VA elect to continue and expand the Community Choice program, the VA could consider any of these models for administering the program. In addition, VA clinicians coordinating with private sector providers may coordinate patient care with entities working under numerous administrative structures. In this diverse environment, it will be important for clinicians to understand the range of payment structures that constrain their counterparts.

2.5 *Evolution of Public Sector and Private Sector Healthcare Responsibilities: Concurrent and Complementary*

The US healthcare system evolved over two centuries as the government and the private sector responded to changes in technologies and changes in political and social pressures. In this subsection, we provide an overview of public sector and private sector contributions to that evolutionary process, in each of three segments of time. This perspective can be useful for assessing predictions about ongoing trends in the healthcare system.

2.5.1 1700–1850

In these early years, the private sector began to train healthcare professionals and organize professional organizations, while the public sector created a system to fund and provide care for one group: seamen (Kaiser Family Foundation [KFF], 2011). Providing healthcare for seamen was a particularly salient issue because these individuals were away from home for extended periods of time, which meant that they were also away from family caregivers. The work of seamen was also difficult and dangerous, but it was an essential activity for the new nation in need of trade and the commodities that were essential for agriculture and for the domestic needs in the new nation. This trade was supported by private merchant marine vessels that required a full complement of seamen to make difficult voyages across the Atlantic to European manufacturing centers. To finance the new law, the 5th Congress created a mandatory tax of approximately 1% of a seaman's gross pay to be deducted from the maritime sailors' wages and paid by the ship's owner upon entry to a US port. This was the first payroll tax created by the new government (Unger, 2011).

2.5.2 1850–1950

Private Sector Initiatives In the 1920s and 1930s, some private sector employers began providing healthcare for employees (such as employees working in remote locations), and Blue Cross and Blue Shield began offering plans allowing individuals to pre-pay for hospital and physician services (KFF, 2011). These plans were initially developed as strategies to address problems posed by unpaid medical bills.

Dramatic changes occurred during the years 1942–1946. The federal government mandated wage freezes to control the costs of manufactured goods needed to support the military conduct of World War II. At the same time, the government was drafting working-age individuals to serve in the armed forces. (In 1945, approximately 9% of the US population was serving in the military (National WWII Museum, n.d.; Dunn et al., 1945).) Employers faced labor shortages as they worked to produce goods purchased by the US military. While employers were not permitted to offer wage increases to attract new employees, they were permitted to offer new types of fringe benefits such as health insurance. The percentage of US residents with medical insurance increased from 9% in 1940 to 50% in 1950 and two-thirds in 1960 (Carroll, 2017).

Public Sector Initiatives During these years, the public sector created systems focused on public health, and it organized care for military personnel. The federal government strengthened public health through laws such as the Federal Quarantine Act of 1878, the Pure Food and Drug Law of 1906, the Public Health Service Act of 1944, and the Occupational Health and Safety Act of 1970. Federal agencies such as the Centers for Disease Control and Prevention (CDC) (founded in 1946) and the National Institutes of Health (formally created in 1930) were charged with oversight of the public's health, and funded to conduct research and development of technologies and interventions to further the resolution of disease and programs needed to foster the improvement of health (US Department of Health and Human Services [HHS], 2021).

In 1935, the Social Security Act created the system for payments to retirees, but it did not include any provision for health insurance or healthcare for these individuals (KFF, 2011). Bills were introduced in 1943 and 1945 to create universal health insurance, but they did not pass. At this point, unions and large employers backed the concept of private sector health insurance. Offering employer-sponsored health insurance helped employers recruit and retain employees, and it allowed unions to provide a useful service in bargaining for employee benefits. In addition, medical associations opposed the concept of national health insurance (Carroll, 2017).

The federal government delegated responsibility for insurance regulation to state governments in the 1945 McCarran-Ferguson Act, and it facilitated expanded access to healthcare by creating a program to provide funds for construction of hospitals and public health centers in the 1946 Hill Burton Act (KFF, 2011).

2.5.3 1950–Present

Private Sector Initiatives From 1950 until the present, the private sector generated significant advances in surgical and pharmaceutical treatments. In recent decades (1999–2017), dramatic improvements have reduced infant mortality rates and mortality rates for cancers and cardiac diseases for adults aged 45–65 (Curtin, 2019). Notably, the number of infant deaths per 1000 live births dropped from 29.2 in 1950 to 5.7 in 2018 (National Center for Health Statistics, 2021). The federal National Institutes of Health funds basic scientific research, but the majority of funds that support downstream development of these advancements has been provided by private sector entities (Mervis, 2017; Chakravarthy et al., 2016; DrugCostFacts, 2016). Increasing use of costly technologies and pharmaceuticals supported clinical interventions that were more effective and more costly than earlier treatments. Large companies responded to concerns about escalating healthcare costs by moving their employees into managed care during the early 1990s, to incentivize providers to develop efficient strategies for delivering patient care (Lesser et al., 2003).

Public Sector Initiatives As medical advances made healthcare more effective, public concern about uninsured individuals increased. The public sector responded by creating programs to cover individuals who are not typically covered by private sector employer-sponsored health insurance. The federal government began providing coverage for military families in 1956 and for federal employees in 1960. Medicaid and Medicare were created in 1965, and the CHIP expanded coverage for children in 1997. The 2010 Affordable Care Act provided funds to states opting to expand Medicaid coverage for adults and created a system for subsidizing premiums for qualifying adults purchasing insurance as individuals (KFF, 2013). The federal government also created a legal framework for managed care plans, and it prohibited private sector health insurance practices such as preexisting conditions exclusions. These prohibitions were applied to group insurance plans in the 1996 HIPAA and extended to individual plans in the 2010 ACA (Rovner, 2019).

2.5.4 Current System

The public and private sectors fill complementary roles in the US healthcare industry. The private sector role includes training healthcare professionals, setting professional standards, providing healthcare, and insuring individuals through employer-sponsored health insurance plans and individually purchased plans.

The federal government role focuses on funding healthcare for individuals who are not covered by employer-sponsored health insurance and providing a legal and regulatory framework for the private sector entities that fund, administer, and provide healthcare. The federal government also funds healthcare for federal employees, active and retired members of the military, members of Native American tribes and Alaskan native people, retired individuals and eligible individuals with disabilities (covered by Medicare), and prisoners in the federal correctional system (who receive care funded by the Federal Bureau of Prisons). The federal government also partners with states to fund Medicaid, which primarily insures individuals with low incomes (CMS, 2021c).

State governments also regulate the healthcare and health insurance systems, specify state licensure requirements for healthcare providers and facilities, and impose patient protection requirements. In addition, healthcare professional associations, for-profit and non-profit health insurers and hospitals, and various private advocacy and professional, religious, and philanthropic groups create policies and standards. A significant quasi-regulatory function is exercised by court systems as judicial decisions in healthcare lawsuits set precedents. Finally, private insurance companies set reimbursement policies and standards of care that structure payment systems.

As this discussion illustrates, the decentralized nature of the healthcare system in the United States has evolved in coordination with the decentralized federalist structure to be described in the following section. The recent debate about a single-payer system could evolve in two ways. It could be narrowly focused to consider how money will be collected and disbursed to pay for healthcare services that continue to be provided under existing payment and provider systems. Alternately, the debate could be more widely focused to consider alternate system strategies for funding, administering, and delivering healthcare. In each case, all costs associated with the part of the system intended to be managed by a single payer have to be considered before comparing total system costs. There is, at present, no clear answer to the question of which system would be less costly (Congressional Budget Office, 2020). However, evaluation of proposals to restructure one or more components of the current system should not focus solely on total expenditures. Instead, evaluations of alternate proposals should consider value created along with expenditures incurred to create that value. One strategy to accomplish this goal would be to focus on the ratios of changes in expenditures to changes in health outcomes (Baicker & Chandra, 2020).

2.5.5 Contrast with European Systems

The US healthcare system differs dramatically from more centralized systems used in other developed countries. This reflects differing philosophies about the roles of citizens and their governments, as well as differing historical circumstances. The relationship between US citizens and their government is based on a social compact described in the Declaration of Independence.

> Governments are instituted among Men, deriving their just Powers from the Consent of the Governed, that whenever any Form of Government becomes destructive of these Ends, it is the Right of the People to alter or to abolish it, and to institute new Government… (United States. Declaration of Independence, 1776)

This social compact between citizens and their government differs from European monarchical models that defined the supreme authority of the monarch and the duty of the citizen to recognize that authority and serve the monarch. The development of governmental roles in a system that holds the people as grantors of power to the government was a significant departure from the centrally controlled governments in Europe.

Under the US philosophy, healthcare was viewed as primarily a private sector responsibility, with a limited role for government. Further, in the decentralized federalist structure of the US government, healthcare was deemed to be a local responsibility rather than a responsibility of the centralized federal government.

This evolutionary process is ongoing, as new technologies and new political and social issues create new pressures for change. Clinicians are affected by ongoing changes in payment structures, quality-based payment incentives, and regulations. Strategists monitor shifts in relationships among industry components and introductions of new technologies and business models that may affect cost structures. They monitor initiatives in both sectors because policies introduced by CMS such as quality-based payment incentives and bundled payment for episodes of care have been selectively adopted by the private sector and strategies initiated in the private sector have been adopted by CMS (such as managed care). They also monitor pilot programs conducted by CMS to test new strategies. Monitoring these programs can provide insights about potential future policy directions under consideration by CMS, which can help clinicians and managers plan new services or consider extending existing services to new populations. (See MedPAC [2021a, b] for a discussion of initiatives currently implemented by the Center for Medicare and Medicaid Innovation.)

One clinical issue of emerging importance is the gaps in healthcare system capacity highlighted during the COVID-19 pandemic. Following strenuous efforts to reduce costs and streamline the system, private sector hospitals do not maintain standby capacity to handle dramatic surges in demand for specific types of care. Private sector hospitals do not typically undertake this function because the cost of maintaining excess capacity is not a billable expense. The pandemic revealed substantial shortages of facilities, equipment, supplies, and personnel. The strategy of relying on federal stockpiles was also shown to be inadequate due to the ongoing evolution of technology and inadequate funding for inventory control and maintenance.

In addition, the pandemic generated shifts in the types of care needed. These shifts strained the financial resources of some types of providers. A recent study of the negative financial effects of the pandemic on healthcare providers concluded that these impacts were more severe in the United States than in other developed healthcare systems (Waitzberg et al., 2021). The study found that much of the problem stemmed from the prevalence of activity-based payment systems that are focused on a clearly described benefit package with narrowly specified allowable costs and minimal direct government control over available provider capacity (Waitzberg et al., 2021). In the current system, healthcare providers optimize capacity to serve payers by offering interventional approaches that are carefully costed and tailored to the exact benefits the payers are willing to fund. It is well known that services such as general patient and community education, family support, and communicable disease control strategies are generally outside the parameters of payer contracts and therefore not included in provider capacity planning. The pandemic highlighted the fact that maintenance of standby capacity is also outside the parameters of payer contracts.

Systems in countries that have a higher percentage of budget-driven payment can be more resilient with respect to demand surges, if they are able to redirect existing budgeted resources in emergency situations. Eventually budgets will have to be supplemented or adjusted to account for emergency resource diversions, but some flexibility provided by drawing on existing budgeted funds in unplanned ways exists in most budgeted systems. This flexibility has also been observed in the VA, one of the few major US healthcare systems that is largely budget-driven. However, as the blended approach expands in the VA system with the projected expansion of community care, attention should be directed to preserving system flexibility. The VA client base is composed of military service members who may develop unexpected needs based on combat exposure effects that are slow to manifest themselves. These maladies cannot be anticipated but may prove to require different services or approaches that cannot be adequately described in community contracts for VA member care. Clearly, VA clinicians are needed to identify, describe, and support such care delivery needs and contribute to private sector contract adjustments that are evidence-based and adequate to handle these needs.

The type of system stress demonstrated during the pandemic could lead to policy initiatives designed to increase the system's standby capacity and flexibility. Policymakers could consider an array of strategies. Medicare payments to providers could include explicit payments for maintaining excess capacity regarding facilities, supplies, and staff. Alternately, they could look at models used for essential industries outside the healthcare industry such as the utility industry. Traditionally, state regulators have required regulated utilities to maintain specific amounts of "reserve capacity," and some rate structures have included specific payments for capacity.

Another important trend, that is often understated, is the evolution of the role of the patient and the family in this complex system. Patients and families face significant financial and informational requirements in this evolving public/private system. Patient choice in this new system is supported in many areas for which information to enable wise choices may be lacking. Development of evidence-based patient education systems and support is needed. These activities may or may not be reimbursed directly; hence, clear evidence of impacts and cost-effectiveness may be needed. This will require program developers to acquire detailed knowledge of payment systems and incentive systems.

A third issue that may generate health system change focuses on the current law prohibiting CMS from negotiating prices with pharmaceutical companies. Policymakers are concerned about current prices paid by patients, Medicare managed care plans, and drug plans that are currently buying drugs. They are also concerned about potential impacts of new regulations and policies on the pace of new drug research and development. Current research efforts may generate new life-saving or life-enhancing treatments for future patients; hence, policies that slow the pace of innovation could harm future patients (Cubanski et al., 2019).

A fourth issue generating health system change focuses on emerging technologies such as telehealth and mobile apps and devices. DeVore (2021) reports recent survey results indicating that 96% of large self-insured employers intend to offer telehealth services (including behavioral health) by 2023. Implementation details may be affected by state decisions on licensure laws and state decisions regarding the Psychology Interjurisdictional Compact (PSYPACT).

3 Payment Systems

Two payment structures are widely used by major publicly funded programs and by private sector insurance companies: fee-for-service (FFS) payment and capitated payment. Each structure is accompanied by an array of variations; however, we will focus on the central features of each structure.

3.1 Fee-for-Service Payment Structure

Under the FFS payment structure, providers are paid for each covered service or procedure they perform. The FFS payment system is also known as a "retrospective" payment system because the payment is computed after the payer receives information about services actually delivered.

3.1.1 Implementing FFS: Tasks and Issues

Implementing the FFS payment structure places substantial responsibilities on the funder. We will discuss two necessary tasks involved in administering an FFS system, including (i) setting rates that facilitate smooth operation of the healthcare system and (ii) structuring incentives that induce provider organizations to design systems that support provision of high-quality care that is also cost effective.

3.1.2 CMS Method to Set Rates

The FFS side of Medicare is a large purchaser in the healthcare market. CMS has established codes for thousands of medical services and procedures, and it must set rates for each coded service delivered to individuals enrolled in Medicare (CMS, 2021a). In addition, state Medicaid programs set rates for services delivered to Medicaid recipients.

CMS has traditionally used a cost-based system to set rates for ambulatory care procedures that reflect three types of costs: clinician work, the practice's expenses associated with the service or procedure, and the cost of malpractice insurance associated with the task. On average, the clinician work component accounts for 50% of these costs. The factors considered in estimating the amount of clinician work are the time and technical skill required to complete the procedure or service, the physical and mental effort and judgment required, and the stress associated with potential risk to the patient (AMA/Specialty Society, 2020).

This focus on setting Medicare fee-for-service payment rates to reflect costs lies at the heart of the current controversy about telehealth reimbursement rates (Ellimoottil, 2021). Under the current cost-based system for setting rates, the rates paid for telehealth versus inpatient visits will be determined by actuarial analyses of costs incurred to provide the two types of visits and the clinical effort required to provide each type of visit. Whether the two sets of costs and efforts are comparable is currently under debate. However, a different perspective is offered by analysts who argue that value-based payment would be a more appropriate strategy for determining rates for telehealth visits. This would require detailed analyses of the impacts of telehealth on patient outcomes, on provider efficiency, and on issues such as health disparities. One organization (Alliance of Community Health Plans) has proposed a multiyear strategy for undertaking these analyses (Morenz & Liao, 2021).

Rate-setting methods are important because system-wide inefficiencies are created when rates do not accurately reflect costs. Because Medicare and Medicaid account for substantial proportions of healthcare expenditures, specific details in the payment systems used by these programs can create inefficiencies in the healthcare system. Provider organizations must continually adjust their financial and administrative systems to accommodate changes in Medicare and Medicaid payment requirements such as prospective payment, diagnosis-related group (DRG) billing, and limits on indirect cost pass-through. In addition, state Medicaid payment rates are typically substantially lower than the rates set by Medicare (Mendoza, 2020). Medicaid payments typically cover the hospital's operating costs for treating Medicaid recipients, but they do not cover the hospital's fixed costs. Part of the reason that some or all indirect costs (including fixed costs) are not covered by Medicaid is that reimbursement rates defined by this payer are set by administrative processes rather than by negotiation between providers and payers. In addition, these Medicaid rate structures frequently contain efficiency incentives that are not always uniformly applicable or equitable for all acute care facilities (Mendoza, 2020). A recent randomized study of hospital cost recovery in one state found that Medicaid and CHIP reimbursement covered 80% of total costs (Mendoza, 2020).

The same study concluded that Medicare reimbursement covered 85% of hospital total costs, and a 2019 report concluded that Medicare payments do not, on average, fully cover the costs hospitals incur to treat patients covered by Medicare (MedPAC, 2019; Goodson et al., 2021).

Privately owned and operated hospitals must ensure, for their continuing survival, that total revenues cover total costs. Hospitals achieve this by setting rates for individuals covered by private insurance that cover both the cost of treating those patients and the loss incurred by treating Medicaid and Medicare patients. (This cross-shift from private sector payers to cover unreimbursed costs incurred treating Medicare and Medicaid patients contributes to the complexities of estimating the financial impacts of shifting to a single payer or Medicare-for-all system.)

A recent review of the literature on healthcare cost recovery noted that private insurers paid nearly double the Medicare rates for hospital services (Lopez et al., 2020). Debate is ongoing about the cost-shift between the public and private sector in healthcare services. Some private insurance companies require hospitals to provide Medicare cost reports during the rate negotiation process, to justify the rates they propose. This cost-shift also contributes to ongoing debates about hospital price transparency and surprise bills. Advocates for new regulations correctly argue that hospital pricing systems are opaque; however, the proposals do not typically address the underlying cost-shift (Rao et al., 2021; Keith et al., 2021). Public systems are subject to political pressures from a variety of constituents, and the prices such systems pay for care are highly debated and frequently adjusted to try to create appropriate incentives as well as fair reimbursement for providers together with efficient and effective care for consumers. For example, there are a variety of Medicare demonstration projects that experiment with and evaluate new payment systems designed to incentivize value rather than volume of healthcare services for Medicare enrollees. If the VA Community Care Program expands, this private sector cost-shifting situation may pose challenges for VA negotiations with private sector providers.

In addition, these rate-setting approaches and changes generate subtle, and sometimes overlooked, impacts because Medicaid and Medicare rates have substantial impacts on healthcare provider business and caregiving strategies. Physician practices and hospitals monitor proportions of patients covered by Medicaid, Medicare, and private sector insurance carefully. (Private sector insurance companies are also known as "commercial payers.") Providers lose money treating patients covered by Medicaid because of the strict control of costs not directly related to the episode of care and their revenues exceed costs when they treat patients covered by private sector insurance, because these payers are more willing to cover indirect costs. Therefore, providers work to ensure an appropriate balance among numbers of patients covered under each of these systems. For example, they may limit numbers of visit slots for patients covered by public payers, to limit the revenue gap that must be covered by charging higher prices to privately insured patients.

The complexity of the streams of revenue earned by private sector providers may affect VA clinician efforts to coordinate care with private sector providers. The team working on coordination will need to identify relevant services that are (and are not) covered under the system used by the VA to compensate private sector providers and by other entities compensating private sector providers. This will require significant information flow and experience using the coverage information developed in the Community Care Program. VA and private sector clinicians will need to understand the constraints and incentives faced by their counterparts, in order to conceptualize realistic care coordination strategies. Capacity constraints in the private sector also need consideration. For example, if the VA Community Care Program agrees to cover a caregiver education program, the private provider will have to be assured that the volume of VA patients is sufficient to support reasonable overhead costs to establish and run the program. Since most private providers do not have such programs, it would also be necessary to consider start-up costs.

VA clinicians working to coordinate with private sector providers will also need to understand the quality-based and value-based incentive systems facing these providers. This knowledge is essential, because an effective clinical intervention in the modern healthcare system must consider the way payment will be made for care, how care will be measured and evaluated by the payer, and impacts of the intervention on provider scores on quality-based incentive systems.

These systems were developed in response to concerns that FFS payment structure may not provide incentives for providers to develop new healthcare delivery strategies to improve patient health or reduce the overall cost of delivering healthcare. Congress addressed this issue in the Medicare Access and CHIP Reauthorization Act (MACRA) of 2015, which specified a system for adjusting payment rates to the quality of care delivered by the practice or the individual clinician. The new system, known as MACRA, replaced an earlier cost-containment strategy that was widely viewed as unworkable (Aaron, 2015; Wah, 2015). Under MACRA, clinicians may elect to enroll in one of two tracks. This discussion will focus on the most widely used track: the Merit-Based Incentive Payment System, known as MIPS. Clinicians who provide services covered under Medicare Part B are eligible to participate in MIPS, including physicians, nurse practitioners, physician assistants, clinical psychologists, and others.

Clinicians and practices are scored on four performance categories, measuring Quality, Cost Performance, Clinical Practice Improvement Activities, and Promoting Interoperability, with the weights detailed in Table 2.2. The Cost Performance category focuses on the total cost of Medicare Part B claims submitted for Medicare patients attributed to the clinician or practice. The Clinical Practice Improvement Activities category focuses on activities designed to improve care such as care coordination, patient engagement, and patient safety. The Promoting Interoperability category focuses on use of certified electronic health record systems and exchanging health information with other provider organizations and with patients.

In 2017, which was the first reporting year, MACRA included only three of these four categories: Quality, Promoting Interoperability, and Clinical Practice Improvement Activities. The Cost Performance category was added to the system in 2018. For the 2022 performance year, the weight for the Quality category was designed to be 30%, the weight for the Cost Performance category was 30%, the weight for Clinical Practice Improvement Activities was 15%, and the weight for

Table 2.2 Components of MACRA and weights used in 2019 and 2021

	Performance year	
	2017	2022
Quality	60%	30%
Cost performance[a]	–	30%
Clinical practice improvement activities	15%	15%
Promoting interoperability[b]	25%	25%

[a]Total cost of Medicare Part B claims for Medicare patients attributed to the clinician or practice
[b]Formerly known as Advancing Care Information

Promoting Interoperability was 25% (qpp.cms.gov, 2021). Notably, the weight for Quality measures was scheduled to decline from 60% in 2017 to 30% in 2022, while the weight for Cost Performance increased from 0% to 30%.

Payments to clinicians and practices with relatively low scores will be reduced, and payments to those with relatively high scores will be increased under MACRA. The MACRA system is self-financing; hence the dollar value of the penalties must be equal to the dollar value of the rewards. The maximum penalty will be 9% of Medicare Part B payments for the 2022 reporting year. (If clinicians and practices report data for the 2022 reporting year, the rewards and penalties will be applied to payments earned in 2024.) Clinicians and practices with high 2022 scores will receive the "base" amount earned plus a possible 9% bonus, while those with the lowest scores will receive the base amount minus 9%. If a low-scoring clinician earned $100,000 providing services and procedures to Medicare Part B enrollees in FFS plans, they could receive as little as $100,000–$9000 = $91,000. If a high-scoring clinician earned the same amount, they could potentially receive $100,000 + $9000 = $109,000. The difference between the highest scoring clinicians and the lowest scoring clinicians is potentially 18% of the earned $100,000. Clinicians with high MIPS scores may also earn an exceptional performance payment adjustment (mymipsscore.com, 2021).

In addition, MACRA mandates that CMS post clinician-level MIPS scores in its online portal, Physician Compare. CMS has created a five-star system for summarizing the MIPCS score information on this website. In addition, CMS has announced that it will provide Physician Compare datasets to third-party websites that provide physician ratings for consumers. Private sector health insurance plans will be able to view these ratings when they are contracting to create physician networks. Finally, a clinician's performance follows that individual if he joins a different group. If he earned a low MIPS score in 2022, for example, and moved to join a new group in 2023, the new practice's 2024 payment adjustment will reflect that clinician's low score in 2022. Thus, the system creates patient-shopping reputation incentives and professional/contracting incentives along with the direct payment incentives (Terry & Muhlestein, 2021). The VA has begun posting hospital performance data on the CMS site. The site does not report as much information for VA hospitals, however, as it does for private sector hospitals at this point.

The MACRA system offers opportunities for entrepreneurial providers to develop programs that will strengthen patient outcomes while also reducing total Medicare Part B expenditures for the provider's patients. This situation also offers opportunities for psychologists aiming to work with primary care practices to provide integrated care. Reaching agreements with primary care practices may, however, require strategies for conducting ongoing cost-effectiveness studies, to verify that the integrated care program is "paying for itself" by generating sufficient improvements in patient health, and consequent increases in Medicare payments.

Providers with successful programs will receive revenue boosts, while revenues will shrink for less successful providers. Providers receiving higher Medicare payments will be able to submit attractive bids for inclusion in managed care provider networks. Thus, the MACRA system for adjusting Medicare payments also creates a new type of financial risk for practices and individual clinicians.

Carefully designed program evaluation analyses will also be needed to help individuals working in both systems assess the impacts of interventions aiming to boost patient health outcomes. One of the recurrent critiques of the MACRA/MIPS strategy is the weak base of evidence that currently exists to support this strategy for strengthening healthcare quality (McGlynn, 2020).

3.2 Capitated Payment and Managed Care

The managed care strategy was initially created by private sector employers, as a cost-containment strategy. Under this strategy, the employer pays a fixed amount per month to the managed care entity for each individual covered under the plan. Because individuals enrolled in the plan are frequently referred to as "plan members," this is known as a per-member-per-month (pmpm) structure. It is also known as a "capitated" rate, because the funder makes payments based on the number of people enrolled in the plan. The payment is essentially a "per capita" payment. It is also known as a "prospective" payment system because the payment is computed before care is delivered. The amount of the payment is based on healthcare expenditure projections, given the characteristics of the managed care plan's enrollees.

The managed care organization contracts with providers, verifies provider licenses, designs rate structures and set payment rates, and administers anti-fraud activities. Evidence indicates that the rate of increase in healthcare expenditures declined when employers began contracting with managed care companies, largely due to the reduction in rates paid to providers (Dranove et al., 2008). Managed care companies created networks of providers. For a provider, a contract with a managed care organization offered a trade-off. In exchange for the large volume of patients who might seek care from this provider, he accepted a payment rate that was lower than the typical FFS rate.

As a result of competition among providers to obtain managed care contracts, payment rates for most hospitals declined during the "high point" of managed care that occurred prior to the year 2000 (Lesser et al., 2003). The only hospitals that did not experience decreases in payment rates were hospitals that were viewed as "must have," in the sense that a managed care company would believe that it must include a well-known hospital in its network (Devers et al., 2003). Managed care also generated concerns about consumer protection; hence, employers began utilizing hybrid systems with some elements of managed care and some elements that permitted more patient choices.

The managed care strategy was adopted by Medicare and Medicaid programs to pursue the same goal. Conceptually, the managed care plan has more flexibility than a publicly funded program to test and incentivize care management or preventive care strategies and to test strategies for structuring quality-based incentives offered to healthcare providers.

Nationally, two-thirds of Medicaid beneficiaries are enrolled in managed care plans (KFF, 2019). In this situation, the state Medicaid program subcontracts with a private sector Medicaid managed care provider.

Similarly, Medicare beneficiaries choose whether to enroll in a FFS plan or a managed care plan (known as a Medicare Advantage Plan). In 2019, 63% of Medicare beneficiaries enrolled in FFS plans, while 37% elected to enroll in managed care plans (CMS, 2020). Enrollment in Medicare Advantage Plans (known as MAPs) has been growing, and projections indicate that half of Medicare beneficiaries are likely to enroll in MAPs by 2030 (Freed et al., 2021b).

As the proportion of Medicare beneficiaries enrolled in Medicare Advantage Plans has grown, the responsibility for conducting administrative tasks has shifted from CMS to the private sector Medicare Advantage Plans. Private sector health insurance administrative costs account for a growing proportion of total administrative expenditures for the three CMS programs (Medicare, Medicaid, and CHIP), as illustrated in Fig. 2.4. This indicates a shift from reliance on the strategy illustrated in row C of Fig. 2.3 to reliance on the strategies illustrated in rows D and E. This trend has been described as the "privatization of Medicare" (Neuman & Jacobson, 2018).

A recent survey of consumers indicates that consumers switch to advantage plans to obtain coverage for services such as dental and vision care, home visits and care, transportation services, and caregiver support (SYKES, 2020). In addition, some Medicare Advantage Plans have no monthly premiums, while individuals choosing to remain in "traditional Medicare" typically pay a monthly premium. An actuarial study concluded that average costs paid by members of advantage plans (including premiums, copayments, and deductibles) are lower than average costs paid by individuals in traditional Medicare (Mike et al., 2019).

3.2.1 Implications of Payment System Design

Provider contracts with managed care companies specify payment levels and payment structures. While the managed care company is paid a capitated rate, the managed care company may pay providers using either FFS or capitated payment structures. Managed care companies initially used FFS as the primary system for

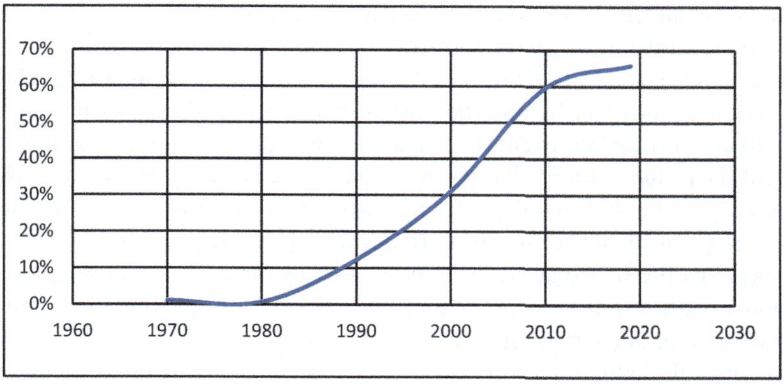

Fig. 2.4 Percent of administration expenditures for CMS programs paid by private health insurance. Note: The CMS programs include Medicare, Medicaid, CHIP. Source: NHE

paying providers. The FFS structure plays a dominant, but declining, role in private sector insurance: a survey of provider organizations indicated that 72% of provider revenue from treating privately insured patients was administered through the FFS structure in 2018, which was projected to decline to 63% of revenue in 2020. The FFS structure plays a smaller role in Medicare and Medicaid: 44% of provider revenue from treating Medicare and Medicaid patients was administered using the FFS structure in 2018, and this percentage was projected to decrease to 36% in 2020 (Speed & Stempniewicz, 2019).

Under the managed care strategy, the provider receives a fixed payment each month for each individual enrolled in the plan. In return, the provider agrees to provide all care required for the enrolled individuals within the categories specified in the managed care contract. In some cases, there are financial strategies for managing catastrophic expenses such as accidents or other major health calamities that exceed the usual healthcare expenses. These situations are usually decided on a case-by-case basis between the provider and the insurer.

If the managed care company owns a provider group or network, such as the Kaiser healthcare system, the providers are usually salaried employees who may also have access to performance bonuses and other incentives for providing quality care.

One of the major implications of these payment arrangements for clinicians is that some useful activities are not covered by health insurance plans, or by managed care plans, because they are not "insurable events." An insurable event is, by definition, an expensive uncertain event. If the event is certain to occur, or if it is not an expensive event, it does not make sense to insure it, because insurance adds additional costs (due to the cost of necessary administrative activities and the risk born by the insurer) to the cost generated by inexpensive or predictable event. The additional cost is known as the "cost of the insurance policy." All insurers incur costs to administer processes for collection of premiums, payment of claims, management of contracts, compliance with all pertinent regulations, and wise stewardship of funds. In order to remain in business, insurers need to set a premium that is sufficient to cover the cost of the event as well as the cost of the administrative tasks and the cost of bearing risk. If the insurer writes a policy to cover a certain event, the insurance for that event will cost more than the event itself due to these charges. A rational consumer or purchaser would not choose to pay the additional premium costs but would rather save the needed funds to pay out-of-pocket for the certain event and essentially self-insure. This logic explains the fact that car insurance policies typically cover damage from collisions, but not routine maintenance such as oil changes. It also explains the fact that car insurance premiums for low-deductible policies are higher than premiums for high-deductible policies: it makes sense to focus on insuring events that are unpredictable and expensive.

Some events such as pregnancy generate some predictable expenditures and some unpredictable expenditures. Insurers build the premium for these events by recognizing the certain costs and estimating the potential costs, weighed by probability that these potential costs will occur, and then adding an administrative fee and a risk premium. A purely rational consumer would choose to pay the certain costs of pregnancy and insure only for the unforeseen event of a complication. However, the convenience of insurance coverage for the entire event and the likelihood that prenatal care may reduce the probability of complications are important reasons that pregnancy and delivery are usually covered in group health insurance policies.

Insurers also consider such issues as the efficacy vs cost of new unproven therapies. New care technology, pharmaceuticals, and therapies such as gene alteration are uncertain and unproven new strategies that, if insurable, would require a high-risk premium since results are very uncertain. Insurers generally avoid covering such therapies until better information decreases uncertainty and risk. Services such as custodial long-term care, costs of family caregiving, and general health education are not typically covered because they are considered to be either uninsurable events or current interventions cannot be clearly quantified or targeted.

The reluctance of payers to cover unproven services or treatments extends to most patient and family education. Evidence that a particular patient education and/or management strategy is effective must be presented to payers to reduce the insurance company's uncertainty about the intervention. There are exceptions to this rule, primarily in the area of chronic diseases such as diabetes and recovery after extensive surgical intervention such as mobility training (CMS, 2021b). However, in general, specific patient counseling and education programs must be proven to "pay for themselves" through cost savings achieved by decreasing financial risk or through revenue increases achieved by strengthening the provider's contract negotiation position or strengthening the provider's performance on incentive payment systems. These justifications hinge on careful cost-effectiveness studies and participation by clinicians skilled in counseling and communication.

Clinicians considering whether to contract to receive FFS payment or capitated payment face an important decision about risk. If they accept capitated payment, they will bear the risk that a small number of covered individuals may incur extraordinary healthcare expenses. If the funder contracts with a managed care company that uses FFS to pay the providers, this risk is incurred by the managed care company. If the managed care company uses capitated payments to pay the providers, some (or all) of this risk is transferred to the provider organization. This risk transference to providers implies that providers need to evaluate each insurance contract carefully to assess the financial risk involved. To the extent that providers accept risk, they must design strategies to manage these risks, and they must verify that the management strategies are evidence-based and effective. Unlike healthcare delivery systems funded from public budgets like the VA, private sector providers face bankruptcy if they are unable to manage within the terms of contracts they sign. According to the statistics provided by the New Generation Research's bankruptcydata.com, 752 healthcare and medical sector companies (including hospitals, physicians' offices and clinics, specialty outpatient facilities, assisted living facilities, and other providers) declared bankruptcy in 2020. Of these, 458 were Chapter 11 filings[7] in which the debtor retains ownership of the assets (Cody & Douglas, 2021). Thus, there is a clear role for healthcare professionals skilled in patient communication, support and education in these organizations, to help ensure financial solvency and provide quality care. Patient communications must equip the patient to understand treatment regimens on an intuitive level and to support patient efforts to comply with these regimens. This is challenging for provider organizations because it is difficult to design these programs to target patients who are most likely to benefit. Clinical psychologists skilled in these interventions may be able to make significant contributions to these efforts.

4 Conclusion

The US system evolved to include public sector and private sector entities, with numerous interactions between the two sets of organizations. The dramatic increase in these interactions, which occurred as Medicaid and Medicare enrollees shifted from FFS to managed care plans, has been described as the "privatization of Medicare."

A similar (but smaller scale) shift could occur if Congress or the VA decide to continue and expand the Community Care Program. If this occurs, VA clinicians

[7] This chapter of the Bankruptcy Code generally provides for reorganization, usually involving a corporation or partnership. A Chapter 11 debtor usually proposes a plan of reorganization to keep its business alive and pay creditors over time. People in business or individuals can also seek relief in Chapter 11. https://www.uscourts.gov/services-forms/bankruptcy/bankruptcy-basics/chapter-11-bankruptcy-basics#:~:text=This%20chapter%20of%20the%20Bankruptcy,and%20pay%20creditors%20over%20time

and private sector providers treating patients under this program will devise new strategies for coordinating care across the VA system and private sector healthcare provider organizations. System-level perspectives and broad knowledge of payment structures, constraints, and incentives in both systems will support efforts to develop and implement coordination strategies that align the business models of the VA and private sector providers.

Many of the concepts discussed in this chapter will be new to the clinical reader, particularly in a budget-supported healthcare system. In such systems, providers usually do not have to consider concepts such as financial risk, cost of an episode of care, or coordination of care across systems with varying financial incentives. Our discussions of some of the clinical implications of these functions have focused on examples of the need for cross-system information to support cross-system coordination efforts and trends that may affect those efforts. The continual evolution of care systems, and the technology that enables systems to support increasingly complex goals and objectives, will be more successful if clinicians understand some key concepts of healthcare industry dynamics, financing, and administration. Conversely, those who finance and administer care will need a basic understanding of the clinical issues that are important to the patients and providers they are serving. The material in this chapter is a first step toward a shared understanding of some of these ideas.

References

Aaron, H. J. (2015). Three cheers for logrolling – The demise of the SGR. *New England Journal of Medicine, 372*(2), 1977–1979. https://doi.org/10.1056/NEJMp1504076

AMA/Specialty Society. (2020). *RVS update process*. American Medical Association. https://www.ama-assn.org/system/files/2020-09/ruc-update-booklet.pdf

Baicker, K., & Chandra, A. (2020). Do we spend too much on health care? *New England Journal of Medicine, 383*(7), 605–608. https://doi.org/10.1056/NEJMp2006099

Berwick, D. M., Nolan, T. W., & Whittington, J. (2008). The triple aim: Care, health, and cost. *Health Affairs. (Millwood)., 27*(3), 759–769. https://doi.org/10.1377/hlthaff.27.3.759

Carroll, A. E. (2017). The real reason the U.S. has employer-sponsored health insurance. *New York Times*. https://www.nytimes.com/2017/09/05/upshot/the-real-reason-the-us-has-employer-sponsored-health-insurance.html

Centers for Medicare & Medicaid Services. (2016). *Veterans health administration hospital performance data: Overview of VA transparency and public reporting on CMS hospital compare*. Retrieved 9 July 2021 from https://www.cms.gov/Medicare/Quality-Initiatives-Patient-Assessment-Instruments/HospitalQualityInits/VA-Data#:~:text=Approximately%2050%20percent%20of%20Veterans,where%20they%20receive%20inpatient%20services

Centers for Medicare & Medicaid Services. (2020). *National health expenditure data: Historical*. https://www.cms.gov/Research-Statistics-Data-and-Systems/Statistics-Trends-and-Reports/NationalHealthExpendData/NationalHealthAccountsHistorical

Centers for Medicare & Medicaid Services. (2021a). *Chapter I: General correct coding policies for National Correct Coding Initiative policy manual for Medicare services*. Retrieved 9 July 2021 from https://www.cms.gov/files/document/chapter1generalcorrectcodingpoliciesfinal112021.pdf

Centers for Medicare & Medicaid Services. (2021b). *Medicare & you 2021: The official U.S. government Medicare handbook.* Department of Health and Human Services. https://www.medicare.gov/Pubs/pdf/10050-Medicare-and-You.pdf

Centers for Medicare & Medicaid Services. (2021c). *Medicaid* (February 2021 Enrollment Report). Retrieved 9 July 2021 from https://www.medicaid.gov/medicaid/index.html

Centers for Medicare & Medicaid Services. (n.d.-a). *Dental services.* Retrieved 9 July 2021 from https://www.medicare.gov/coverage/dental-services

Centers for Medicare & Medicaid Services. (n.d.-b). *Medicare & other health benefits: Your guide to who pays first* (p. 26). Retrieved 9 July 2021 from https://www.medicare.gov/Pubs/pdf/02179-medicare-coordination-benefits-payer.pdf

Chakravarthy, R., Cotter, K., DiMasi, J., Milne, C.-P., & Wendel, N. (2016). Public- and private-sector contributions to the research and development of the most transformational drugs in the past 25 years: From theory to therapy. *Therapeutic Innovation & Regulatory Science, 50*(6), 759–768. https://doi.org/10.1177/2168479016648730

Cody, M. A., & Douglas, M. G. (2021, February). *Focus on health care provider bankruptcies.* Jones Day Publications, Insights. https://www.jonesday.com/en/insights/2021/02/focus-on-health-care-provider-bankruptcies

Cohen, R. A., Terlizzi, E. P., Cha, A. E., & Martinez, M. E. (2021). *Health insurance coverage: Early release of estimates from the National Health Interview Survey, January–June 2020.* National Center for Health Statistics. https://doi.org/10.15620/cdc:100469

Congressional Budget Office. (2020). *How CBO analyzes the costs of proposals for single-payer health care systems that are based on Medicare's fee-for-service program* (Working Paper series). Washington, DC. https://www.cbo.gov/system/files/2020-12/56811-Single-Payer.pdf

Cubanski, J., Neuman, T., True, S., & Freed, M. (2019, October 17). *What's the latest on Medicare drug price negotiations?* Kaiser Family Foundation. https://www.kff.org/medicare/issue-brief/whats-the-latest-on-medicare-drug-price-negotiations/

Curtin, S. C. (2019). *Trends in cancer and heart disease death rates among adults aged 45–64: United States, 1999–2017* (National Vital Statistics Reports, Volume 68, Issue 5). Centers for Disease Control and Prevention. https://www.cdc.gov/nchs/data/nvsr/nvsr68/nvsr68_05-508.pdf

Devers, K. J., Casalino, L. P., Rudell, L. S., Stoddard, J. J., Brewster, L. R., & Lake, T. K. (2003). Hospitals' negotiating leverage with health plans: How and why has it changed? *Health Services Research, 38*, 419–446. https://doi.org/10.1111/1475-6773.00123

DeVore, S. (2021, January 20). Health care in 2021: Five trends to watch. *Health Affairs Blog.* https://doi.org/10.1377/hblog20210119.724670

Dodaro, G. L. (2021). *High-risk series: Dedicated leadership needed to address limited progress in most high-risk areas* (Report to congressional committees). U.S. Government Accountability Office. https://files.gao.gov/reports/GAO-21-119SP/index.html

Dranove, D., Lindrooth, R., White, W. D., & Zwanziger, J. (2008). Is the impact of managed care on hospital prices decreasing? *Journal of Health Economics, 27*(2), 362–376. https://doi.org/10.1016/j.jhealeco.2007.05.004

DrugCostFacts. (2016). *What role does private sector R&D play compared to the National Institutes of Health?* https://www.drugcostfacts.org/public-vs-private-drug-funding

Dunn, H. L., Grove, R. D., Moriyama, I. M., Moore, F. E., Jr., Greville, T. N. E., Newman, S. C., Bailey, A. E., Morrison, F. S., & West, H. (1945). *Vital statistics of the United States 1945: Part 1.* Centers for Disease Control and Prevention. https://www.cdc.gov/nchs/data/vsus/vsus_1945_1.pdf

Ellimoottil, C. (2021). Understanding the case for telehealth payment parity. *Health Affairs Blog.* https://www.healthaffairs.org/do/10.1377/hblog20210503.625394/full/

Farmer, C. M., Hosek, S. D., & Adamson, D. M. (2016). Balancing demand and supply for Veterans' health care: A summary of three RAND assessments conducted under the Veterans Choice Act. *RAND Health Quarterly, 6*(1), 12.

Freed, M., Damico, A., & Neuman, T. (2021a, January 13). A dozen facts about Medicare Advantage in 2020. *KFF Issue Brief.* https://www.kff.org/medicare/issue-brief/a-dozen-facts-about-medicare-advantage-in-2020/

Freed, M., Biniek, J. F., Damico, A., & Neuman, T. (2021b, June 21). *Medicare advantage in 2021: Enrollment update and key trends*. Kaiser Family Foundation. https://www.kff.org/medicare/issue-brief/medicare-advantage-in-2021-enrollment-update-and-key-trends/

Furukawa, M. F., Machta, R. M., Barrett, K. A., Jones, D. J., Shortell, S. M., Scanlon, D. P., Lewis, V. A., O'Malley, A. J., Meara, E. R., & Rich, E. C. (2020). Landscape of health systems in the United States. *Medical Care Research and Review, 77*(4), 357–366. https://doi.org/10.1177/1077558718823130

Gaal, M., & Gusland, C. (2019). *Is direct-to-provider contracting a potential silver bullet for achieving value-based care for employer-sponsored plans?* Milliman. https://www.milliman.com/en/insight/is-direct-to-provider-contracting-a-potential-silver-bullet-for-achieving-value-based-care

Goodson, J. D., Shahbazi, S., & Song, Z. (2021, July 8). Medicare's 2021 physician fee schedule: A redistribution that requires further refinement. *Health Affairs Blog*. https://www.healthaffairs.org/do/10.1377/hblog20210706.220969/full/

Huang, G., Muz, B., Kim, S., & Gasper, J., (2018). *2017 survey of Veteran enrollees' health and use of health care data findings* (Data findings report by Westat). U.S. Department of Veterans Affairs. https://www.va.gov/healthpolicyplanning/soe2017/va_enrollees_report_data_findings_report2.pdf

Kaiser Family Foundation (KFF). (2011). *Timeline: History of health reform in the United States.* https://www.kff.org/wp-content/uploads/2011/03/5-02-13-history-of-health-reform.pdf

Kaiser Family Foundation (KFF). (2013). *Summary of the Affordable Care Act.* https://www.kff.org/health-reform/fact-sheet/summary-of-the-affordable-care-act.

Kaiser Family Foundation (KFF). (2019). *Medicaid managed care tracker*. https://www.kff.org/other/state-indicator/total-medicaid-mco-enrollment/?currentTimeframe=0&sortModel=%7B%22colId%22:%22Location%22,%22sort%22:%22asc%22%7D

Kaiser Family Foundation (KFF). (n.d.). *Health insurance coverage of the total population.* https://www.kff.org/other/state-indicator/total-population/?currentTimeframe=0&sortModel=%7B%22colId%22:%22Location%22,%22sort%22:%22asc%22%7D

Keith, K., Hoadley, J., & Lucia, K. (2021, July 6). Banning surprise bills: Biden administration issues first rule on the No Surprises Act. *Health Affairs Blog.* https://www.healthaffairs.org/do/10.1377/hblog20210706.903518/full/

Lesser, C. S., Ginsburg, P. B., & Devers, K. J. (2003). The end of an era: What became of the "managed care revolution" in 2001? *Health Services Research, 38*, 337–355. https://doi.org/10.1111/1475-6773.00119

Lopez, E., Neuman, T., Jacobson, G., & Levitt, L. (2020). *How much more than Medicare do private insurers pay? A review of the literature* (Issue brief). Kaiser Family Foundation. https://www.kff.org/medicare/issue-brief/how-much-more-than-medicare-do-private-insurers-pay-a-review-of-the-literature/

McGlynn, E. A. (2020). Improving the quality of U.S. health care – What will it take? *New England Journal of Medicine, 383*(9), 801–803. https://doi.org/10.1056/NEJMp2022644

Medicare Payment Advisory Commission. (2019). *Medicare and the health care delivery system* (p. 66) (Report to congress). http://www.medpac.gov/docs/default-source/reports/mar19_medpac_entirereport_sec_rev.pdf?sfvrsn=0

Medicare Payment Advisory Commission. (2021a, March). *Medicare and the health care delivery system* (p. 18) (Report to congress). https://www.medpac.gov/wp-content/uploads/import_data/scrape_files/docs/default-source/reports/mar21_medpac_report_to_the_congress_sec.pdf

Medicare Payment Advisory Commission. (2021b, June). *Medicare and the health care delivery system* (p. 50) (Report to congress). http://www.medpac.gov/docs/default-source/default-document-library/jun21_medpac_report_to_congress_sec.pdf?sfvrsn=0

Mendoza, R. L. (2020). Cost-shifting and cost-cutting as joint and mutually reinforcing strategies in the financial management of hospitals and similar healthcare organizations. *Journal of Health Care Finance, 47*(1), 1–25.

Mervis, J. (2017). Data check: U.S. government share of basic research funding falls below 50%. *American Association for the Advancement of Science*. https://www.sciencemag.org/news/2017/03/data-check-us-government-share-basic-research-funding-falls-below-50

Mike, D., Friedman, J., & Yilmaz, G. (2019). Average annual beneficiary health care costs for various Medicare coverage options (Milliman Client Report). *UnitedHealth Group*. https://milliman-cdn.azureedge.net/-/media/milliman/pdfs/articles/medicare-advantage-ffs-benefit-value.ashx

Miller, B., Moffit, R., Ficke, J., Marine, J., & Ehrenfeld, J. (2021, April 12). Reversing hospital consolidation: The promise of physician-owned hospitals. *Health Affairs Blog*. https://doi.org/10.1377/hblog20210408.980640

Morenz, A., & Liao, J. (2021, August 2). Payment to resolve the debate about telehealth payment parity. *Health Affairs Blog*. https://doi.org/10.1377/hblog20210726.882779

mymipsscore.com. (2021). *How is MIPS Score calculated?* Accessed 20 Sept 2021.

National Center for Health Statistics. (2021). *Health, United States, 2019* (Trend tables). National Institute of Health. https://www.ncbi.nlm.nih.gov/books/NBK569311/?report=reader

National WWII Museum. (n.d.). *Research starters: U.S. military by the numbers*. https://www.nationalww2museum.org/students-teachers/student-resources/research-starters/research-starters-us-military-numbers

Neuman, P., & Jacobson, G. A. (2018). Medicare advantage checkup. *New England Journal of Medicine, 379*(22), 2163–2172. https://doi.org/10.1056/NEJMhpr1804089

Paterson, M. A., & Wendel, J. (1996). Managing risk in a changing health care system. *Journal of Health Care Finance, 22*(3), 15–22.

Quality Payment Program. (2021). *Explore measures & activities*. Centers for Medicare & Medicaid Services. https://qpp.cms.gov/mips/explore-measures?tab=costMeasures&py=2021

Rao, P., Fischer, S., Vaiana, M. E., & Taylor, E. A. (2021). *Barriers to price and quality transparency in health care markets* (Research report). The RAND Corporation. https://www.rand.org/pubs/research_reports/RRA1158-1.html

Roe, D. P. (2019, February 27). *VA 2030: Vision for the future of VA: Hearing before the Committee on Veterans' Affairs U.S. House of Representatives, One Hundred Sixteenth Congress, First Session, Serial No. 116–1* (Opening statement). Printed for the use of the Committee on Veterans' Affairs. https://docs.house.gov/meetings/VR/VR00/20190227/108891/HMTG-116-VR00-Transcript-20190227.pdf

Rovner, J. (2019, May 21). Did the ACA create preexisting condition protections for people in employer plans? *Kaiser Health News & Politifact Healthcheck*. https://khn.org/news/did-the-aca-create-preexisting-condition-protections-for-people-in-employer-plans/

Sawyer, B., & Claxton, G. (2019, January 16). How do health expenditures vary across the population? *Peterson-KFF Health System Tracker*. https://www.healthsystemtracker.org/chart-collection/health-expenditures-vary-across-population/#item-start

Speed, C. A., & Stempniewicz, N. (2019). *Taking risk, 4.0: Clearing a pathway to value-based care* (AMGA Fourth Annual Risk Survey). American Medical Group Association. https://www.amga.org/amga/media/pdfs/about%20amga%20family/family/consulting/riskpaper2019.pdf

Stone, R. (2019, February 27). *VA 2030: Vision for the future of VA: Hearing before the Committee on Veterans' Affairs U.S. House of Representatives, One Hundred Sixteenth Congress, First Session, Serial No. 116–1* (Opening statement). Printed for the use of the Committee on Veterans' Affairs. https://docs.house.gov/meetings/VR/VR00/20190227/108891/HMTG-116-VR00-Transcript-20190227.pdf

SYKES. (2020, October 23). *2020 consumer survey insights: Medicare enrollment decisions*. https://www.sykes.com/resources/blog/medicare-open-enrollment-consumer-survey-insights/

Terry, K., & Muhlestein, D. (2021, March 11). Medicare advantage for all? Not so fast. *Health Affairs Blog*. https://www.healthaffairs.org/do/10.1377/hblog20210304.136304/full/

Tollen, L., & Keating, E. (2020, August 3). COVID-19, market consolidation, and price growth. *Health Affairs Blog*. https://doi.org/10.1377/hblog20200728.592180

U.S. Department of Health & Human Services. (2021). *HHS historical highlights.* https://www.hhs.gov/about/historical-highlights/index.html

U.S. Department of Veterans Affairs. (2020). *VA dental care.* Retrieved 9 July 2021 from https://www.va.gov/health-care/about-va-health-benefits/dental-care/

Unger, R. (2011, January 7). Congress passes socialized medicine and mandates health insurance – In 1798. *Forbes.* https://www.forbes.com/sites/rickungar/2011/01/17/congress-passes-socialized-medicine-and-mandates-health-insurance-in-1798/?sh=111b83eb53ff

Wah, R. M. (2015, May 4). *How we overcame the SGR hurdle.* American Medical Association. https://www.ama-assn.org/about/leadership/how-we-overcame-sgr-hurdle

Waitzberg, R., Quentin, W., Webb, E., & Glied, S. (2021). The structure and financing of health care systems affected how providers coped with COVID-19. *The Milbank Quarterly, 99*(2), 542–564. https://doi.org/10.1111/1468-0009.12530

Zhang, J., Chen, Y., Einav, R., Levin, J., & Bhattacharya, J. (2021). Consolidation of primary care physicians and its impact on healthcare utilization. *Health Economics, 30*, 1361–1373.

Chapter 3
Clinical Practice and Financial Management

Mary Paterson

1 Introduction to Clinical Financial Management in Public Systems

Clinical managers need to be familiar with two main financial issues: (1) the money the clinic expects to receive for providing care and (2) the cost of quality care delivery. Because clinical treatment and patient management decisions are fundamental drivers of the cost of care, clinical staff need to have a general understanding of these financial issues and the clinical influences on them. In a fee-for-service system, the cost of care is passed through to the patient or the patient's insurance company. In these systems if a patient is insured, the limits to provider charges are largely determined by the insurer's pre-negotiated fee schedules. These schedules are normally developed by analyzing the usual and customary provider fees in a geographic area and negotiating discounts. These discounts from usual and customary fees are negotiated by each insurer based on factors such as the expected number of patients, benefits design, and the insurer's size and risk management strategies. The revenue expected for providing care is estimated based on the number and demographic characteristics of insured individuals as well as estimates of the revenue that can be recovered from uninsured individuals who pay directly for care. Payment is guaranteed for insured patients as long as the insurer remains solvent, and the provider is compliant with the insurance contract. If the provider also accepts uninsured patients who pay out-of-pocket, the financial transactions between the provider and the uninsured patient are regulated by market forces and government regulation rather than by insurers. The private provider who is not paid for services to the uninsured can and usually does enlist the help of collection agencies as well as legal options to access any property or wages the patient has in payment.

M. Paterson (✉)
Conway School of Nursing, Catholic University of America, Washington, DC, USA
e-mail: paterson@cua.edu

L. C. James et al. (eds.), *Clinical Health Psychology in Military and Veteran Settings*, https://doi.org/10.1007/978-3-031-12063-3_3

Public care delivery systems usually provide budgets for the care required for the entitled patient. Budget-driven healthcare systems manage cost and revenue in fundamentally different ways. In these systems an overall final budget is determined for the clinical unit for a certain budget period. This budget is developed and finalized through negotiation with the public funding authority. The provider of care in a budget-defined system is subject to constraints determined by the negotiated budget including the allowable total costs of care defined by the budget. In these systems budget shortfalls require additional funds, or delivery of care must be deficit-financed. If additional funds are not provided, costs must also be constrained. In extreme cases providers may have to accept delayed salaries and possibly employment interruptions such as layoffs or furloughs. Support staff may also be affected further threatening quality of care. There is clearly a strong incentive for providers to ensure accurate budget projections and to practice within the costs allowed by the budget. This means that unplanned shocks to the delivery system such as unexpected patients needing service or unplanned changes in the services to be delivered are difficult to accommodate and may and usually do result in budget shortfalls. Clinical managers need to be consulted when such shocks occur so that care can be safely delivered regardless of unplanned system change. Contingency planning of this sort is an important process, and clinical staff must have a basic understanding of the budget in order to contribute to clinical adaptation to unexpected demand or other unanticipated conditions affecting care.

The 2015 budget shortfall in the Veterans Healthcare Administration, a budget-driven healthcare system, is a good example of this. In 2015 the Veterans Health Administration initiated an urgent supplemental funding request. In a letter to the Senate Committee on Veterans' Affairs that accompanied this request, the Deputy Secretary of Veterans Affairs stated that if Congress did not act on this supplemental request, the VA would "face shutting down hospital operations by August 2015" (Gibson, 2015). As a result of this budget problem, the Government Accountability Office (GAO) was requested by Congress to investigate the 2015 projected budget shortfall of 2.75 billion dollars that triggered the supplemental request. The GAO concluded that 85% of the budget shortfall was accounted for by higher-than-expected obligations under the well-established Care in the Community (CIC) program (US Government Accountability Office [GAO], 2016). This program was used in preference to the newly established but underused Veterans Choice Program. The causal chain for this large cost overrun in CIC shows that many veterans were newly qualified to use community rather than VA providers because they could not easily obtain VA care due to the distance from the veteran's home or long wait times at their nearest VA facility. The newly enacted Veterans Choice Program allowed these individuals to use community providers instead. Many veterans who tried to access care using the new Choice program in 2015 found that the program was not yet well established. Private provider networks that were required to provide care under the Choice Act were incomplete, and VA clinical staff did not know how to use these new networks. Thus, veterans were referred to the long-standing and more familiar CIC program which lacked adequate funding to serve the volume of patients newly determined eligible for community provider care under the new Community Choice Program.

Much of this problem developed due to the long planning horizon required for VA budget development that did not adequately forecast the number of veterans newly eligible for community care. Additionally, time was needed to establish the administrative structures and contracts required for the new choice program and familiarize clinical staff with the new program. Due to quickly rising demand by veterans newly qualified for community care, there was little choice available to VA providers but to refer newly eligible veterans for community care to the established and familiar CIC program.

The problem was compounded due to slow identification of the budget deficit. The VA did not realize that they were facing a significant shortfall in the CIC program until 6 months of the 2015 budget-year had elapsed. The realization of the imminent shortfall of funds caused the emergency budget request to Congress in June 2015. The essential problem in this delay was the inadequacy of the centralized VA financial management system to deal with projections and expenditure management of claims from private providers under the CIC system. As a result of this severe budget problem and subsequent GAO investigation, the GAO categorized VA healthcare as a high-risk financial program for the following reasons: (1) ambiguous policies and inconsistent processes, (2) inadequate oversight and accountability, (3) information technology challenges, (4) inadequate training for VA staff, and (5) unclear resource needs and allocation priorities. VA healthcare has retained the high-risk designation since 2015 and remains on the 2021 GAO high-risk list (Dodaro, 2021).

Clinical staff rely on financial managers to administer the budget and to manage the patient volume to assure that the budget will cover the cost of the care delivered. However, as the previously discussed VA 2015 budget shortfall illustrates, clinical staff need to be informed about the budget process, timelines, and budget terms and provisions since their patients' welfare and their own livelihood directly depend on sound budget management. Additionally, timely and accurate projections of patient demand in response to proposed legislative and program changes are vital to clinical financing and care. In public care delivery systems, budget matters usually do not disrupt clinical activities unless routine budget projections and monitoring are inadequate. Clinicians can help protect against these situations by helping program planners understand the clinical implications of new programs and by having enough knowledge to contribute in a meaningful way to the development of impact assessments before program initiation. This is particularly true in veteran's health since new programs initiated in this highly visible budget-driven system are usually justified either by potential clinical cost savings or increased quality of care. VA clinicians involved in new programs need to understand how the costs of the program are calculated when asked to participate in initiating or evaluating such programs. The VA Directive 1043 (US Department of Veterans Affairs [VA], 2016) on the restructuring of VHA clinical programs outlines clear requirements and responsibilities for clinical managers in restructuring or starting new programs. Part of the requirements outlined in this directive includes clinician involvement in a business plan, infrastructure requirements for the new or expanded program, and a well-specified evaluation plan including a description of evaluation parameters for quality, cost, patient satisfaction, and program effectiveness.

This chapter will provide an overview of concepts of public budgeting and provide a description of strategies to manage clinical care within a public budget. It will also address principles of budget planning, management, and operational control important to public system clinical managers and direct care providers. Throughout the chapter, examples will be provided specific to budget-defined public healthcare delivery systems. These systems have a unique set of characteristics because of the political environment in which they operate and the constituency they serve. After reading this chapter, clinicians will gain enough familiarity with these topics to knowledgeably participate in budget discussions and planning with financial and accounting professionals.

2 Public Budget Concepts and Characteristics

Budgets require three distinct management functions in both public and private organizations: strategic planning, management control, and operational control (Schick, 1966). Not all these management functions are the concern of the clinical staff; however, all of these functions will require clinical input and management at some level. For example, during budget planning clinical staff will be asked for information on clinical strategic planning which includes but is not limited to knowledge of standards and guidelines for care as well as emerging pharmaceuticals and treatment technologies. Once the budget is approved, clinical staff focus shifts from strategic planning to operational issues such as clinical staffing, case management using available technology, and control of clinic operations. Clinical managers and providers also need to provide some of the information needed to understand and manage external environmental influences through all stages of the budget cycle, as was clearly shown in the 2015 budget problem described earlier.

The larger organization that contains the clinical unit is linked to the community through a web of influences that include the availability of health professionals, the political and social position of the organization within the community, and the opinions of the population in need of and qualified for the organization's services. The public sector exerts influence on the public sector clinician in the form of public regulation, management of the political agenda, and political power shifts that affect the amount and availability of public funds and the spending priorities for these funds. In the previously discussed VA 2015 budget crisis, new popular political initiatives that invited veterans to increase their access to community providers resulted in an increased demand for services that VA healthcare could not accommodate with existing systems. Providers in both private and VA healthcare needed better information and preparation to help VA patients and private providers successfully navigate the newly defined access requirements. Because this information was not yet available, use of the relatively small previously available CIC program was the only option available to referring VA clinical staff facing client demand for the promised access to private sector providers.

The strategic management tools used to understand and manage environmental impacts include stakeholder analysis, development of accurate volume projections, and sensitive monitoring systems that alert clinical managers early when existing projections are proven incorrect. These tools will be discussed in more detail in the sections on clinical inputs to budget management and budget variance management and reporting. Subsequent chapters on data systems and evaluation systems such as cost-effectiveness analysis are also important to develop necessary budget management and monitoring skills.

Stakeholder analysis is an important clinical management tool and explicitly required in any VA proposal for new clinical services or expansion of existing services. Aaron Wildavsky (1988), a public budget theorist, argued that the political dimension of public budgeting, an expression of the stakeholder's will, is the major driver of public budget formation because public budgets apportion governmental resources to reflect the priorities and will of stakeholders who, in a democracy, elect the government. The assumption is that elected officials will faithfully reflect the will of their constituents and make the compromises necessary when there is conflict among competing constituent interests. The public budget reflects the resolution of this struggle. Political concerns pervade the public healthcare clinical environment and affect both management and operational control of clinical services. That is why clinicians need a general understanding of the political dimension of public budgeting as well as the opinions of the end users of services and organizations that represent them.

In the United States, there are four healthcare delivery organizations that are directly funded with federal dollars: (1) the Defense Health Agency for those on active military duty administered by the Department of Defense (DOD) through five DOD divisions, (2) the Indian Health Service for Native Americans entitled to federal healthcare by treaty provisions and congressional mandates administered by the Bureau of Indian Affairs in the Department of the Interior, (3) federal prisoner healthcare administered by the Federal Bureau of Prisons housed in the Department of Justice, and (4) veterans' healthcare for military service-related injuries and illnesses administered by the Veterans Administration (VA). The VA has the largest direct healthcare provision budget of these four organizations and is the focus organization for this chapter. These four programs are not the only federal programs concerned with individual health. The federal Medicare program insures eligible individuals over 65. The federal government also provides funds to states to administer the State Health Insurance Program for children and the Medicaid program for qualified state residents. These large programs are not direct delivery programs; rather, they are public insurance programs operated by federal and state government. In this chapter we will consider only federally funded organizations that are budgeted to directly deliver healthcare.

The VHA organizes care delivery in 22 regional healthcare sectors known as Veterans Integrated Service Networks (VISNs). Currently, these geographic regions must manage multiple revenue sources in order to pay for care. One of the tasks for clinical managers and clinicians in the VA system is to understand the revenue sources that contribute to the clinical budget and to understand the general strategic interests of each contributor to the clinical budget.

3 Strategic Planning and the Budget

The clinical manager and provider in the VHA serve a variety of clients using two main funding sources: federal funds provided through an annual budget and funds provided through the Medical Care Collections Fund (MCCF). These collections include third-party payment for services provided by the VHA as well as direct patient billing for copays and deductibles as allowed. Federal funding for the VA is divided into mandatory funding and discretionary funding. Mandatory federal funding is determined by the legislative mandates that enable the VA to fulfill the promise made by Abraham Lincoln to care for those who have borne the battle and for their dependents. Funds needed to support the basic services guaranteed to veterans by federal law are not subject to the annual congressional appropriations process. The VA services included in mandatory funding for FY 2022 are compensation and pensions, readjustment benefits, and veterans' insurance and indemnities (VA, 2021a). These programs amounted to a 145.3-billion-dollar budget request in the FY 2021 budget submission. Discretionary funding is programmatic funding for the VA to support their core mission; all healthcare services including services such as the community care program established by the VA Maintaining Systems and Strengthening Integrated Outside Networks Act commonly known as the Mission Act passed in 2018 are examples of discretionary spending (McCain et al., 2018). Discretionary funding is subject to the congressional annual appropriations process and to any domestic spending requirements or limits in effect at the time of budget negotiations. Annual budget proposals from federal agencies are subject to Congressional Budget Office review 2 years in advance of congressional action on the appropriations. This implies that most of the budget planning within the VISNs must take place at a minimum of 30 months before funding is received. Figure 3.1 shows a 10-year trend in appropriations and projected appropriation for the VA in billions of dollars divided into mandatory funding, discretionary funding, and medical collections.

Appropriations history and trends such as these provide a useful strategic planning indicator for clinical managers in public healthcare organizations. Additionally, the clinical manager in the VHA system needs to appreciate the interdependence of mandatory and discretionary funding since some mandatory spending impacts directly on planned discretionary spending on veteran's healthcare services. For example, the growth of appropriations over time can provide clinical managers with insights into changes in the funding approach. Figure 3.1 shows the growth in the three types of appropriations from 2011 to 2021. All appropriations have grown over time; however, the growth in discretionary programs has been steadily positive and trending upward. Some of that recent growth has been due to the reclassification

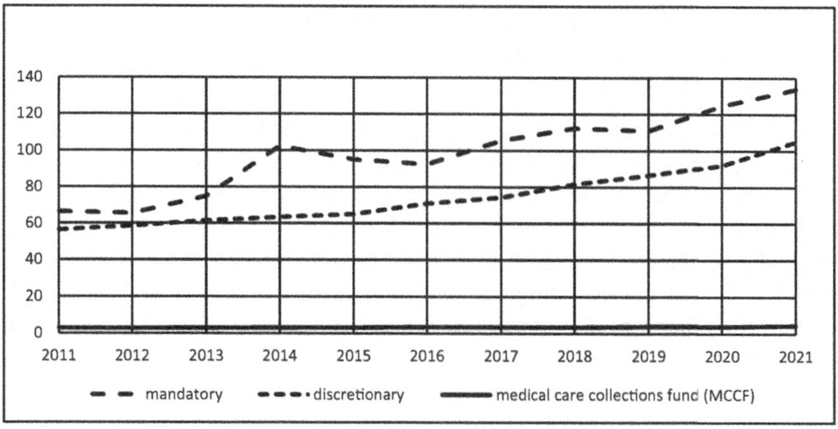

Fig. 3.1 VA appropriations by type.
Source: US Government. Department of Veterans Affairs (2020). Budget in Brief. Retrieved from https://www.va.gov/budget/docs/summary/fy2021VAbudgetInBrief.pdf
Note: Mandatory amounts include $15 billion provided by the Veterans Choice Act in 2014, $2.1 billion in 2017, and $7.3 billion in 2018

of the Veterans Choice Program from mandatory to discretionary in the 2021 budget. This reclassification is an example of the impact of decisions made about mandatory spending that impacts VHA healthcare planning. The Congressional Budget Office periodically recommends to Congress adjustments in mandatory spending that can impact government deficit spending to control the amount of federal debt. One such recommendation is to increase the amount of disability required for a veteran to receive disability payments. If the recommendation is adopted into law by Congress, disabled veterans no longer eligible for disability payments may need help managing their in-home care, required equipment and medications to manage their conditions, and nutritional support. This will impact the kind and intensity of medical treatments that they can receive and may also increase their need for healthcare. Since healthcare is generally part of VA discretionary spending, this change in eligibility in the mandatory spending criteria for disabled vets will directly impact the VA healthcare discretionary budget. Clinical managers and staff need to be aware of these changes and anticipate the increased resource requirements in their budget submissions. As we have seen, supplemental requests may be needed if changes in mandatory programs take place after the regular 24-month budget cycle.

In general, managers viewing these appropriation trends including prospective cuts or reclassification of spending in the mandatory area of the budget should, at the least, be aware that discretionary programs requiring full congressional budget review are likely to increase or change with the need to control mandatory spending. Discretionary programs require annual budget planning and need ongoing data justification. These justifications will require clinical input and evidence, underlining the need for ongoing strategic financial planning as well as program evaluation, and financial and impact data at the clinical level.

4 The Basic Components of Financial Strategy in Clinical Applications

We have established that clinical staff in publicly budgeted systems need to be aware of the public budget cycle as well as the type of budget justifications required for the major financial flows within the organization. These flows will vary somewhat depending on the nature of the public healthcare organization, so the first step in formulating the clinical financial strategy is to understand the budget cycle and major revenue categories within the budget. In the VA example, we have seen that there are three appropriation categories that comprise the major revenue streams into the organization: (1) mandatory funding that is determined by legislative mandates directly related to the VA's core mission to support those who retired after a career in military service and also those who incurred a service-related injury leading to a significant disability while on active military duty. The amount of money provided for the portions of the VA budget that are in the mandatory spending category depends on the number of individuals who meet the criteria for the program, not on the annual budgetary allocation provided in the federal budget. Mandatory programs are not subject to annual budgetary limits such as zero growth and will continue from year to year unless they have been proposed to end or "sunset" after a given period has elapsed. Changing a mandatory spending program to a discretionary program is possible, but difficult. Mandatory program changes are in effect new legislation and are subject to all the requirements necessary to pass a new Federal law. Medicare is a good example of a mandatory healthcare program, while most Indian Health Service and VA health programs are not. The Veterans Choice Program is one health program that was initially a mandatory program with a specific end (sunset) date. When that date passed, the program was eventually renewed by Congress as a discretionary spending program subject to Congressional Budget Office review and annual budget congressional approval.

Fundamental financial strategic planning in the public sector needs to be based, in part, on the type of program that is being planned. We have seen that mandatory programs must be designed to serve all who are eligible and are funded based on eligibility in a given budget period. Discretionary programs such as the VHA must operate within the budgetary limits set during annual budget negotiations. This is a fundamental consideration for the VA clinical financial manager. A foundational question for mandatory program strategic planning is how many enrollees may be expected, while for discretionary programs, the planner must know what budgetary limits have been set. If budgets are not sufficient, the number of recipients for a discretionary program must be decreased by changing eligibility requirements or by planned service delays such as queuing or delayed entry into the program. We will consider each of these challenges in more detail.

Access is one of the most important planning considerations for the mandatory programs that are part of a clinical manager's responsibility. Since all enrollees who meet the criteria for program eligibility must be served, strategic planning needs a primary focus on how many enrollees might be expected and what services must be delivered to them. One of the risks in mandatory programs is expansion of the program to provide costly extra services to enrollees. Since all who are eligible for a mandatory program must be served, program expansion without additional funds increases program financial risk. Data that supports access, cost, and service analysis is vital to the planner focused on these programs. Additionally, deploying financial resources to assure quality processes and outcomes within the allowable budget envelope is both socially and politically important. The federal government is, in a sense, a purchaser of these services for a defined group of citizens. If the citizens meet the legislated criteria for service under the program, they must be served well, or there will be significant political concerns voiced. Elected representatives of these citizens will not hesitate to hold the clinical manager responsible for poor outcomes, as will the citizens themselves and their advocates. Thus, the planning focus for mandatory programs must assure access and provide acceptable process and outcomes for all eligible program participants.

Quality is no less important in discretionary programs. However, a different financial planning focus is required. When considering these programs, the planner needs to prioritize program design and process to manage cost-effective delivery of services with acceptable quality. Careful consideration must be given to how many program participants can be adequately served given the proposed program design. Good costing data that provides the planner with an accurate per capita program cost should be prioritized. This costing data can form a basis for program enrollment design to avoid over or under enrollment and the resulting dissatisfactions that may follow. Planners need to consider outcomes that reflect the intentions of those budgeting resources for the program as well as delivering these outcomes both on time and on budget.

The financial management control of both types of clinical programs will be discussed in the next section. There we will discuss tools and strategies to move from program planning to delivery of service, analysis of outcomes, and assurance of adequate financial data to plan and evaluate both mandatory and discriminatory programs.

5 Budgetary Management in Clinical Programs

Once the clinical budget has been determined, clinical managers turn their attention to budget monitoring. Budgetary control of a clinical program or department requires three important financial functions: (1) managerial accounting that creates and monitors objective data on budget allocations and spending, (2) internal management evaluation and feedback on budget performance, and (3) consultation with and management of external financial stakeholders with an interest in the clinical area's services and activities. The principles which are the basis of each of these financial control operations are (1) budget allocation strategies such as cost classification using tools such as fund accounting, (2) budget monitoring strategies such as variance reporting, and (3) external financial stakeholder identification, outreach, and monitoring. Public organizations usually centralize cost classification, budget monitoring, and reporting so that the financial data collection and analysis is not an autonomous clinical department responsibility. However, it is important that clinicians understand the principles that underlie these activities so that clinical accountability for budget results is supported with knowledge of budgetary process. The Health Economics Resource Center (HERC) (https://www.herc.research.va.gov) provides excellent background data and analysis on VA clinical costs and should be a primary resource to understand VA health cost structure.

6 Cost Classification and Fund Accounting

Private organizations are generally responsible to the owners of the enterprise, which may be privately held or publicly traded through stock shares. In either case, workers in private organizations try to maximize value for the owners as measured by return on the owner's investment. To track these results, companies usually partition their financial data by product or service line so that they can quickly understand which products or services earn revenue in excess of costs and which do not. The most common way to accomplish this is a practice referred to as fund accounting. The cost of labor, materials, and managerial inputs supporting a revenue-producing product or service is allocated to a specific expense fund, so that all costs of production for that product or service are collected. These costs may be further classified into recurrent costs such as labor and consumable supplies and capital costs such as buildings, major equipment, and computer systems. Capital costs are generally depreciated over time to allow organizations to create depreciation accounts that enable carry-over of depreciation funds until the useful life of major equipment is reached. At this point these retained depreciation funds are used to purchase new equipment.

Financial professionals are careful to define the costs important to monitor budget compliance and earnings from services delivered. The following table provides an overview of the common financial definitions of cost. It should be noted that these technical cost definitions are quite different from the definitions economists and program evaluators use to determine overall costs of a given program. Financial and accounting cost categories and definitions are linked to the end product or service produced by the organization and accounted for in operational budget planning. Costs that are not considered include opportunity costs, costs shifted to other organizations, and costs borne by the household or society. Deferred costs that the organization recognizes will occur in the future but are not part of the current financial obligation and are also not part of operations cost accounting. Examples of this type of cost would be future technology or developing pharmaceuticals that are not yet available. All of these costs must be considered in applications such as program evaluations or future planning but are not part of the organization's operational cost analysis (Table 3.1).

Table 3.1 Operational cost definitions

Type of cost	Definition	Example
Cost object	The unit that is the focus of the cost analysis	Administrative units such as mental health services or medical surgical services, units of delivery such as a patient day, a surgery, or a treatment
Direct cost	Costs that are traceable or attributable to the cost object	Direct care personnel, medications, sterile supplies, patient treatments, diagnostic equipment
Indirect cost	Costs that are associated with but not directly traceable to the cost object	Information systems, utilities, administrative staff, security staff, multipurpose equipment such as dietary or general diagnostic or surgical equipment
Fixed cost	Costs that do not change with the volume of services delivered	Facility rent or mortgage expense, communication systems, physical plant fixtures, dietary equipment
Variable cost	Costs that change with service volume	Treatment services, supplies, drugs, direct care personnel
Semi-variable costs	Costs that change after a specific amount of services are delivered	Information systems, administrative staff, housekeeping staff, dietary services
Depreciation cost	The allocation of the cost of a significant asset over its useful life	Assets over a threshold amount that must be periodically replaced due to use or obsolescence such as computers, imaging equipment, communication equipment, or furniture
Capitol cost (Not a direct issue for public agencies; the federal government must consider these costs in the overall budget)	Costs associated with borrowing money, acquiring money through bond or stock issue, or seeking venture capital	Interest and loan origination fees, bond or stock issuance costs, and dividend or interest charges
Recurrent costs	Costs that repeat in a predictable way	Annual or quarterly interest payments, annual dividend payments to stock or bond holders, taxes, and fees

Revenue earned from the sale of the product or service or, in the case of public organizations, the receipt of an appropriation made by Congress is reported in a separate but linked revenue or receipt fund. In the case of profit-making firms, profit is calculated by the simple formula *Total revenue – Total expense = Profit*. The time period used for this calculation also must be specifically stated, to ensure that the calculation includes all revenue earned and expenses incurred over the defined time period. In the case of public organizations, the critical issues for the receipt of budget funds are:

- Purpose of the appropriation (bona fide need of the specified term for which the appropriation is made).
- Time (period of availability).
- Amount (money that is available in the appropriation).

Expense accounts must be linked to the receipt or budget account that matches the budget authorization. Continuing expenses such as depreciation of equipment are handled as part of operating expenses, so that the cost of major investments authorized by Congress is recovered over a stated time period. Public organizations develop the practices of cost classification, fund accounting, and depreciation in accordance with policies and practices such as those developed by the Governmental Accounting Standards Board (GASB). The GASB fund accounting standards are available from the GASB website (www.gasb.org) which is updated as new policies and practices are defined. Information about the practices used to establish funds to monitor government expenditures is important when issues of program costs are addressed. GASB standards are one authority on cost definitions and cost reporting in governmental organizations. Clinical staff conducting cost evaluations requiring financial data should refer to the GASB definitions, Department of Treasury policies, and agency policies to clearly understand program cost classification within overall government accounts. For example, Volume 2 of the Department of Veterans Affairs Financial Policy Manual contains a list of Veterans Health Administration general funds consistent with the appropriations budgetary cycle.

Public organizations also use fund accounting to account for clinical labor costs against allocations provided for the service or product that is delivered. Service providers in public organizations are asked to allocate their time to various activities, each of which may be reported under a different fund or charge code. In some cases, the provider's time is completely allocated to the delivery of one authorized service, and no charge code for fund reporting at the provider level is needed. The organization's financial systems will automatically aggregate the entire provider's salary to one expense fund for financial reporting purposes. In other cases, the providers time is divided according to predetermined criteria. When program cost evaluations are done, it is important to verify that such allocations of clinical time are, in fact, accurate. This is usually done by targeted time and motion studies intended to verify the allocation strategy.

Overhead costs pose a challenge for all fund accounting systems since these materials and services are used in the production of many product or service lines. Allocation of these costs across all the funds related to them introduces reporting and analytical complexity. For example, the cost of complex electronic medical records system that supports all services delivered by a healthcare organization is not what the organization is funded or authorized to do; rather, it is an essential supportive service that makes the delivery of care possible. To illustrate this idea, consider a public sector organization like the VA that is funded to deliver healthcare services to qualified veterans. In order to do this, an electronic medical records system is needed. The cost of this system may appear as a separate congressional appropriation and budget line in the VA budget; however, the calculation of the cost of services delivered to veterans must include the cost of the medical records system. Therefore, the cost of the electronic medical records system must be allocated to each service budgeted for and delivered to VA clients. Financial analysts consider allocation of supportive services to end products or services a problem of indirect cost allocation. Determining the cost of a unit of care, such as a primary care encounter or a diagnostic procedure, must include some allocation of the indirect costs that make care delivery possible. The allocation of a portion of the indirect costs of separately appropriated administrative services needs to be addressed to assure correct estimates of the total cost of an episode of care. Large public organizations such as the Veterans Administration centralize these accounting procedures and practices; the VA Managerial Accounting Office (MCAO) develops and implements indirect cost allocation procedures for VA-authorized services.

7 Cost Allocation

Costs are classified by traceability to the cost object. For example, the cost of clinical supplies needed to provide care is directly traceable to the care provider and the service delivered. Traceable costs are categorized as direct costs. Indirect costs, on the other hand, are those that are not directly traceable either to the provider or to the service. Indirect costs include items such as electronic medical records systems, physical plant systems such as heating and lighting, sanitation services, administrative support services, diagnostic technology services, and security services. Financial systems use various algorithms to allocate a portion of these indirect costs to each of the services the organization produces, so that the total cost for the budgeted service can be correctly allocated, reported, and evaluated. As discussed in the previous section, in the case of public organizations, congressional authorizations may be made to directly support large indirect costs such as a VA-wide medical records system. In this case, the managerial accounting system will maintain a separate account to track expenses for this system. However, computation of the total cost of a patient care encounter will still have to allocate the cost of the medical records system to the encounter before a correct total cost computation can be made. In all systems, allocation of indirect costs uses various algorithms which use estimators to assign costs to units that provide care. These algorithms can introduce distortions in costs since they estimate usage rather than directly observe it. Increased computing capacity has made the use of more precise algorithms for cost accounting and tracing possible so that indirect cost allocation in modern financial systems eliminates most of the allocation distortions. However, no allocation system is as precise as directly observing resource use. Direct observation of all costs, making all the costs of an episode of care traceable, is done in systems known as activity-based costing systems.

Activity-based costing (ABC) methods are often used when precision is required to evaluate cost-effectiveness of new programs or to justify older programs that may be in question. The GASB term for these types of studies is "Service Effort and

Accomplishment Studies" or SEA studies. These studies require precise input cost calculations which may involve a period of activity-based cost observation and data collection. Unlike indirect cost allocation algorithms, activity-based costing traces and documents all program input by real-time observation or documentation. For example, to trace costs such as clinical labor, the clinician is either asked to keep a diary of activities to document the actual time spent in each aspect of care delivery, or an objective observer conducts a time and motion study to independently record clinician's effort. Data from electronic medical records systems (EMRs) may also be used in these studies.

It is easy to appreciate the additional time required to develop costing of activities when observational or direct reporting methods are required. Computer time-tracking programs are available and lessen the manual labor required for ABC cost documentation; however, such costing studies generate large amounts of data that must be managed and verified. For this reason, the duration of costing studies is usually limited to a brief data collection period that may be repeated at appropriate intervals if program characteristics require periodic direct sampling of clinical staff. Guidelines are available to support such micro-costing studies, as, for example, the VA Health Economics Research Center's Microcost Methods Guidebook (https://www.herc.research.va.gov/files/BOOK_458.pdf).

In contrast to specific evaluative cost studies, clinical administrators generally receive routine financial and budget reporting data by fund for which they are responsible with indirect costs already aggregated and charged to each budgeted service provided. If the organization is required to report the cost per visit produced, the financial system can aggregate indirect costs and allocate them to each visit cost according to algorithmic procedures such as step-down analysis. It should be emphasized that these routine reports are estimates of indirect resource use rather than directly observed data. The illustration that follows illustrates the estimation process called step-down analysis. In this example, the indirect cost of clinic administration is allocated to its two clinical departments both of which produce patient visits: primary care and diagnostic testing. The basis of the allocation is the number of visits observed during the costing period converted to percent of total departmental visits. Primary care accounts for 38% of the departmental clinical visits, and diagnostic testing accounts for 62%; thus, primary care is allocated $226,579.00 or

Table 3.2 Allocation of "administration" cost to clinical departments costs

		Allocation of "administration" costs		
Cost center	Direct costs	Percent	Amount	Total costs
Administration	596,734			
Primary care	2,147,687	38%	226,759	2,374,446
Diagnostic testing	617,282	62%	369,975	987,257
Total	**3,361,703**	100%	**596,734**	**3,361,703**
Discrepancy			*0*	*0*

38% of the $596,734.00 cost of administration, while diagnostic testing is allocated 62% of the administrative cost or $396,975.00 (Table 3.2).

Methods for assigning the share of indirect costs to departments that directly serve the organization's client base are the subjects of debates in financial policy. Recent studies of indirect cost allocations in private hospitals report that these allocated indirect costs represent up to 50% of the cost of a hospital day and have consistently risen faster than overall medical inflation (Kalman et al., 2015). Equipment and processes that generate Indirect costs are necessary to support clinical care, but they are not generally overseen by clinical staff. Many debates within the healthcare organization concern the cost, clinical necessity, and quality of these indirect services to the final clinical service or product.

In the case of public healthcare systems such as the VA, indirect costs are allocated by the step-down method using an algorithm developed in the VA Managerial Accounting Office (MCA) and applied to all VA healthcare facilities (Phibbs et al., 2015). The allocation basis of indirect costs in large systems such as the VA may not be transparent and may not appear equitable to clinical managers. Therefore, when costing precision is required, as in the case of evaluative studies of new programs, clinical financial managers will critically assess cost reports provided to them to clearly understand the allocation basis of indirect costs and the percentage of program cost represented by indirect cost allocations. When these assessments are required, it is helpful to have a systematic approach to evaluation of cost reports. For example, each fund that is reported against should be clearly defined so that the manager is aware of what direct costs are contained in the fund, what indirect costs are allocated to the fund, and how the allocation is done. The Department of Veterans' Affairs Financial Policy Manual Chap. 13 outlines the policies used to allocate indirect costs (VA, 2021b). This is an example of indirect cost management information available for use in most large public budget organizations at the federal as well as the state and local level. Understanding of these indirect allocations and policies is essential before program cost evaluation is completed.

Collecting, evaluating, and summarizing clinical budget resources and expenses are the first steps for a clinical financial manager to undertake in developing an understanding of budgets and cost behavior. The next step is to define the services delivered and how they relate to the budget. This step is important to determine costs per service delivered by the department. The clinical department may need to construct internal reports that subdivide the departmental budget into smaller units that directly relate to services provided, or they may find that the department report is sufficient to use in the aggregate. This decision is best made by examining department utilization data to determine whether the departmental cost report is directly related to utilization or not. For example, a unit that provides three discrete services may receive a cost report that is not divided by each service. The clinical manager may need to create some internal department reports that disaggregate the cost data into these discrete service lines. These reports will enable clinical managers to understand more clearly the cost of each service they provide and how best to optimize departmental resources for efficiency and cost-effectiveness. Evaluative studies of clinical programs will usually require a breakdown of standard budget and cost reports to the specific services included in the program. The goal of these analytical activities is to enable cost analysis that relates directly to program goals and objectives. Many such analytic studies have been done to assess cost of care for large federal programs. An example of such studies can be found in the 2018 guidebook for VA inpatient care (Wagner et al., 2018).

Careful identification of the cost object is very important in operational costing. For example, much concern has been expressed in recent reports concerning the cost of mental health services for veterans. A 2011 evaluation of the VA mental health programs noted that veterans with mental health and substance abuse disorders account for a high share of VA healthcare costs (Watkins et al., 2011). This type of costing analysis is not the same as that discussed above since the operations cost of a specific mental health program is only one piece of information contributing to the overall cost of a particular mental health or substance abuse diagnosis. The importance of the cost object, the starting point of any costing study, cannot be overstated in this context. For example, a 2020 analysis noted that in 2020 PTSD constituted 65% of service-related injuries reported by veterans. This finding does not directly translate into VA mental health program costs since a veteran who served in combat or combat support activities is likely to require some type of intervention that can range from simple stress management to more acute problems such as substance abuse or suicidal ideation or attempts. In addition, individuals with PTSD are likely to need other medical interventions that are not classified as mental health services as well as individual and family support services that are not classified as healthcare services. In order to understand the total cost of the reported PTSD injury, the costs of all these services would need to be included. This is the reason that the number of veterans with a particular type of service-related injury does not directly translate to operational costs of mental health services. Much more information is required before cost projections can be made based on the number of veterans reporting a particular type of injury.

8 Monitoring Spending: Principles of Budget Variance Analysis

In addition to using fund accounting and cost allocation to understand department and program costs, clinical staff need a basic understanding of the relationship of spending to budgets. Large publicly budgeted healthcare delivery organizations face significant challenges when trying to accomplish this goal. The purpose of this discussion is to outline the conceptual framework that supports financial monitoring of budgets, explain the possible causes of budget variation within organizations, and provide suggestions for public sector clinical managers to gain an actionable understanding of the relationship between departmental spending and departmental budgets.

The practice of monitoring spending against allocated budgets is familiar to most private sector financial managers. The financial reporting framework is usually designed to produce monthly budget reports that report any variance, either positive or negative, from the budget allocation. These systems may also present some analysis of the reasons for the variance. Actual performance can be affected by changes in the volume of services as well as changes in the cost or amount of resources required to deliver these services. Some of these cost variations can be managed at the clinical level and some cannot. Clinical managers need to understand which variances are within their control so that they can recommend or initiate appropriate clinical actions. Variance analysis is one of the main financial tools to gain some understanding of the reason over or underspending occurs so that appropriate decisions can be made.

Some of the potential drivers of cost variation are:

- The cost of inputs required for the clinical service being provided.
- The quantities of inputs required to support departmental services.
- The type of inputs needed such as technology, drug therapy, or qualifications and types of personnel.
- Interdependent inputs that are not in the direct control of the department such the allocation and cost of nursing or ancillary personnel, medical record system changes that impact clinical time and/or staffing, or any other external department change that impacts departmental clinical management and cost.
- Events in the environment that affect departmental volume or process.

In highly centralized public healthcare systems, department managers may lack information on some of these cost drivers. For example, bulk purchasing of necessary departmental supplies is usually done by a central purchasing authority that does not provide detailed supply cost information to departmental mangers. Sudden changes in the availability or type of clinical supplies can certainly affect clinical time and effort. However, budget reports that identify the clinical supply cost variance may lack the details necessary to account for significant variations at the level of detail needed to understand changes. Detailed cost data is usually available for a focused study of significant department cost changes; however, the manager must determine whether the department effort needed for the study is justified. Controllability of increases that relate to direct costs of care is the first step in this determination. Significant cost increases that persist over time and cannot be easily accounted for within the department merit further analysis to define the source of the cost increase and examine the feasibility of managing it. This was certainly the case in the earlier example of the 2015 VA health-wide excess spending due to use of an existing program (CIC) over the newly established Veterans Choice Program. VA physicians providing care may have provided referrals to CIC because they were familiar with that community referral program. Newly empowered veterans seeking community care exerted pressure on VA departmental clinical or managerial staff to provide referrals to which they were newly entitled; absent clear understanding of the new VA choice program the familiar CIC program was used. Cost escalation in the CIC program was certainly noted in budget reports; however, the systemic cause of the increased costs was not identified until late in the budget cycle. Careful analysis of the root cause of the CIC budget variance would have uncovered this problem sooner.

A simple analysis of a monthly budget variance report may clarify these basic concepts (Table 3.3).

Based on the example above, a clinical manager can see that given the number of RVUs delivered this month, the cost of each RVU in provider's time exceeded the budgeted RVU cost for this number of visits by $30,500.00; the other negative variances seen are technology cost and indirect costs. Most clinical managers would accept a budget variance that is within 1% of allowable cost without further investigation. Therefore, in this case the variances in providers time and technology cost deserve some explanation. The positive variance in supply cost, if too large, might also merit some inquiry. In this example, the manager decides to accept the positive variance in supplies for this month, but she will watch the future trend. The budget overruns in provider's time and technology cost should be the subject of clinical management review to determine what is happening in these areas. Explanation may inform future planning, as, for example, if providers' salary expenditures exceed the allowable amount or inexperienced providers increase the cost of labor. It is also possible that the budgeted RVU cost has become unrealistic due to competition in the labor market resulting in periodic periods of understaffing followed by higher salary expectations. Changes in the technology mix can also affect provider costs since clinical effort is immediately affected by technology. Budget variation analysis is very helpful to future planning as well as stakeholder analysis. For example, in the above case, it would be useful to understand any changes in the external environment that may be affecting the kind of patient being seen in the clinic as well as the technology mix generally required. As in the example of the CIC cost overrun, sicker patients may have elected to remain with VA providers rather than switch to more convenient community providers; the increasing acuity of the VA patient base may have contributed to the overall cost overruns experienced in the 2015

Table 3.3 Example of monthly budget variance report

Cost category	# RVUs this month[a]	Budgeted cost of 1 RVU Unit[b]	Budgeted monthly cost	Actual monthly cost	Variance
Provider's time	4650	$30.00	139,500.00	170,000.00	(30,500.00)
Technology cost	4650	$10.00	46,500.00	50,000.00	(3500.00)
Supply cost	4650	$ 7.00	32,550.00	25,000.00	7550
Indirects	4650	$ 6.00	27,900.00	28,000.00	(100)
Total		$53.00	246,450.00	273,000.00	(26,550)

[a]In this example, we will assume that the volume of RVUs delivered is budgeted for at the rate of $53.00 for each RVU

[b]In this example, care units are based on relative value units (RVU). One RVU unit is costed based on a 15-minute provider encounter plus average costs of supplies, technology, and allocated indirect costs consumed during a 15-minute provider encounter. Development and costing of RVUs based on unit of care are a common way to allocate budget resources

budget. Significant changes in the environment can result in a change in the patient population requiring care. This, in turn, can affect month-to-month budget variances. Since clinical managers must plan future departmental resource requirements at least 30 months in the future, early signals of future trends such as significant budget variances are solid planning aids.

In summary, we have seen that some attention to the nature of costs, the type of costs allocated to the clinical department, and departmental variances from budgeted resources provide useful evidence for clinical administration, planning, and evaluation. The last topic to be considered in this discussion of clinical financial and budget policy is the evidence that can be gathered about the external environment through stakeholder analysis.

9 Stakeholder Analysis in Financial Program Planning and Evaluation

Stakeholder analysis in healthcare management is a systematic way to understand the opinions, preferences, needs, and influence of organizations and individuals who are important to the organization's survival. As public healthcare organizations gained prominence and influence, they also began to use stakeholder analysis to define the relationship of influential individuals and organizations to their organization and mission. In the case of the VA, a Survey of Enrollees has been conducted 17 times since 1999. This survey uses stakeholder analysis techniques to survey a nationally representative sample of VA enrollees to understand such issues as health status, satisfaction with VA services, knowledge and attitudes concerning VA services, and patterns of healthcare utilization. The most recent survey results were released in March 2020 and are publicly available (Wang et al., 2020).

As illustrated by the VA enrollee survey, health services managers may use stakeholder analysis for a variety of reasons such as to understand the relationships between the network of healthcare organizations who serve a population. A hospital may use stakeholder analysis to determine the satisfaction of the physician practices who refer patients to them. Since the source of the hospital's revenue is dependent on the satisfaction of referring physicians, the results of this type of stakeholder analysis is central to the hospital's survival in a competitive marketplace. Stakeholder analysis can also be used to understand the demographics, health status, and use of healthcare services for end users of a healthcare organization's services.

In the case of healthcare organizations supported by federal funding, influential stakeholders might include not only the end users of care but also those public and nongovernmental organization officials whose opinions shape the organization's budget. In the specific case of the Veterans Administration, the influence of the end users of care was, until recently, mainly indirect. This was true because the VA was the only supplier of insured care for those veterans qualified to receive it. End users could influence the quality of care they received by appeal to the VA itself, their elected representatives, or to the organizations that represent them. An important change occurred with the passage of the Veterans Access, Choice, and Accountability Act of 2014 because veterans were approved under certain conditions to seek care from community providers (VA, 2014). This Act was supported by mandatory funding for an initial 3-year period, at the end of which the mandatory program was discontinued. It was replaced with the Veterans Choice Program in 2019. This program, funded by discretionary money, was similar to the 2014 Veterans Access, Choice, and Accountability Act, in that it opened direct access to private providers for qualified veterans under certain conditions. Establishment of this type of program introduced limited competition between the VA and the community providers. Thus, the satisfaction of the veteran with VA care was, in some cases, directly important to the VA clinical community. As previously noted, veterans have always had influence over the care delivered to them through their organizations, their elected congressional representatives, and direct feedback to the VA itself. However, with the passage of the Veterans Access, Choice, and Accountability Act in 2014 and the Choice Program in 2019, they could also seek care from private providers in some circumstances and thus exert significant influence over the VA provider by "voting with their feet."

Since the passage of the Veterans Access, Choice, and Responsibility Act of 2014, consultation by VA providers with end users about their satisfaction with and opinion of VA care has appeared more frequently in the literature. For example, a 2017 research study examining the opinion of female users of primary care at the VA is an excellent example of stakeholder analysis conducted by interested clinicians to assess the perceived quality of an evidence-based approach to women's primary healthcare at the VA (Hamilton et al., 2017). The use of such studies to provide evidence for future clinical program proposals and budget planning is one way for VA caregivers to shape new program proposals as well as ongoing funding requests for resources to support care delivery.

The stakeholder analysis as an internal planning or evaluation tool may be a very limited sample of direct program end user's opinions, or it may be a more ambitious project that samples opinions from many levels of external stakeholders, some of whom are in positions of influence and some who are direct beneficiaries of the program's services. The World Health Organization provides a Stakeholder Analysis Toolkit[1] which provides useful guidance and templates for organizing, implementing, and analyzing such an expanded stakeholder analysis in the healthcare sector.

At the start of this discussion, we noted that clinical staff in publicly funded healthcare delivery systems did not historically concern themselves with financial management. In such organizations, financial management was usually highly centralized and required specialized knowledge not only of accounting and finance but also of the intricacies of government budgets and fiscal reporting. In the private sector, on the other hand, clinical staff have become much more aware of financial management strategies because of the highly competitive nature of private

[1] https://www.who.int/workforcealliance/knowledge/toolkit/33.pdf

healthcare markets and the necessity of compliance with the clinical requirements of multiple payers. Practices such as the requirement of second opinions or the preference for generic pharmaceuticals force clinical awareness of reimbursement requirements that was not the case in earlier eras of practice.

As the largest publicly funded healthcare delivery organization, the VA is an important provider of care for over nine million veterans enrolled in the VA health program. A program of this size will inevitably attract a great deal of political and consumer attention. As the VA health program expands, increased clinical staff awareness of funding policy and operational finance is inevitable. A basic understanding of the concepts of public budgeting and strategies to manage clinical care within a public budget has become a necessary part of the clinician's toolkit. In fact, improving the management of risks and the quality of VA health is one recommendation the General Accounting Office has made to VA health to reduce the high-risk status of their program (Dodaro, 2021).

The skills and practices introduced in this chapter will provide a foundation for further development and application of clinical financial management in large publicly funded healthcare organizations and will ensure that clinical staff are fully involved in important financial decisions that directly impact cost and quality of VA healthcare.

References

Dodaro, G. L. (2021). *High-risk series: Dedicated leadership needed to address limited progress in most high-risk areas* [Testimony before the committee on oversight reform, house of representatives]. United States Government Accountability Office. https://www.gao.gov/assets/gao-21-383t.pdf

Gibson, S. D. (2015). *Letter to U.S. House of Representatives chairman Jeff Miller about the 2015 fiscal year budget for the Department of Veterans Affairs*. https://www.va.gov/budget/docs/signed_letters_to_congress.pdf

Hamilton, A. B., Brunner, J., Cain, C., Chuang, E., Luger, T. M., Canelo, I., Rubenstein, L., & Yano, E. (2017). Engaging multilevel stakeholders in an implementation trial of evidence-based quality improvement in VA women's health primary care. *Translational Behavioral Medicine, 7*(3), 478–485. https://doi.org/10.1007/s13142-017-0501-5

Kalman, N. S., Hammill, B. G., Schulman, K. A., & Shah, B. R. (2015). Hospital overhead costs: The neglected driver of health care spending? *Journal of Health Care Finance, 41*(4), 1–15.

McCain, J. S., III., Akaka, D. K., & Johnson, S. R. (2018). *VA maintaining internal systems and strengthening Integrated Outside Networks Act of 2018 or the VA MISSION Act of 2018* [Public law no. 115–182]. https://www.congress.gov/bill/115th-congress/senate-bill/2372

Phibbs, C. S., Barnett, P. G., & Fan, A. (2015). *Research guide to the managerial cost accounting national cost extracts* [Guidebook]. U.S. Department of Veterans Affairs. https://www.herc.research.va.gov/include/page.asp?id=guidebook-mca-nde

Schick, A. (1966). The road to PPB: The stages of budget reform. *Public Administration Review, 26*(4), 243–258. https://doi.org/10.2307/973296

U.S. Department of Veterans Affairs. (2014). *Fact sheet: Veterans access, choice, and accountability act of 2014*. Office of Public Affairs and Media Relations. https://www.va.gov/opa/choiceact/documents/choice-act-summary.pdf

U.S. Department of Veterans Affairs. (2016). *VHA directive 1043: Restructuring of VHA clinical programs* [Policy brief]. https://www.va.gov/vhapublications/ViewPublication.asp?pub_ID=3292
U.S. Department of Veterans Affairs. (2021a). *Annual budget submission: President's budget request—Fiscal year 2022*. Office of Budget. https://www.va.gov/budget/products.asp
U.S. Department of Veterans Affairs. (2021b). *Managerial cost accounting, volume XIII, chapter 3* [Financial policy]. VA Financial Policy Manual. https://www.va.gov/finance/docs/VA-FinancialPolicyVolumeXIIIChapter03.pdf
U.S. Government Accountability Office. (2016). *VA's health care budget: In response to a projected funding gap in fiscal year 2015, VA has made efforts to better manage future budgets* [Report to the Committee on Veterans Affairs, House of Representatives]. https://www.gao.gov/assets/gao-16-584-highlights.pdf
Wagner, T., Chow, A., Su, P., & Barnett, P. G. (2018). *HERC's average cost datasets for VA inpatient care* [Guidebook]. U.S. Department of Veterans Affairs. https://www.herc.research.va.gov/include/page.asp?id=guidebook-inpt-ac
Wang, Z. J., Dhanireddy, P., Prince, C., Larsen, M., Schimpf, M., & Pearman, G. (2020). *2019 Survey of Veteran enrollees' health and use of health care* [Data findings report]. U.S. Department of Veterans Affairs. https://www.va.gov/HEALTHPOLICYPLANNING/SOE2019/2019_Enrollee_Data_Findings_Report-March_2020_508_Compliant.pdf
Watkins, K. E., Pincus, H. A., Smith, B., Paddock, S. M., Mannle, T. E., Jr., Woodroffe, A., Soloman, J., Sorbero, M. E., Farmer, C. M., Hepner, J. A., Adamson, D. M., Forrest, L., & Call, C. (2011). *Veterans health administration mental health program evaluation* [Capstone report]. The RAND Corporation. http://www.rand.org/pubs/technical_reports/TR956.html
Wildavksy, A. B. (1988). *The new politics of the budgetary process*. Scott.

Chapter 4
Social Circumstances and Behavioral Patterns: Impacts on Health and Initiatives to Mitigate These Impacts

Aina Katsikas

1 Introduction

Social circumstances, behavioral patterns, environmental exposures, and genetic predispositions generate significant impacts on health. The substantive nature of these impacts is garnering increasing attention from health policy analysts, health insurance plan administrators, Medicare and Medicaid program administrators, and clinicians. This chapter focuses on the two factors that are particularly relevant for psychologists working in integrated care: social circumstances and behavioral patterns. Statistical analyses indicate that these two factors account for at least half of all preventable deaths (McGinnis et al., 2002). We provide an overview of statistical work indicating both causal and associative relationships[1] of these factors on health, and we discuss implications for clinicians.

While healthcare is an important tool for strengthening health and preventing adverse health outcomes, other factors may generate larger impacts on health. McGinnis et al. (2002) concluded that gaps in healthcare account for only 10–15% of preventable deaths, while social circumstances and behavioral patterns account for more than half of all preventable deaths (McGinnis et al., 2002). Advances in pharmaceutical and surgical treatments for cardiac diseases, cancers, and conditions responsible for infant mortality have generated improved outcomes for patients;

[1] Causal relationships are identified via experimental design methods. Associative relationships are established via basic regression analysis.

A. Katsikas (✉)
University of Nevada, Reno, NV, USA
e-mail: akatsikas@unr.edu

L. C. James et al. (eds.), *Clinical Health Psychology in Military and Veteran Settings*, https://doi.org/10.1007/978-3-031-12063-3_4

however, social circumstances and behavioral patterns continue to affect health in significant ways.

Social circumstances and behavioral patterns can also have significant implications for healthcare providers. Medical professionals are held accountable for health outcomes, yet these factors exert larger influences on health than medical care. Providers working under value-based payment (VBP) models face incentives to generate good health outcomes. While clinicians face incentives to develop strategies to mitigate these impacts, they cite numerous barriers that hinder these efforts, including lack of control over relevant decisions and processes in healthcare organizations and in social service agencies (Winfield et al., 2018). Finally, the complexity of the web of factors affecting health makes it difficult to identify and implement effective programs.

Several terms are used to describe the set of factors encompassing social circumstances and behavioral patterns, including "social determinants of health" and "health-related social needs." In this chapter we focus on four components of these constructs: income, education, housing security, and food security.

This chapter has four sections. The section following this introduction summarizes evidence describing the relationship between social circumstances, behavioral patterns, and health. We discuss this relationship that occurs at three stages in the life cycle: adulthood, childhood, and infancy. The third section of the chapter explores intervention strategies and discusses strategic issues facing clinicians as they work to mitigate the health impacts of social circumstances and behavioral patterns.

2 Factors That Affect Health

This section summarizes the results of statistical analyses designed to yield evidence about impacts of social circumstances and behavioral patterns on health. We focus on studies that examine relationships between social circumstances and health or between behavioral patterns and health. The body of evidence is substantial. Many studies document associations between social circumstances, behavioral patterns, and health, while others used experimental design strategies to generate evidence of causal links between social circumstances, behavioral patterns, and health.

Evidence indicates intergenerational relationships of income, education, and health. Adult health is affected by the adult's own social circumstances and behavioral patterns and by her health as an infant and then as a child. When this adult becomes a parent, her health behaviors and social circumstances can affect the health of her children – who will be part of the next generation of adults. The relationship between social circumstances and health may also reflect two-way causality between income and health: income can affect one's health, and one's health can affect income if poor health limits one's work hours.

Because studies typically focus on impacts that occur at a specific life stage, this section includes three subsections that summarize evidence about impacts on adults, children, and infants. We include overviews of studies that address four components of the social circumstances construct: housing security, food security, education, and income. We also include overviews of studies that address socioeconomic components of health behavior patterns. There are strong interactions between social circumstances and behavioral patterns. For example, education is typically categorized as a social circumstance. However, it is associated with behavioral patterns. Similarly, income is associated with the availability of safe outdoor recreation spaces, which could be a factor shaping propensity to exercise.

2.1 Health as an Adult

Adult health can be affected by the individual's health as an infant and child and by the adult's social circumstances and behavioral patterns. This subsection begins by summarizing evidence about the impacts of adult social circumstances and behavioral patterns on health.

Social circumstances and health behaviors are intertwined. Exercise can reduce the effect of age-related losses in muscle mass and strength (Distefano & Goodpaster, 2018). However, access to exercise resources such as equipment and safe outdoor spaces can be a product of socioeconomic factors. High-quality diets that entail good nutrition are associated with better physical functioning in older ages (Artaud et al., 2017; Hagan et al., 2016; Robinson, 2018). However, good nutrition requires convenient and affordable access to nutritious food and basic knowledge of nutrition and cooking strategies.

In this subsection, we examine the impacts of social circumstances on adult health. The first subsection reviews evidence on the impacts of housing security and housing quality on health outcomes. The second focuses on the associations of food insecurity with health concerns and higher medical expenditures. The third section reports evidence on the impact of education on health behaviors, cognitive ability, and the management of chronic illnesses. The last section explores impacts of income on health, through pathways shaped by access to transportation, ability to fund copayments, financial access to good nutrition, and financial access to long-term services and supports (LTSS).

2.1.1 Housing Security and Quality

Housing security and housing quality affect health. Homelessness is associated with infectious diseases, mental illness, mortality, a higher need for medical services, and longer hospital stays (McCormick & White, 2016; Morrison, 2009; Williams & Bryant, 2018). Low-quality housing is linked to poor health and higher mortality rates. This section will explore associations between housing and health.

The incidence of tuberculosis, hepatitis C virus (HCV), and human immunodeficiency virus (HIV) is higher among homeless individuals than among those with secure housing. In population-dense homeless groups, such as those living in downtown Los Angeles, 26.7% of sampled adults tested positive for HCV, and almost half of them were unaware of the infection (Beijer et al., 2012; Gelberg et al., 2012).

In addition to infectious diseases, homeless groups also suffer from mental illnesses. About 26% of all sheltered persons who are homeless have a severe mental illness, and almost 35% of all sheltered, homeless adults have a chronic substance abuse issue (Substance Abuse and Mental Health Services Administration, 2011).

The high prevalence of disease and mental illness contributes to the high mortality rates for homeless individuals. Homelessness carries an all-cause mortality hazard ratio of 1.6 compared to non-homeless cohorts, after controlling for age, sex, prior hospital admissions, and contributing socioeconomic conditions. Hospital admissions for drug-related causes raise the hazard ratio of death by 3.9 for the general population, but for homeless individuals, this statistic is 7.2 (Morrison, 2009).

Homeless individuals require more medical services. This can be a costly burden. Housing insecurity is associated with longer hospital stays, more emergency department visits, and higher in-hospital mortality rates (Hunter et al., 2017; McCormick & White, 2016). Homeless individuals who did not achieve residential stability, had higher rates of unmet physical care needs compared to those who did not achieve residential stability (Jaworsky et al., 2016). Individuals with insecure housing also report delaying physician visits due to financial issues (Stahre et al., 2015). These patterns are also observed among veterans (Kushel et al., 2002). Veterans in the United States without a home are four times more likely to visit the emergency room within 1 year than non-homeless veterans (Tsai et al., 2013).

There are federal resources available to secure housing for homeless veterans. The Veterans Affairs (VA) implements evidence-based programs such as the Housing and Urban Development-Veterans Affairs Supportive Housing vouchers (HUD-VASH). The HUD-VASH program utilizes the "housing first" model in which veterans are given a housing choice voucher. The individual is then paired with a VA case manager and supportive services to assist in sustaining the housing agreement and recovering from physical or mental health problems. Another program similar to this is the Grant and Per Diem (GPD) Program which are VA grants awarded to community-based agencies to create transitional housing programs (National Conference of State Legislatures, 2020).

Homeless patients also have more lengthy and more frequent hospital stays and higher in-hospital mortality rates. The average length of stay per hospital admission is longer for individuals with no fixed abode compared to those with stable housing, even after controlling for the severity of diagnosis (McCormick & White, 2016). The overall in-hospital mortality rate for homeless groups is 10% higher compared to those with housing. This higher mortality rate is mostly due to more severe diagnoses for homeless individuals.

While attention tends to focus on the housed vs. homeless dichotomy, it is also useful to consider housing as a continuous variable. Inadequate housing is associated with chronic illness, higher mortality rates, and infectious diseases (Butler et al., 2017; Desmond & Bell, 2015; Hood, 2005; Johnson, 2012; Martinez et al., 2018).

Neighborhood plumbing and insulation problems are each associated with a 3.9 point lower index of General Health Status (Johnson, 2012). (See Box 4.1 for a definition of General Health Status.)

Box 4.1:
Definition: General Health StatusGeneral Health Status (GHS) is based on one question asked of household heads: "Would you say your health in general is excellent, very good, good, fair, or poor?" This question was asked at each wave of data collection between 1984 and 2005. It is highly predictive of morbidity measured in clinical surveys. A decrease in the GHS Index signifies a decrease in overall health. For more information, see Johnson, (2012).

Areas with a higher prevalence of poor housing conditions also have higher mortality rates. Rural low-income populations are susceptible to poor living conditions. Poor housing conditions are a health concern because they are associated with asthma, lead poisoning, heart disease, and developmental delays. From 2005 to 2009, rural households had a 13% higher mortality rate compared to that of metropolitan households (Martinez et al., 2018).

2.1.2 Food Security

Food insecurity is a barrier to attaining optimum physical health. This concern is most prevalent among low-income households. This subsection will explore how food insecurity is associated with health concerns and higher healthcare expenditures.

Individuals facing food insecurity have higher rates of chronic disease, disability, and health concerns. In 2019, 10.5% of US households faced food insecurity (Coleman-Jensen et al., 2020). Food-insecure households include those facing low and very low food security (see Box 4.2 for a definition of food insecurity). These households have higher rates of illnesses such as hypertension, coronary heart disease, asthma, diabetes, and other illnesses. Adults in households reporting very low food security are 15.3% more likely to have a chronic illness compared to adults reporting very high food security (Gregory & Coleman-Jensen, 2017).

Box 4.2:
Definition: Food InsecurityHouseholds are defined to have food insecurity if they have difficulty providing food for themselves at some time during the year due to a lack of resources (Coleman-Jensen et al., 2014). Households facing low food security report reduced quality, variety, or desirability of diet. There is little to no indication of reduced food intake. Households facing very low food security report multiple indications of disrupted eating patterns and reduced food intake (Coleman-Jensen et al., 2021).

Food-insecure households incur higher healthcare expenditures (by $1863 per year) than households with food security. The extra spending stems from more ED visits, longer and more frequent hospital stays, and higher expenditures for prescriptions among food-insecure individuals than among food-secure households. This association is robust after controlling for potential confounders like age, race, education, income, and health insurance (Berkowitz et al., 2017; Nord, 2008). Food-insecure individuals are 1.47 times more likely to visit an ED than food-secure individuals (Berkowitz et al., 2017). The greatest divide was found among those enrolled in public health insurance. Among Medicare and Medicaid enrollees, food-insecure individuals are likely to have more emergency visits and hospital stays than food-secure enrollees.

2.1.3 Education

Education affects health through several pathways. It influences health behaviors, alters cognitive ability, and improves the health management of chronic illness. One additional year of schooling reduces rates of self-reported poor health by 4–6.4% points for women and 4.5–5.4% points for men (Brunello et al., 2016).

More years of schooling are linked to healthier lifestyles. Health behaviors encompass obtaining vaccinations, utilizing contraceptives, practicing good nutrition, and avoiding smoking and heavy drinking. Educated populations are associated with higher vaccination rates and contraceptive use (Brunello et al., 2016; Cutler & Lleras-Muney, 2010; Nagata et al., 2013; Rosenzweig & Schultz, 1989). This could be due to the fact that groups with more schooling also have better access to preventive healthcare. This positive association with education also occurs in couples with regard to contraceptive use. Couples with more schooling are more likely to know how to use various forms of contraception compared to couples with less education (Rosenzweig & Schultz, 1989). Cohorts with more years of schooling are less likely to smoke, practice heavy drinking, or be obese (Cutler & Lleras-Muney, 2010). An estimated 50% of all deaths in the United States are attributable to behaviors like smoking, exercise, diet, and heavy drinking (Mokdad et al., 2005). These behaviors are affected by numerous factors including individual choices and behavior patterns (Centers for Disease Control and Prevention [CDC], 1999; McGinnis & Foege, 1999). These behaviors also affect health. Diet choices, for example, are associated with coronary heart disease, stroke, diabetes, and various cancers (Walker & Walker, 1989). Similarly, a lack of exercise is associated with an increased risk for heart disease, dementia, osteoporosis, and diabetes (Manley, 1996). Smoking, another modifiable behavior, also contributes to a large portion of preventable premature deaths.

Another mechanism by which education influences health is that it alters cognitive ability (Cutler & Lleras-Muney, 2010). For example, educated individuals are more likely to implement medical recommendations for managing diabetes and the human immunodeficiency virus (HIV) (Goldman & Smith, 2002).

Educational attainment improves the management of chronic illnesses. There is a positive relationship between years of schooling and quality of at-home management of chronic conditions. Educated individuals are more likely to be aware of a diabetic condition, monitor key health metrics related to diabetes, and adhere to clinician guidelines (Goldman & Smith, 2002; Smith, 2007). In a sample of adult men with diabetes, 38% of those with a high school diploma were unaware of their diabetic condition compared to only 21% of those with more than a high school diploma (Smith, 2007). This study defined diabetes as having an HbA1c value of 6.5% or greater (see Box 4.3 for more detail). Self-management activities follow a similar gradient. More schooling is associated with higher rates of monitoring blood glucose levels and exercise and lower rates of missed insulin injections and smoking (Smith, 2007).

Box 4.3:
Definition of Diabetes Used in Smith, 2007 The lab exam for diabetes in this study measures the glycosylated hemoglobin A1c (HbA1c) test. This is a measure of the percent of hemoglobin molecules bound to glucose. HbA1c is highly correlated with fasting plasma glucose levels. Smith (2007) uses the standard convention of values greater than or equal to 6.5% to indicate clinical diabetes for the purpose of this study. The results of the study are not sensitive to the specific threshold chosen.

2.1.4 Income

An individual's income can affect health through several pathways including access to reliable transportation, ability to fund copayments, financial access to nutritious foods, and financial access to long-term services and supports (LTSS).

Unreliable transportation weakens a patient's ability to show up for appointments and implement clinician instructions and advice (Baren et al., 2001; Heiman & Artiga, 2015; Syed et al., 2013; Virapongse & Misky, 2018). In a study of 189 Hispanic and Latino women who were recommended to receive a follow-up mammogram, over a third did not pursue follow-up care within 3 months of the recommended time frame (Parra, 2016). Breast cancer is the leading cause of cancer mortality among Hispanic and Latino women (American Cancer Society, 2018). Unreliable transportation was frequently cited as an inhibiting factor for women who were dependent on public transportation. This issue can be important for low-income, uninsured, or underinsured women. Low-income individuals are far more likely to utilize "active transportation" such as biking, walking, or public transportation, which can pose a barrier to attendance at scheduled medical appointments (McKenzie, 2014). Transportation vouchers are successful in reducing readmissions when included in hospital discharge programs (Coleman et al., 2006). Fewer providers located near a patient result in longer travel distances and consequently higher transportation costs. This is linked to significantly fewer visits (Sloan et al., 2004).

Copayments and the cost of medications can also deter proper medical follow-up. Men facing copayments over $10 or with deductibles over $250 are significantly less likely to receive a prostate cancer screening compared to men facing lower copayments (Liang et al., 2004). The cost of medication is commonly cited as a factor affecting care transitions after a hospital visit (Virapongse & Misky, 2018).

Financial access to long-term services and supports (LTSS) can be an impediment to good health for patients struggling with activities of daily living. LTSS caregivers assist with medication management, prescription adherence, and care management. They can also help monitor vital health metrics and support care logistics for older adults (Fineberg, 2008; Gitlin & Wolff, 2011; Williams et al., 2012; Wolff et al., 2016). LTSS services can be provided in an institutional or residential facility, such as a skilled nursing facility or assisted living facility, or in the home. Caregivers are essential for older adults with chronic illnesses that require self-management, such as diabetes or coronary heart disease. A lack of LTSS can pose a barrier to implementing healthcare recommendations, with adverse health consequences for the patient.

2.2 *Childhood Health*

The income and food security of a child's household can affect that child's health. This subsection will report evidence of associations of income and food security with childhood health.

Childhood health is an important factor in contributing to long-term health status in adulthood. Case et al. (2005) found that children who report poor health have significantly lower educational status, lower health status, and lower income in adulthood, even after controlling for parental income and education. Chronic conditions developed before age 7 that persist to age 16 have a significant association with health status at age 42 (Case et al., 2005). A child's height at age 16 is significantly associated with better health at ages 23, 33, and 42. However, a child's height is also correlated with her father's education and income.

Childhood health is influenced by numerous factors, including family income and food security. The following sections will discuss evidence of the impacts of these two factors on childhood health.

2.2.1 Family Income

Children from low-income households report poorer health than those in high-income households (Curtis et al., 2001). For families in the $15,000–50,000 income bracket, a $10,000 increase in annual income is associated with a 0.53% point increase in the average General Health Status of the children living in these families

(Johnson & Schoeni, 2011). Doubling family income generates a four percentage point increase in the probability that a young child (ages 0–3) will have excellent or very good health (Case et al., 2002). The strength of this effect increases as the child ages: doubling family income generates a 6.4 percentage point increase in the probability that a teenager (ages 13–15) will have excellent or very good health (Currie & Stabile, 2003). One possible explanation for this result stems from the higher incidence of health shocks among children living in low-income versus higher-income families (Currie, 2009). For example, only 11% of high-income children (ages 0–3) have chronic conditions (asthma and mental health problems) compared to 23% of low-income children (Currie et al., 2007). Children from low-income households also have a higher probability of being limited by these chronic conditions during adolescence compared to others with the same chronic conditions from high-income households (Currie, 2009). One of the reasons for this is that children living in low-income families are less likely to efficiently manage their asthma than children living in high-income families, resulting in consequences lasting through their teenage years (Currie, 2009). These longer-term consequences affect the subsequent health of that individual when he becomes an adult.

2.2.2 Food Security

Household food security is associated with childhood health. Adolescents raised in food-unstable households have lower health status and higher rates of chronic illness. Children from food-insecure homes are twice as likely to report being in fair or poor health and 1.4 times more likely to have asthma compared to children raised in food-secure homes (Gundersen & Ziliak, 2015). Compared to children in food-secure homes, children enduring food insecurity are more likely to have anemia (Eicher-Miller et al., 2009; Skalicky et al., 2006). They also more likely to have depression or anxiety between the ages of 4 and 8 years old (Melchior et al., 2012). Food insecurity in childhood is also associated with a higher risk of hospitalization over the course of the child's lifetime (Cook et al., 2006). Hunger experienced in childhood is also a strong predictor of depression, anxiety, and suicide ideation in later teenage and early adult years (McIntyre et al., 2013; Melchior et al., 2012).

2.3 Health at Birth

A child can be affected by his or her preceding health status at birth. Infant health has implications for health conditions later in adolescence and even adulthood. The following sections will discuss evidence documenting relationships between family income, mother's education, and infant health.

Many studies demonstrate that health at birth has long-term implications for health in adulthood. For example, low birthweight is associated with developing coronary heart disease and hypertension as an adult, and it is also associated with insulin resistance syndrome in adulthood (Barker et al., 1989, 1993; Law & Shiell, 1996).

The following sections will discuss two factors that influence infant health: family income and mother's education.

2.3.1 Family Income

Infants born into higher-income families have more favorable birth outcomes (Conley & Bennett, 2000; Currie & Lin, 2007). Data from 1985 British birth records indicate a higher prevalence of low birthweight infants whose fathers were in low-prestige occupations compared to those of high-prestige occupations (6.4% vs. 5%) (Currie & Hyson, 1999). California birth records from the 1970s found the same association when comparing birth outcomes in high-income and low-income zip codes (6% vs. 7%) (Currie, 2009). Even in countries with universal health insurance (Canada and the United Kingdom), the income gap in childhood health is present.

2.3.2 Mother's Education

The mother's education can influence the health of her infants by influencing her health behaviors. Maternal education is associated with lower smoking rates and higher rates of prenatal care utilization (Currie & Moretti, 2003). These health behaviors affect gestational age and the infant's birthweight (Evans & Ringel, 1999). College-educated mothers have lower rates of smoking and higher rates of participating in prenatal care compared to mothers with less than a high school diploma (Currie & Moretti, 2003). This pattern was identified during the expansion of colleges in the United States in the early 1940s that provided educational opportunities for women. From the sample of college-educated mothers, only 2% smoked during pregnancy compared to 34% from the sample of mothers with less than a high school education. Even after the 1964 Surgeon General's Report on Smoking and Health established that smoking is detrimental to the mother's health while pregnant, there was an educational divide in the reaction to this new information. The smoking habits of educated pregnant women immediately dropped following the report compared to those of less educated pregnant women (Aizer & Stroud, 2010). Smoking during pregnancy is concerning because it increases the risk that an infant will have a low birthweight by a factor of two. Infant birthweight and gestational age increase with higher rates of college attendance among women. An extra year of college education reduces the likelihood of the mother having a low birthweight child by 20% and a preterm birth by 15% (Currie & Moretti, 2003). Maternal education is a key indicator of infant health because of its effects on health behaviors. An excise tax on cigarettes can increase average birthweight. A one-cent increase in the state tax rate of cigarettes leads to an increase in average birthweight by 0.21 g (Evans & Ringel, 1999).

2.3.3 Maternal Health During Pregnancy

Statistical evidence indicating impacts of parental health, income, and behavioral patterns on infant health is important because it clarifies pathways by which parental health and income can be transmitted to the next generation via two pathways: gestational health and the health behaviors of parents.

Gestational health can influence the development of the embryo in utero. Exposure to adverse health events in utero can indirectly affect the weight and overall health of the infant (Roseboom et al., 2000). The embryo relies on a stream of oxygen and nutrients. Anything that tampers with this mechanism (e.g., smoking while pregnant or poor nutrition) can have a significant effect on the infant's health. Amsterdam records show that infants exposed to the Dutch famine while in utero from 1944 to 1945 exhibited lower glucose tolerance as adults and higher rates of coronary heart disease (Ravelli et al., 1998; Roseboom et al., 2000). The risk of lower respiratory illness before the age of 2 is greatest among children whose parents had childhood lower respiratory illness and smoked (Mann et al., 1992). Smoking while pregnant poses a moderate risk factor for preterm delivery and is a major risk factor for intrauterine growth retardation (Case & Paxson, 2002).

3 Initiatives to Mitigate the Impacts of Social Circumstances and Behavioral Patterns

Social circumstances and individual behaviors can generate adverse impacts on individual health, and these factors can weaken the impacts of clinician efforts to strengthen individual health (McGinnis et al., 2002). Healthcare organizations have two strategic options to mitigate the adverse impacts of inadequate education, insecure food and housing, and unhealthy behaviors: (i) healthcare organizations can assume primary responsibility for implementing programs within healthcare settings to offset potential adverse impacts of these factors on patient health outcomes, or (ii) these organizations can play a supporting role by strengthening coordination between healthcare entities and social service agencies and between healthcare organizations and education agencies and by advocating for increased funding to support the work of these entities. This section of the chapter describes three types of efforts currently undertaken by healthcare organizations and agencies, and it poses strategic questions raised by these efforts. Clinicians can enrich the analysis and discussion of these questions by engaging with health policy analysts and health policy makers.

3.1 Initiatives in Health Services

Some healthcare organizations are offering programs designed to offset potential adverse health impacts of low education and insecure food and housing and to help individuals adopt more healthy behavior patterns. This subsection discusses three examples of programs aiming to achieve these goals: pharmacist-led interventions, hospital discharge coordination programs, and integrated care.

First, pharmacist-led interventions provide individualized care such as medication management, programs to resolve drug therapy issues, and patient education. These programs were implemented following passage of the Affordable Care Act of 2010, which led to expansions in pharmacist scope of practice in some states (Smock, 2013; Wachino, 2017). Targeted education, pharmacotherapeutic monitoring, and health screenings led by pharmacists have been shown to cut medical costs while improving health. These programs generated an increase in medication costs that were offset by reductions in medical costs from reduced hospitalization and emergency department (ED) visits (Wang et al., 2016). Medication adherence programs successfully helped patients adhere to recommended medication regimes (Smith, 2009); achieve reductions in average lipid levels, HbA1c values, and systolic blood pressure readings (Cranor et al., 2003); prevent diabetes-related cerebrovascular or cardiovascular events (Wang et al., 2016); and reduce the number of days absent from work (Cranor et al., 2003; Fera et al., 2009). Evidence also indicates that the strategy used to provide pharmacist counseling may be important: one study concluded that counseling provided in retail settings is more effective than counseling provided during telephone calls (Brennan et al., 2012).

Second, healthcare organizations are developing and implementing comprehensive hospital discharge programs (also known as transitional care interventions) to improve health outcomes. These programs may include monitoring patient status following hospital discharge, or they may utilize nurse advocates who arrange follow-up patient appointments, confirm medication reconciliation, and conduct patient education. These strategies can effectively reduce hospitalization following the initial hospital discharge (Jack, 2009).

Some programs focus on specific populations, such as high-risk patients, elderly patients, or adults with chronic homelessness. Transitional care interventions focused on high-risk patients have reported reductions in readmissions, hospital days, and medical costs. A 2008 North Carolina transitional care program for Medicaid recipients with chronic conditions was successful in reducing readmissions with care that involved comprehensive medication management, face-to-face medication education, and outpatient follow-up (Jackson et al., 2013).

For elderly patients with chronic conditions, comprehensive discharge programs demonstrate a reduction in short-term readmission rates, medical expenditures, and number of rehospitalizations (Naylor et al., 1999).

Chronically homeless adults also benefit from transitional care including transition coaches and emphasizing patient-centered communication (Buchanan et al., 2006). Programs that provide housing and case management are linked to reduced inpatient hospitalizations and ED visits for these populations (Sadowski et al., 2009).

Third, integrated care can be a cost-effective strategy for improving quality of care. Compared with patients who received care in traditional settings, integrated care patients enjoyed better adherence to treatment recommendations and fewer symptoms. Insurers benefited from lower total medical care expenditures, and clinicians reported increased satisfaction (Blount, 2003; Katon, 1995; Lenz et al., 2018).

Integrated care programs can deliver medical and behavioral care via coordinated, co-located, or integrated strategies (Blount, 2003; Coleman et al., 1979; Cummings et al., 2009). All methods require communication between primary and behavioral healthcare providers. Coordination requires significant time and effort from both medical and behavioral health providers. Nonetheless, the Hawaii Project I, led by Nicholas A. Cummings and Herbert Dorken implemented widespread coordinated care for Hawaii Medicaid beneficiaries in the 1980s (Cummings, 1990). The program improved patient adherence to recommended medical regimens and prompted significant patient lifestyle changes.

In the co-located model, behavioral and primary care providers are physically located in the same suite of offices to facilitate collaboration. The first widespread HMO implementation of this strategy demonstrated a rich exchange of information between providers. Patients were more likely to keep their behavioral health appointments if they were introduced to the behavioral health provider during the primary care visit (Blount, 2003). Co-located settings can also mitigate barriers of access to care for patients who lack reliable transportation to visit providers. Primary care providers in co-located settings reported feeling more comfortable to ask about psychosocial issues knowing that they could readily refer the patient to an expert (Blount, 2003).

The integrated care model offers an additional advantage: the patient receives a unified treatment plan that includes both behavioral and medical elements. This integration can be useful for patients with both chronic illness and depression (Blount, 2003).

Implementation of these programs highlights the importance of determining whether each program is cost-effective in each specific setting. Useful programs that are not cost-effective use organization resources that could have been deployed to fund alternate programs. This situation requires careful analyses to assess whether each program generates sufficient benefits to justify allocating resources away from other programs. The question of whether a program is cost-effective in a specific setting requires site-specific analysis. Program costs and benefits can vary across settings due to differences in the characteristics of patient populations, differences in professional compensation and facility costs, and differences in the local availability of complementary or substitute resources and programs.

In addition to these efforts, some states are exploring strategies to incentivize nonprofit hospitals to design and implement "community benefit" programs that address key health equity issues (NASHP, 2021). Federal Internal Revenue Service regulations mandate that these hospitals must engage in community benefit activities as a prerequisite for maintaining tax-exempt status. Some states are considering strategies to require hospitals to focus these activities on social determinants of health and to audit the impacts of these activities on health and health disparities.

3.2 *Initiatives to Address Gaps in Education, Food Security, and Housing Security*

Instead of focusing on implementing programs to offset the health effects of income, healthcare organizations could focus on addressing gaps in education, food security, and housing security directly. Healthcare organizations could consider two strategies for undertaking this work: (i) provide food and housing to high-risk individuals or (ii) partner with community organizations that focus on education, food security, and housing security. Some healthcare organizations are implementing the first strategy. For example, some managed care companies provide housing for individuals with chronic conditions who also experience chronic homelessness. Some nonprofit hospitals invest in affordable housing to meet federal requirements, stating that tax-exempt hospitals must generate community benefits (Tanumihardjo et al., 2021). These programs typically target individuals with high healthcare expenditures and frequent visits to hospital emergency departments. While these programs can demonstrate good results, the magnitudes of these programs tend to be small relative to the magnitude of the population of homeless individuals.

In contrast, the federal Department of Housing and Urban Development provides subsidized housing on a larger scale. Even this is not sufficient: only 25% of individuals eligible for this assistance actually receive it due to funding limitations (Katch & Bailey, 2020). Nonetheless, some Medicaid programs partner with state housing authorities to develop systems for housing individuals with complex health conditions or individuals who need help with activities of daily living.

This raises the question: How should healthcare organizations direct their efforts and resources? Should they continue to develop targeted small-scale programs or should they invest resources to build partnerships with social service and education agencies and advocate for increased funding for these agencies?

Healthcare organizations considering these options will note that the strategy of providing housing for limited numbers of individuals faces several challenges. First, Medicaid programs cannot reimburse organizations for providing housing due to constraints imposed by federal law. Second, adult membership in a specific health plan, or a Medicaid managed care plan, can be short term if the adult gains or loses Medicaid eligibility or if the adult chooses a new health plan at the end of a plan year. It is not clear how housing provided by a healthcare organization would be affected by changes in health plan coverage. Finally, healthcare organizations may not have experience and expertise in managing housing programs (Katch & Bailey, 2020).

Preschool programs for disadvantaged children illustrate two additional dilemmas facing healthcare providers. Programs such as the Perry Preschool and Head Start yield positive effects on adult outcomes (Deming, 2009; Heckman et al., 2010). For example, evaluation of the Perry Preschool Program indicates that participants enjoyed higher education and earnings and increased participation in healthy behaviors at age 40 compared to children who were not enrolled in the program (Heckman et al., 2010). Despite the positive impact on adult health, however, these programs are not likely to be cost-effective for healthcare organizations due to the long lag between the educational investment and the subsequent improvement in adult health. In addition, evidence indicating that health is affected by an array of factors suggests that it may not be realistic to expect the healthcare system to assume a primary role in addressing each of the factors (McGinnis et al., 2002). Instead, it might be more useful for healthcare organizations to assume supporting roles in addressing these issues.

The Centers for Medicare & Medicaid Services (CMS) is testing one strategy to help healthcare organizations assume an effective supporting role. CMS funded a set of Accountable Health Communities (AHCs) beginning in 2017 as pilot programs.[2] AHCs build information technology infrastructure to facilitate partnerships between healthcare and community organizations (Alley et al., 2016; Brown et al., 2020). The partnerships develop and implement systematic processes to link Medicare and Medicaid beneficiaries with community resources offering services designed to address health-related social needs including housing and food security, reliable transportation, and paying for home utility bills. The partnerships are designed to solve a two-part problem: First, some individuals who are eligible for assistance do not apply for it. Second, some healthcare organizations employ social workers to help individuals identify likely sources of assistance and complete applications, but these efforts are not typically supported by an efficient referral and communication system. For example, a social worker might refer a patient to a specific social service agency. In many communities, that social worker will not receive feedback about this referral to indicate whether the patient applied for assistance, whether the patient was deemed to be eligible, and whether the patient renewed the application in a timely manner. Without this information, the social worker is not equipped to organize an efficient referral system.

The AHC model links traditional healthcare systems with a "bridge organization" that provides referrals to community services. Bridge organizations serve as system hubs that implement a three-step process: awareness, assistance, and alignment. The first step screens beneficiaries for unmet health-related social needs, the second provides community service referrals, and the last aligns community service partners with healthcare providers.

Bridge organizations can include health networks, hospitals, healthcare payers, or academic institutions. For example, St. Joseph's, a nonprofit healthcare system in Syracuse, New York, implemented the AHC model in 2018. It serves as the hub or bridge organization. St. Joseph's screens eligible beneficiaries for unmet social needs and refers these individuals to appropriate community services. Preliminary results show a 9% reduction in ED visits in the first year after screening. Program evaluation, to be conducted at the end of the 5-year period in 2022, will provide insights about (i) the relationship between unmet social needs and health and (ii) and the usefulness of this strategy for meeting those needs.

---

[2] See Sheingold et al. (2021) for a discussion of additional steps CMS could take to support efforts to strengthen health equity.

Some analysts argue that healthcare organizations should also provide vigorous support for increased government funding for social service agencies, for education, and for other government-provided services that boost health. Unless these organizations also support tax increases, this strategy requires careful consideration of the trade-offs facing federal and state lawmakers. While this issue is important at both the federal and state levels, it is most clear at the state level. In fiscal year 2019, before states were affected by the economic effects of COVID-19, states spent 38% of state general revenue on education and 16% on Medicaid (Kaiser Family Foundation, 2019). With these two expenditure categories accounting for more than half of state expenditures, substantial increases in expenditures for social services would pose difficult trade-offs for state lawmakers.

3.3 Initiatives to Adjust Provider Quality Metrics

Because social circumstances and behavioral patterns can impact patient health, they can also affect provider performance on quality metrics. Performance on these metrics can affect provider revenue when payment systems include a quality-based incentive. They can also affect the provider's reputation when the quality scores are publicly available. To the extent that low education and insecure food and housing exert adverse impacts on patient implementation of medical recommendations and patient health outcomes, providers treating disproportionate numbers of patients with low income (SES) are likely to have lower quality scores than comparable providers treating more affluent patients (Kassel, 2014). In this situation, providers treating disproportionate numbers of patients with low SES will receive lower payments than clinicians providing comparable services to more affluent patients. This scenario has generated concern that quality-based incentive payment systems could generate the unintended consequence of reducing resources available to practices focusing on patients with low SES.

In this subsection, we will describe (i) the value-based payment system currently used to adjust Medicare payments, (ii) potential reputation impacts of publicly available quality scores, and (iii) the current policy discussion about differential impacts of value-based payment systems on providers treating more (versus fewer) patients with low SES.

Payments to clinicians for providing care to patients covered by Medicare are adjusted to reflect performance on four types of quality metrics. The system was mandated by Congress in the 2015 Medicare Access and CHIP Reauthorization Act (MACRA). Under the most widely used MACRA track, four types of quality metrics are used to assess clinician or practice performance: traditional quality metrics, total healthcare expenditures for patients attributed to the clinician (or the practice), engagement in quality improvement activities, and the use of interoperable electronic systems to record, store, and exchange health information. Under MACRA, payments to clinicians with low-quality scores are reduced by as much as 9%, while payments to clinicians with high scores are increased by as much as 9% (Centers for

Medicare & Medicaid Services, 2020). Top-performing clinicians can receive additional bonus payments (The National Council, 2017).

In addition to this monetary incentive system, Medicare posts clinician-level and practice-level scores online. This creates an additional reputation incentive to earn high scores in the four areas. In addition, many states are creating all-payer claims databases (APCD) which are large state-run databases that include information on the treatments and procedures that generated all healthcare claims submitted to public and private insurers in the state. In many situations, the information will be made available to insurers and researchers to conduct analyses to support efforts to improve healthcare affordability, efficiency, and cost transparency. These databases will contain sufficient data to support analyses of efficiency and quality at the practice level. Currently, more than 30 states maintain an APCD or are developing one (Agency for Healthcare Research and Quality, 2017).

Publicly available performance data are not new. CMS has been posting organization-level data on managed care organization performance on quality measures specified in the Healthcare Effectiveness Data and Information Set (HEDIS) system. These measures provide a broad set of standardized performance measures, to support consumer efforts to select high-quality managed care plans.

These efforts to incentivize healthcare organizations to deliver high-quality healthcare are designed to pursue an important goal. However, the potential adverse – and unintended – consequences for providers treating high numbers of patients with low SES are concerning. Providers affected by value-based payment incentives, such as MACRA, may avoid serving disadvantaged populations and shift to serving more affluent populations. Incentivizing providers to implement strategies to boost patient compliance has also led to discussions of whether providers should be able to "fire" noncompliant patients.

In 2014, the National Quality Forum convened a panel of 26 national experts to consider whether CMS should set a lower performance threshold for providers treating a disproportionate number of patients with low SES, to avoid this unintended consequence (Kassel, 2014). This policy option offers both benefits and costs. The proposal's key benefit is that it would reduce or eliminate the expected adverse impact of the MACRA system on providers treating disproportionate numbers of patients with low SES. On the other hand, however, the proposal would create a two-tiered definition of quality in which providers can earn comparable rewards by providing lower-quality care to patients with low SES or higher-quality care to patients with patients with higher SES.

Sheingold et al. (2021) suggest that it will be useful to frame the discussion as consideration of two competing viewpoints:

(i) Payment incentives are designed to incentivize providers to deliver high-quality care that is evidence-based and consistent with medical guidelines. Statistical evidence indicates, however, that patients with moderate or high SES receiving this care are likely to experience better health outcomes than patients with low SES who receive the same care. The incentive system should be adjusted to avoid penalizing providers who treat disproportionate numbers of individuals with low SES.

(ii) The payment incentive system should be designed to incentivize providers to generate good health outcomes for all patients. While all patients should receive high-quality care, individuals with low SES may require additional services, including social services, to achieve good health outcomes. Physicians treating disproportionate numbers of these individuals should receive the additional resources needed to achieve these results.

The difference between these two viewpoints highlights the importance of the question of whether those additional services should be funded by healthcare payers and delivered by healthcare provider organizations, or whether it would be more effective to channel those resources directly to agencies responsible for providing social services. It also highlights the limited scope of using payment incentive risk adjustment, as a key strategy for addressing the role of SES in generating health disparities.

4 Conclusion

Evidence indicates that social circumstances and individual health behaviors affect health directly, and they mediate the impact of clinician efforts on patient health. Healthcare organizations face two types of strategic choices. Healthcare organizations could implement programs to mitigate the effects of social circumstances on health, or they could work to address the underlying gaps in social services. If they opt to address gaps in social services, they can either implement programs to address the gaps themselves or they can assume a supportive role by partnering with social service agencies.

Each strategy presents a dilemma that requires careful consideration. If healthcare organizations opt to implement programs designed to mitigate the effects of social circumstances on health, it is important to determine whether these programs are cost effective. If they do not generate sufficient financial benefits to offset the costs, these programs use organizational resources that could be allocated to other programs or services. Organization administrators and clinicians must weigh the trade-offs between programs designed to mitigate the effects of social circumstances on health and competing programs that may serve the same set of patients or different sets of patients.

Second, if the organization opts to focus on the underlying gaps in social services, they face two strategic questions. Can they utilize their resources more effectively by providing services such as housing directly, or should they use these resources to build partnerships with existing social service agencies? In addition, they face an associated question. Should they advocate for increased funding for social service agencies, even if that might encourage lawmakers to reduce funding for healthcare expenditures? Given the interactions among healthcare and other factors that affect health, it is possible that transferring funds from healthcare to social services might strengthen population health. Essentially, healthcare organizations face the question of whether the social service agencies can administer assistance programs more effectively than healthcare organizations.

Finally, current emphasis on value-based payment initiatives poses a difficult question: Should these systems include a more lenient performance standard for providers who treat disproportionate numbers of patients with low income (SES)? This is a thorny question, with logical arguments supporting both sides of the issue. To the extent that social circumstances affect patient health and mediate the health impacts of clinician efforts, applying the same performance standards to practices that do (and do not) treat disproportionate numbers of patients with low SES will shift resources from practices treating disproportionate numbers of low-income patients to practices treating more affluent patients. On the other hand, reducing the performance standard for providers who treat disproportionate numbers of patients with low incomes raises concerns about the implications of a two-tiered quality standard. Recognizing that both of these options pose substantive issues, some analysts argue that it would be useful to enlarge the discussion to consider alternate payment structures.

References

Agency for Healthcare Research and Quality. (2017, March). *All-payer claims databases*. https://www.ahrq.gov/data/apcd/index.html

Aizer, A., & Stroud, L. (2010). *Education, knowledge and the evolution of disparities in health*. National Bureau of Economic Research. https://doi.org/10.3386/w15840

Alley, D. E., Asomugha, C. N., Conway, P. H., & Sanghavi, D. M. (2016). Accountable health communities-Addressing social needs through Medicare and Medicaid. *New England Journal of Medicine, 374*(1), 8–11. https://doi.org/10.1056/nejmp1512532

American Cancer Society. (2018). *Cancer facts & figures for Hispanics/Latinos 2018–2020*. American Cancer Society, Inc. https://www.cancer.org/content/dam/cancer-org/research/cancer-facts-and-statistics/cancer-facts-and-figures-for-hispanics-and-latinos-2018-2020.pdf

Artaud, F., Sabia, S., Dugravot, A., Kivimaki, M., Singh-Manoux, A., & Elbaz, A. (2017). Trajectories of unhealthy behaviors in midlife and risk of disability at older ages. *Innovation in Aging, 1*(Suppl_1), 75–75. https://doi.org/10.1093/geroni/igx004.311

Baren, J. M., Shofer, F. S., Ivey, B., Reinhard, S., DeGeus, J., Stahmer, S. A., Panettieri, R., & Hollander, J. E. (2001). A randomized, controlled trial of a simple emergency department intervention to improve the rate of primary care follow-up for patients with acute asthma exacerbations. *Annals of Emergency Medicine, 38*(2), 115–122. https://doi.org/10.1067/mem.2001.116593

Barker, D. J., Osmond, C., Golding, J., Kuh, D., & Wadsworth, M. E. (1989). Growth in utero, blood pressure in childhood and adult life, and mortality from cardiovascular disease. *BMJ, 298*(6673), 564–567. https://doi.org/10.1136/bmj.298.6673.564

Barker, D. J., Hales, C. N., Fall, C. H., Osmond, C., Phipps, K., & Clark, P. M. (1993). Type 2 (non-insulin-dependent) diabetes mellitus, hypertension and hyperlipidaemia (syndrome X): Relation to reduced fetal growth. *Diabetologia, 36*(1), 62–67. https://doi.org/10.1007/bf00399095

Beijer, U., Wolf, A., & Fazel, S. (2012). Prevalence of tuberculosis, hepatitis C virus, and HIV in homeless people: A systematic review and meta-analysis. *The Lancet Infectious Diseases, 12*(11), 859–870. https://doi.org/10.1016/s1473-3099(12)70177-9

Berkowitz, S. A., Seligman, H. K., & Basu, S. (2017). *Impact of food insecurity and SNAP participation on healthcare utilization and expenditures*. University of Kentucky Center for Poverty Research Discussion Paper Series. https://uknowledge.uky.edu/ukcpr_papers/103/

Blount, A. (2003). Integrated primary care: Organizing the evidence. *Families, Systems & Health: The Journal of Collaborative Family Healthcare, 21*(2), 121–133. https://doi.org/10.1037/1091-7527.21.2.121

Brennan, T. A., Dollear, T. J., Hu, M., Matlin, O. S., Shrank, W. H., Choudhry, N. K., & Grambley, W. (2012). An integrated pharmacy-based program improved medication prescription and adherence rates in diabetes patients. *Health Affairs, 31*(1), 120–129. https://doi.org/10.1377/hlthaff.2011.0931

Brown, J. A., Berzin, O., Clayton, M., Cluff, L., Derzon, J., Evans, L., Farrel, K., Fraze, T., Haber, S., Hessler, D., Husick, C., Liu, E., Parish, W., Payne, J., Renaud, J., Smith, L., Stockdaye, H., & Vincent, A. (2020). *Accountable health communities (ahc) model evaluation first evaluation report*. RTI International. https://innovation.cms.gov/data-and-reports/2020/ahc-first-eval-rpt

Brunello, G., Fort, M., Schneeweis, N., & Winter-Ebmer, R. (2016). The causal effect of education on health: What is the role of health behaviors? *Health Economics, 25*(3), 314–336. https://doi.org/10.1002/hec.3141

Buchanan, D., Doblin, B., Sai, T., & Garcia, P. (2006). The effects of respite care for homeless patients: A cohort study. *American Journal of Public Health, 96*(7), 1278–1281. https://doi.org/10.2105/ajph.2005.067850

Butler, S. M., Matthew, D. B., & Cabello, M. (2017, February 15). *Re-balancing medical and social spending to promote health: Increasing state flexibility to improve health through housing*. Brookings Institution. https://www.brookings.edu/blog/usc-brookings-schaeffer-on-health-policy/2017/02/15/re-balancing-medical-and-social-spending-to-promote-health-increasing-state-flexibility-to-improve-health-through-housing

Case, A., & Paxson, C. (2002). Parental behavior and child health. *Health Affairs, 21*(2), 164–178. https://doi.org/10.1377/hlthaff.21.2.164

Case, A., Lubotsky, D., & Paxson, C. (2002). Economic status and health in childhood: The origins of the gradient. *The American Economic Review, 92*(5), 1308–1334. https://doi.org/10.1257/000282802762024520

Case, A., Fertig, A., & Paxson, C. (2005). The lasting impact of childhood health and circumstance. *Journal of Health Economics, 24*(2), 365–389. https://doi.org/10.1016/j.jhealeco.2004.09.008

Centers for Disease Control and Prevention (CDC). (1999). Cigarette smoking among adults–United States, 1997. *MMWR. Morbidity and Mortality Weekly Report, 48*(43), 993–996.

Centers for Medicare and Medicaid Services. (2020, March 23). *Quality payment program*. https://www.cms.gov/Medicare/Quality-Initiatives-Patient-Assessment-Instruments/Value-Based-Programs/MACRA-MIPS-and-APMs/MACRA-MIPS-and-APMs

Coleman, J. V., Patrick, D. L., Eagle, J., & Hermalin, J. A. (1979). Collaboration, consultation and referral in an integrated health-mental health program at an HMO. *Social Work in Health Care, 5*(1), 83–96. https://doi.org/10.1300/j010v05n01

Coleman, E. A., Parry, C., Chalmers, S., & Min, S.-J. (2006). The care transitions intervention: Results of a randomized controlled trial. *Archives of Internal Medicine, 166*(17), 1822–1828. https://doi.org/10.1001/archinte.166.17.1822

Coleman-Jensen, A., Gregory, C., & Singh, A. (2014). *Household food security in the United States in 2013*. U.S. Department of Agriculture, Economic Research Service. www.ers.usda.gov/publications/err-economic-research-report/err173.aspx

Coleman-Jensen, A., Rabbitt, M., Gregory, C. A., & Singh, A. (2020). *Household food security in the United States in 2019*. U.S. Department of Agriculture, Economic Research Service. https://www.ers.usda.gov/publications/pub-details/?pubid=99281

Coleman-Jensen, A., Rabbitt, M. P., & Gregory, C. A. (2021, March 21). *Food Security in the U.S.* US Department of Agriculture, Economic Research Service. https://www.ers.usda.gov/topics/food-nutrition-assistance/food-security-in-the-us/.

Conley, D., & Bennett, N. G. (2000). Is biology destiny? Birth weight and life chances. *American Sociological Review, 65*(3), 458–467. https://doi.org/10.2307/2657467

Cook, J. T., Frank, D. A., Levenson, S. M., Neault, N. B., Heeren, T. C., Black, M. M., Berkowitz, C., Casey, P. H., Meyers, A. F., Cutts, D. B., & Chilton, M. (2006). Child food insecurity increases risks posed by household food insecurity to young children's health. *The Journal of Nutrition, 136*(4), 1073–1076. https://doi.org/10.1093/jn/136.4.1073

Cranor, C. W., Bunting, B. A., & Christensen, D. B. (2003). The Asheville project: Long-term clinical and economic outcomes of a community pharmacy diabetes care program. *Journal of the American Pharmaceutical Association, 43*(2), 173–184. https://doi.org/10.1331/108658003321480713

Cummings, N. A. (1990). *The impact of psychological intervention on healthcare utilization and costs: The Hawaii Medicaid project.* Biodyne Institute.

Cummings, N. A., O'Donohue, W. T., & Cummings, J. L. (2009). The financial dimension of integrated behavioral/primary care. *Journal of Clinical Psychology in Medical Settings, 16*(1), 31–39. https://doi.org/10.1007/s10880-008-9139-2

Currie, J. (2009). Healthy, wealthy, and wise: Socioeconomic status, poor health in childhood, and human capital development. *Journal of Economic Literature, 47*(1), 87–122. https://doi.org/10.1257/jel.47.1.87

Currie, J., & Hyson, R. (1999). Is the impact of health shocks cushioned by socioeconomic status? The case of low birthweight. *The American Economic Review, 89*(2), 245–250. https://doi.org/10.1257/aer.89.2.245

Currie, J., & Lin, W. (2007). Chipping away at health: More on the relationship between income and child health. *Health Affairs, 26*(2), 331–344. https://doi.org/10.1377/hlthaff.26.2.331

Currie, J., & Moretti, E. (2003). Mother's education and the intergenerational transmission of human capital: Evidence from college openings. *The Quarterly Journal of Economics, 118*(4), 1495–1532. https://doi.org/10.1162/003355303322552856

Currie, J., & Stabile, M. (2003). Socioeconomic status and child health: Why is the relationship stronger for older children? *The American Economic Review, 93*(5), 1813–1823. https://doi.org/10.1257/000282803322655563

Currie, A., Shields, M. A., & Price, S. W. (2007). The child health/family income gradient: Evidence from England. *Journal of Health Economics, 26*(2), 213–232. https://doi.org/10.1016/j.jhealeco.2006.08.003

Curtis, L. J., Dooley, M. D., Lipman, E. L., & Feeny, D. H. (2001). The role of permanent income and family structure in the determination of child health in Canada. *Health Economics, 10*(4), 287–302. https://doi.org/10.1002/hec.591

Cutler, D. M., & Lleras-Muney, A. (2010). Understanding differences in health behaviors by education. *Journal of Health Economics, 29*(1), 1–28. https://doi.org/10.1016/j.jhealeco.2009.10.003

Deming, D. (2009). Early childhood intervention and life-cycle skill development: Evidence from Head Start. *American Economic Journal: Applied Economics, 1*(3), 111–134. https://doi.org/10.1257/app.1.3.111

Desmond, M., & Bell, M. (2015). Housing, poverty, and the law. *Annual Review of Law and Social Science, 11*(1), 15–35. https://doi.org/10.1146/annurev-lawsocsci-120814-121623

Distefano, G., & Goodpaster, B. H. (2018). Effects of exercise and aging on skeletal muscle. *Cold Spring Harbor Perspectives in Medicine, 8*(3). https://doi.org/10.1101/cshperspect.a029785

Eicher-Miller, H. A., Mason, A. C., Weaver, C. M., McCabe, G. P., & Boushey, C. J. (2009). Food insecurity is associated with iron deficiency anemia in US adolescents. *The American Journal of Clinical Nutrition, 90*(5), 1358–1371. https://doi.org/10.3945/ajcn.2009.27886

Evans, W. N., & Ringel, J. S. (1999). Can higher cigarette taxes improve birth outcomes? *Journal of Public Economics, 72*(1), 135–154. https://doi.org/10.1016/s0047-2727(98)00090-5

Fera, T., Bluml, B. M., & Ellis, W. M. (2009). Diabetes ten city challenge: Final economic and clinical results. *Journal of the American Pharmacists Association, 49*(3), 383–391. https://doi.org/10.1331/japha.2009.09015

Fineberg, H. V. (2008). Retooling for an aging America. *Medscape Journal of Medicine, 10*(8), 188.

Gelberg, L., Robertson, M. J., Arangua, L., Leake, B. D., Sumner, G., Moe, A., Andersen, R. M., Morgenstern, H., & Nyamathi, A. (2012). Prevalence, distribution, and correlates of hepatitis C virus infection among homeless adults in Los Angeles. *Public Health Reports, 127*(4), 407–421. https://doi.org/10.1177/003335491212700409

Gitlin, L. N., & Wolff, J. (2011). Family involvement in care transitions of older adults: What do we know and where do we go from here? *Annual Review of Gerontology & Geriatrics, 31*(1), 31–64. https://doi.org/10.1891/0198-8794.31.31

Goldman, D. P., & Smith, J. P. (2002). Can patient self-management help explain the SES health gradient? *Proceedings of the National Academy of Sciences of the United States of America, 99*(16), 10929–10934. https://doi.org/10.1073/pnas.162086599

Gregory, C. A., & Coleman-Jensen, A. (2017, July 31). *Food insecurity, chronic disease, and health among working-age adults*. Economic Research Service U.S. Department of Agriculture. https://ageconsearch.umn.edu/record/261813/

Gundersen, C., & Ziliak, J. P. (2015). Food insecurity and health outcomes. *Health Affairs, 34*(11), 1830–1839.

Hagan, K. A., Chiuve, S. E., Stampfer, M. J., Katz, J. N., & Grodstein, F. (2016). Greater adherence to the alternative healthy eating index is associated with lower incidence of physical function impairment in the nurses' health study. *The Journal of Nutrition, 146*(7), 1341–1347. https://doi.org/10.3945/jn.115.227900

Heckman, J. J., Moon, S. H., Pinto, R., Savelyev, P. A., & Yavitz, A. (2010). The rate of return to the HighScope Perry Preschool Program. *Journal of Public Economics, 94*(1), 114–128.

Heiman, H. J., & Artiga, S. (2015). *Beyond health care: The role of social determinants in promoting health and health equity* (Issue brief Vol. 4). The Kaiser Commission on Medicaid and the Uninsured. https://www.issuelab.org/resources/22899.pdf

Hood, E. (2005). Dwelling disparities: How poor housing leads to poor health. *Environmental Health Perspectives, 113*(5). https://doi.org/10.1289/ehp.113-a310

Hunter, S., Harvey, M., Briscombe, B., & Cefalu, M. (2017). *Housing for health: A state-of-the-art program for reducing homelessness in Los Angeles County*. RAND Corporation. https://www.rand.org/pubs/research_briefs/RB10000.html

Jack, B. W. (2009). A reengineered hospital discharge program to decrease rehospitalization. *Annals of Internal Medicine, 150*(3), 178. https://doi.org/10.7326/0003-4819-150-3-200902030-00007

Jackson, C. T., Trygstad, T. K., DeWalt, D. A., & DuBard, C. A. (2013). Transitional care cut hospital readmissions for North Carolina Medicaid patients with complex chronic conditions. *Health Affairs, 32*(8), 1407–1415. https://doi.org/10.1377/hlthaff.2013.0047

Jaworsky, D., Gadermann, A., Duhoux, A., Naismith, T. E., Norena, M., To, M. J., Hwang, S. W., & Palepu, A. (2016). Residential stability reduces unmet health care needs and emergency department utilization among a cohort of homeless and vulnerably housed persons in Canada. *Journal of Urban Health: Bulletin of the New York Academy of Medicine, 93*(4), 666–681. https://doi.org/10.1007/s11524-016-0065-6

Johnson, R. C. (2012). Health dynamics and the evolution of health inequality over the life course: The importance of neighborhood and family background. *The B.E. Journal of Economic Analysis & Policy, 11*(3). https://doi.org/10.1515/1935-1682.2823

Johnson, R. C., & Schoeni, R. F. (2011). The influence of early-life events on human capital, health status, and labor market outcomes over the life course. *The B.E. Journal of Economic Analysis & Policy, 11*(3). https://doi.org/10.2202/1935-1682.2521

Kaiser Family Foundation. (2019). *Distribution of state expenditures (in millions)*. https://www.kff.org/other/state-indicator/distribution-of-state-spending/?currentTimeframe=0&sortModel=%7B%22colId%22:%22Location%22,%22sort%22:%22asc%22%7D

Kassel, C. (2014, March 27). *Should provider performance measures be risk-adjusted for sociodemographic factors?* Health Affaris Blog. https://www.healthaffairs.org/do/10.1377/hblog20140327.038175/full/

Katch, H., & Bailey, P. (2020, January 17). Medicaid doesn't pay for housing. Here's what it can do to help meet enrollees' social needs. *Health Affairs Blog*. https://www.healthaffairs.org/do/10.1377/hblog20200110.134351/full/

Katon, W. (1995). Collaborative care: Patient satisfaction, outcomes, and medical cost-offset. *Family Systems Medicine, 13*(3–4), 351–365. https://doi.org/10.1037/h0089387

Kushel, M. B., Perry, S., Bangsberg, D., Clark, R., & Moss, A. R. (2002). Emergency department use among the homeless and marginally housed: Results from a community-based study. *American Journal of Public Health, 92*(5), 778–784. https://doi.org/10.2105/ajph.92.5.778

Law, C. M., & Shiell, A. W. (1996). Is blood pressure inversely related to birth weight? The strength of evidence from a systematic review of the literature. *Journal of Hypertension, 14*(8), 935–941. https://doi.org/10.1097/00004872-199608000-00002

Lenz, A. S., Dell'Aquila, J., & Balkin, R. S. (2018). Effectiveness of integrated primary and behavioral healthcare. *Journal of Mental Health Counseling, 40*(3), 249–265. https://doi.org/10.17744/mehc.40.3.06

Liang, S.-Y., Phillips, K. A., Tye, S., Haas, J. S., & Sakowski, J. (2004). Does patient cost sharing matter? Its impact on recommended versus controversial cancer screening services. *The American Journal of Managed Care, 10*(2 Pt 1), 99–107.

Manley, A. F. (1996). *Physical activity and health: A report of the surgeon general*. DIANE Publishing.

Mann, S. L., Wadsworth, M. E., & Colley, J. R. (1992). Accumulation of factors influencing respiratory illness in members of a national birth cohort and their offspring. *Journal of Epidemiology and Community Health, 46*(3), 286–292. https://doi.org/10.1136/jech.46.3.286

Martinez, O., Jr, Poepsel, M. S., Rolf, M. K., Taylor, B., Dfaapa, P., Wergin, R. L., & Wheeler, P. (2018). *National Advisory Committee on rural health and human services*. U.S. Department of Health and Human Services. https://uscopdcoalition.org/wp-content/uploads/2020/06/Rural-COPD-Report-December-2018.pdf

McCormick, B., & White, J. (2016). Hospital care and costs for homeless people. *Clinical Medicine, 16*(6), 506–510. https://doi.org/10.7861/clinmedicine.16-6-506

McGinnis, J. M., & Foege, W. H. (1999). Mortality and morbidity attributable to use of addictive substances in the United States. *Proceedings of the Association of American Physicians, 111*(2), 109–118. https://doi.org/10.1046/j.1525-1381.1999.09256.x

McGinnis, M. J., Williams-Russo, P., & Knickman, J. R. (2002). The case for more active policy attention to health promotion. *Health Affairs, 21*(2), 78–93. https://doi.org/10.1377/hlthaff.21.2.78

McIntyre, L., Williams, J. V. A., Lavorato, D. H., & Patten, S. (2013). Depression and suicide ideation in late adolescence and early adulthood are an outcome of child hunger. *Journal of Affective Disorders, 150*(1), 123–129. https://doi.org/10.1016/j.jad.2012.11.029

McKenzie, B. (2014). *Modes less traveled-Bicycling and walking to work in the United States: 2008–2012*. American Community Survey Reports. United States Census Bureau. https://www2.census.gov/library/publications/2014/acs/acs-25.pdf

Melchior, M., Chastang, J.-F., Falissard, B., Galéra, C., Tremblay, R. E., Côté, S. M., & Boivin, M. (2012). Food insecurity and children's mental health: A prospective birth cohort study. *PLoS One, 7*(12), e52615. https://doi.org/10.1371/journal.pone.0052615

Mokdad, A. H., Marks, J. S., Stroup, D. F., & Gerberding, J. L. (2005). Correction: Actual causes of death in the United States, 2000. *JAMA: The Journal of the American Medical Association, 293*(3), 293–294. https://doi.org/10.1001/jama.293.3.293

Morrison, D. S. (2009). Homelessness as an independent risk factor for mortality: Results from a retrospective cohort study. *International Journal of Epidemiology, 38*(3), 877–883. https://doi.org/10.1093/ije/dyp160

Nagata, J. M., Hernández-Ramos, I., Kurup, A. S., Albrecht, D., Vivas-Torrealba, C., & Franco-Paredes, C. (2013). Social determinants of health and seasonal influenza vaccination in adults ≥65 years: A systematic review of qualitative and quantitative data. *BMC Public Health, 13*(1), 388. https://doi.org/10.1186/1471-2458-13-388

National Conference of State Legislatures. (2020). *Veteran homelessness: Overview of state and federal resources*. https://www.ncsl.org/research/military-and-veterans-affairs/veteran-homelessness-an-overview-of-state-and-federal-resources.aspx

National Conference of State Legislatures. (2021, March 16). *How states can leverage hospital community benefit policies to advance health equity*. https://www.nashp.org/how-states-can-leverage-hospital-community-benefit-policy-to-advance-health-equity/

Naylor, M. D., Brooten, D., Campbell, R., Jacobsen, B. S., Mezey, M. D., Pauly, M. V., & Schwartz, J. S. (1999). Comprehensive discharge planning and home follow-up of hospitalized elders: A randomized clinical trial. *JAMA: The Journal of the American Medical Association, 281*(7), 613–620. https://doi.org/10.1001/jama.281.7.613

Nord, M. (2008, February 1). *Disability is an important risk factor for food insecurity*. Economic Research Service U.S. Department of Agriculture. https://www.ers.usda.gov/amber-waves/2008/february/disability-is-an-important-risk-factor-for-food-insecurity/

Parra, S. (2016). *Predictors of inadequate follow-up of screening mammograms in Hispanic/Latinas in the Northeastern United States*. Public Health Theses Yale University. https://elischolar.library.yale.edu/ysphtdl/1223/

Ravelli, A. C., van der Meulen, J. H., Michels, R. P., Osmond, C., Barker, D. J., Hales, C. N., & Bleker, O. P. (1998). Glucose tolerance in adults after prenatal exposure to famine. *The Lancet, 351*(9097), 173–177. https://doi.org/10.1016/s0140-6736(97)07244-9

Robinson, S. M. (2018). Improving nutrition to support healthy ageing: What are the opportunities for intervention? *The Proceedings of the Nutrition Society, 77*(3), 257–264. https://doi.org/10.1017/s0029665117004037

Roseboom, T. J., van der Meulen, J. H. P., & Osmond, C. (2000). Coronary heart disease after prenatal exposure to the Dutch famine, 1944–45. *Heart, 84*(6), 595–598. https://doi.org/10.1136/heart.84.6.595

Rosenzweig, M. R., & Schultz, T. P. (1989). Schooling, information and nonmarket productivity: Contraceptive use and its effectiveness. *International Economic Review, 30*(2), 457–477. https://doi.org/10.2307/2526657

Sadowski, L. S., Kee, R. A., VanderWeele, T. J., & Buchanan, D. (2009). Effect of a housing and case management program on emergency department visits and hospitalizations among chronically ill homeless adults: A randomized trial. *JAMA: The Journal of the American Medical Association, 301*(17), 1771–1778.

Sheingold, S., Zuckerman, R., DeLew, N., & Sommers, B. (2021, July 28). Health equity and value-based payment systems: Moving beyond social risk adjustment. *Health Affairs Blog*. https://doi.org/10.1377/hblog20210726.546911

Skalicky, A., Meyers, A. F., Adams, W. G., Yang, Z., Cook, J. T., & Frank, D. A. (2006). Child food insecurity and iron deficiency anemia in low-income infants and toddlers in the United States. *Maternal and Child Health Journal, 10*(2), 177–185. https://doi.org/10.1007/s10995-005-0036-0

Sloan, F. A., Brown, D. S., Carlisle, E. S., Picone, G. A., & Lee, P. P. (2004). Monitoring visual status: Why patients do or do not comply with practice guidelines. *Health Services Research, 39*(5), 1429–1448. https://doi.org/10.1111/j.1475-6773.2004.00297.x

Smith, J. (2007). *Diabetes and the rise of the SES health gradient*. National Bureau of Economic Research. https://doi.org/10.3386/w12905

Smith, M. (2009). Pharmacists' role in improving diabetes medication management. *Journal of Diabetes Science and Technology, 3*(1), 175–179. https://doi.org/10.1177/193229680900300120

Smock, N. (2013, January 14). *Affordable Care Act regards pharmacists as health care providers, not just prescription dispensers*. Pharmacy Times. https://www.pharmacytimes.com/view/affordable-care-act-regards-pharmacists-as-health-care-providers-not-just-prescription-dispensers

Stahre, M., VanEenwyk, J., Siegel, P., & Njai, R. (2015). Housing insecurity and the association with health outcomes and unhealthy behaviors, Washington State, 2011. *Preventing Chronic Disease, 12*, E109. https://doi.org/10.5888/ped12.140511

Substance Abuse and Mental Health Services Administration. (2011). *Current statistics on the prevalence and characteristics of people experiencing homelessness in the United States* (Vol. 201). Substance Abuse and Mental Health Services Administration.

Syed, S. T., Gerber, B. S., & Sharp, L. K. (2013). Traveling towards disease: Transportation barriers to health care access. *Journal of Community Health, 38*(5), 976–993. https://doi.org/10.1007/s10900-013-9681-1

Tanumihardjo, J. P., Gunter, K. E., & Peek, M. E. (2021, June 23). As they take on food insecurity, community-based health care organizations have found four strategies that work. *Health Affairs Blog*. https://www.healthaffairs.org/do/10.1377/hblog20210616.615098/abs/

The National Council. (2017). *MACRA's quality payment program: What does it mean for your agency's Medicare reimbursement?* The National Council.

Tsai, J., Doran, K. M., & Rosenheck, R. A. (2013). When health insurance is not a factor: National comparison of homeless and nonhomeless US veterans who use Veterans Affairs Emergency Departments. *American Journal of Public Health, 103*(S2), S225–S231. https://doi.org/10.2105/ajph.2013.301307

Virapongse, A., & Misky, G. J. (2018). Self-identified social determinants of health during transitions of care in the medically underserved: A narrative review. *Journal of General Internal Medicine, 33*(11), 1959–1967. https://doi.org/10.1007/s11606-018-4615-3

Wachino, V. (2017, January 17). *State flexibility to facilitate timely access to drug therapy by expanding the scope of pharmacy practice using collaborative practice agreements, standing orders or other predetermined protocols*. Center for Medicaid and CHIP Services. https://www.medicaid.gov/federal-policy-guidance/downloads/cib011717.pdf

Walker, A. R., & Walker, B. F. (1989). The surgeon general's report on nutrition and health. *The American Journal of Clinical Nutrition, 50*(4), 884–886. https://doi.org/10.1093/ajcn/50.4.884

Wang, Y., Yeo, Q. Q., & Ko, Y. (2016). Economic evaluations of pharmacist-managed services in people with diabetes mellitus: A systematic review. *Diabetic Medicine: A Journal of the British Diabetic Association, 33*(4), 421–427. https://doi.org/10.1111/dme.12976

Williams, S. P., & Bryant, K. L. (2018). Sexually transmitted infection prevalence among homeless adults in the United States: A systematic literature review. *Sexually Transmitted Diseases, 45*(7), 494–504. https://doi.org/10.1097/olq.0000000000000780

Williams, S. W., Zimmerman, S., & Williams, C. S. (2012). Family caregiver involvement for long-term care residents at the end of life. *The Journals of Gerontology. Series B, Psychological Sciences and Social Sciences, 67*(5), 595–604. https://doi.org/10.1093/geronb/gbs065

Winfield, L., DeSalvo, K., & Muhlestein, D. (2018). *Social determinants matter, but who is responsible? 2017 survey of physicians on social determinants of health.* 2018 Annual Research Meeting. https://academyhealth.confex.com/academyhealth/2018arm/meetingapp.cgi/Paper/24695

Wolff, J. L., Spillman, B. C., Freedman, V. A., & Kasper, J. D. (2016). A national profile of family and unpaid caregivers who assist older adults with health care activities. *JAMA Internal Medicine, 176*(3), 372–379. https://doi.org/10.1001/jamaintermed.2015.7664

Chapter 5
Using Computer Technology to Support Clinical Decision-Making

Dana Edberg

1 Introduction

Helping patients maintain a healthy body and mind requires that healthcare professionals[1] understand the differing problems of each patient and then make decisions over time that will affect the health of that patient. It takes many healthcare professionals working together to help patients stay healthy, and computer technology can serve as the crucial coordination method for those people. This chapter describes the data currently used to coordinate healthcare and explores how that data might evolve in the future to accomplish high-quality, cost-effective patient-centered care. This chapter investigates how data are used to create meaningful information to support healthcare professionals in their challenging work and explores how the data collected for coordinated, integrated healthcare can also be used to support research that will help healthcare professionals work more effectively with patients in the future.

[1] The term "healthcare professional" is used generally in this chapter to represent people such as physicians, nurses, and clinical psychologists. More specifically, using the definitions provided by the Office of the National Coordinator for Health Information Technology (referred to as "ONC") (ONC, 2015), the term "physician" is used to reference an individual with an MD, and "practitioner" includes such healthcare professionals as physician assistant, clinical psychologist, registered dietician, etc. As per the ONC, the term "healthcare provider organization" or "healthcare provider" represents an organization (rather than an individual person) such as a hospital, skilled nursing facility, home health entity, community mental health center, or ambulatory surgical center.

D. Edberg (✉)
Department of Information Systems, University of Nevada, Reno, NV, USA
e-mail: dte@unr.edu

L. C. James et al. (eds.), *Clinical Health Psychology in Military and Veteran Settings*, https://doi.org/10.1007/978-3-031-12063-3_5

1.1 Example 1: Predicting and Preventing Suicide

Information can help a professional understand a problem and take appropriate action. Without information, a professional's decisions are guided by opinions which can be biased by such factors as an overreliance on the first piece of evidence we receive (anchoring) or the last (recency), a tendency to see only evidence that supports favored beliefs (confirmation), a tendency to see patterns in random events (clustering), an inability to view the evidence within a greater context (representative), the drive to ignore dangerous or negative evidence (ostrich effect), or just plain overconfidence in our abilities to evaluate the evidence and make an appropriate decision (Dimara et al., 2020). With information, professionals can acknowledge and overcome biases to make more effective decisions. Technology helps us create information to guide decision-making in ways that were previously considered too time-consuming and tedious to be possible. For example, researchers have long tried to predict and prevent suicide. Suicide is the tenth leading cause of death overall in the USA taking the lives of over 47,500 people in 2019; even more heartbreaking, suicide is the second leading cause of death for people between the ages of 10 and 34. This is an important public health issue: policy makers need to evaluate the allocation of resources when we contemplate that there were nearly two and half times more suicides in the USA (47,511) than homicides (19,141) in 2019 (NIMH, 2021). While the factors that cause a person to contemplate suicide are complex and diverse, past literature has shown that young people disclose risk factors for suicide in social media that they might hesitate to tell a healthcare professional (Lee & Kwon, 2018; Pourmand et al., 2018). This insight and the awareness of the use of technology made researchers wonder if it would be possible to predict suicide attempts with machine learning algorithms using integrated social media posts, demographics, and current events. The results were promising in determining actual suicide behavior and helped provide more information about the timing between suicide ideation and attempt (Roy et al., 2020). This is a small step forward but has the potential to help identify those in most need of intervention.

In the past, we would have to read the text in the tweets used for this research first searching through each for terms such as "hopeless" that would indicate suicide ideation and then identifying and classifying the appropriate adjectives to modify the terms. It would be unthinkable to conduct an in-person review of over three million tweets, as were evaluated for this study. This type of work would be impossible without technology able to identify the terms in unstructured text (text mining), classify the appropriate words and modifiers (sentiment analysis), and identify the patterns based on supervised and unsupervised statistical algorithms (neural networks).

1.2 Example 2: Predicting and Preventing Human Trafficking

Technology also helps us create new information by integrating evidence from multiple sources that were previously not possible to relate. For example, the US Department of Homeland Security is addressing human trafficking by integrating evidence from multiple sources (HSA, 2020). Human trafficking is a large (over 25 million victims worldwide in 2020) and profitable enterprise (billions of dollars) that is difficult to identify, trace, and prosecute. The evidence for this crime is not easy to pinpoint and usually requires participation from many different law enforcement jurisdictions, as well as social welfare agencies. Much of the evidence is contained in unstructured statements from law enforcement officers that must be compared with other text in order to identify patterns correctly (Sabo, 2019). It is especially difficult to identify the patterns unless physical locations of the events are also included. This effort requires combining evidence from differing sources such as various law enforcement agencies (including international agencies), social media sources (i.e., Facebook and Twitter), news sources, classified ads (both in print and online), and recovered victim testimony in order to create information that can be used to identify patterns. This work also requires the translation of digital images by facial recognition algorithms to identify victims more accurately. The Department of Homeland Security uses machine learning programs (i.e., neural networks) to identify the patterns of the criminal groups and has had some success in preventing some trafficking activity (HSA, 2020).

1.3 Defining Data and Information

Both examples have a common thread – they are using technology to accomplish what people alone cannot do. They are using technology to read through reams of text and create meaning from the text, compare that text to other evidence, and identify patterns. Ultimately, a person must interpret the patterns first to fully understand the problem and second to design solutions to mitigate the identified problem; people using the technology must understand its capabilities and limitations to use it effectively. Both examples rely on *data* as the input source. In this chapter, the term "data" means any characters, symbols, or numbers that are capable of being stored on a computer and transmitted in the form of electrical signals. Examples of data include a person's last name, a pain level measure of "1–10," a diagnosis code (ICD-10), a Beck Depression Inventory measurement, a practitioner's typed notes about an encounter with a patient, or a picture of a person's face. A tweet (used as input data for the first example describing an exploratory research project attempting to predict suicide) is a piece of data that contains relatively unstructured text that must be analyzed to create information.

Data are used to create *information*, which is compiled, aggregated, and summarized data that are used to support human actions. In the second example, notes from law enforcement officers were searched by text mining software and then combined with locational data to create meaningful information. That information by itself was useful to inform law enforcement actions because it was possible to create maps that showed the physical patterns of human trafficking (Sabo, 2019). But then that information was combined with social media postings to create integrated sets of data from multiple sources. These integrated data from multiple diverse sources have the potential to produce richer information. These data were then processed further to create additional information to support predictive models that are used to anticipate human trafficking events and take preventive actions (Sabo, 2019).

1.4 Integrated Care Requires Integrated Data

Integrated care is a concept that has no clear single definition (Goodwin, 2016; Kodner, 2009). From a healthcare system perspective, this means that health services are:

> managed and delivered so that people receive a continuum of health promotion, disease prevention, diagnosis, treatment, disease-management, rehabilitation, and palliative care services, coordinated across the different levels and sites of care within and beyond the health sector, and according to their needs throughout life. (Goodwin, 2016, p. 1)

From a patient's perspective, integrated care means that the patient can plan "my care with people who work together to understand me and my carer(s), allow me control, and bring together services to achieve the outcomes important to me" (Lewis et al., 2010, p. 11).

Patient-centered integrated care requires collaboration among multiple healthcare professionals. While integrating behavioral health with primary care continues to grow as healthcare systems recognize the importance of treating the whole patient (Stephens et al., 2020), this collaboration does not mean that all healthcare professionals will be co-located and sharing the same systems. What it does mean is that there must be a way to manage, integrate, and share data effectively (Stephens et al., 2020). Fast and efficient data management is crucial to enable all members of a patient's healthcare team to work together.

Health-related data are captured into an electronic patient record that is frequently referred to as an electronic health record (EHR). This chapter next describes what data are commonly found in the electronic health record (EHR), how these data can be used based on how they are input, and the issues involved with using an EHR system to capture behavioral health data. The third section discusses how data are interrelated among multiple healthcare professionals. The fourth section explores how the data might be used for patient care, analytics, and research. The final section describes the role a healthcare professional should assume as a subject matter expert to ensure that behavioral health data are captured efficiently and correctly for the ongoing enhancement of patient-centered care.

2 Collecting Data: The Electronic Health Record (EHR)

An EHR is a digital record of a patient's encounters with a healthcare provider organization. The EHR is maintained by a healthcare provider organization rather than a specific healthcare professional. This record serves as a detailed description of the healthcare events experienced by a specific patient over time (Kohli & Tan, 2016). The acronym EHR is used to represent both the application programs that capture, store, and process data and the data that are stored about the encounters with patients. EHRs are customized to fit the needs of specific types of healthcare provider organizations; an acute care hospital will most likely have different needs than a small primary care practice.[2] Figure 5.1 provides a general overview of an EHR depicting the stored data categorized by the application program systems that are used to input and/or process that data.

The 2009 Health Information Technology for Economic and Clinical Health (HITECH) Act funded programs to incentivize widespread adoption of EHRs to facilitate data sharing (ONC, 2016b). This funding was viewed as an investment to improve healthcare quality, safety, and efficiency through the promotion of more consistent and reliable health-related data. A 2008 Congressional Budget Office (CBO) report (CBO, 2008) asserted that EHR systems can enable providers to

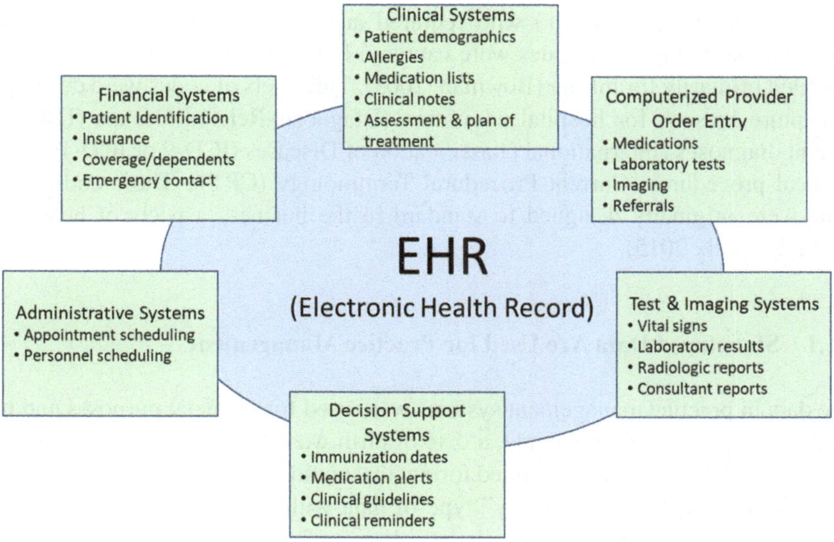

Fig. 5.1 Overview of generalized EHR systems

[2]EHR systems are available in various formats. It is possible to purchase or lease an EHR system from a vendor and run it on an organization's computers. It is also possible to run an EHR system via a cloud-based application or as a service from an EHR vendor. Pricing for EHR systems varies depending on the format, the complexity of the application program systems that are incorporated in the EHR, the number of other systems to which it must interface, and sometimes the number of healthcare professionals using the system.

deliver healthcare more efficiently. The CBO report stated that, for example, an EHR can:

- Eliminate the use of medical transcription and allow a physician to enter notes about a patient's condition and care directly into a computerized record
- Identify harmful drug interactions or possible allergic reactions to prescribed medicines
- Reduce the duplication of diagnostics tests
- Remind physicians about appropriate preventive care
- Help physicians manage patients with complex chronic conditions

Adoption of EHR systems exploded after the date of that report – between 2008 and 2016, EHR implementation among primary care physicians jumped from 7% to 84%, and non-federal acute care hospitals leaped from 9% to 96% (Maisto, 2016).

2.1 *Evolution of EHR Affected the Type of Data Stored*

Many EHR's grew from practice management systems that focused on claims and payments to handle the accounting and billing needs of practices (AMA, 2014). The original practice management systems served a small set of stakeholders (administrative personnel and payers) who required accurate coding to support billing. Procedure and diagnostic codes were captured in standardized, structured formats intended primarily for billing (Bowman, 2005). Three sets of codes were developed to capture reasons for hospital admission (Diagnosis-Related Groups (DRGs[3])), patient diagnoses (International Classification of Diseases (ICD-9 or ICD-10)), and medical procedures (Current Procedural Terminology (CPT)). These coding systems were originally designed to standardize the business aspects of healthcare (Colligan et al., 2015).

2.1.1 Structured Data Are Used for Practice Management

The data in practice management systems were used for financial purposes and had predictable formats. For example, a date of birth was always a "date" type of data with a fixed length and a pre-defined format that could be recognized by a computer. A financial charge was a "money" type of data with a pre-defined format, and a person's last name was a "variable-length character" type of data. This type of data are referred to as *structured data*; each stored data item has a pre-defined format, meaning, and size and can be both stored and accessed readily by computer systems (Hoffer et al., 2019). Structured data are most often stored in tables in a computer system and managed by a relational database management system. For example, a

[3] A DRG is a system to classify patient cases in a hospital into pre-defined groups to identify the products that are provided by a hospital (HMSA, 2018).

row in a patient table represents a unique patient and a column represents a field of data, such as a patient's date of birth.

Structured data can be used to create vivid information visualizations that help healthcare professionals make decisions. People have a highly tuned ability to see patterns, spot trends, and identify outliers if that information is presented using an appropriate visualization method (Ware, 2019). Reports, graphs, infographics, and other information visualization methods can help summarize and categorize structured data in such a way as to create simplified information and help people focus on what is different between two situations. A dashboard is a method of information visualization that combines multiple graphs and narratives into a single computer screen and is based on a set of pre-defined key performance indicators. These indicators are defined by a subject matter expert as important to a particular decision space. Historically, dashboards in practice management systems reflected key performance indicators for such information as the percentage of billings collected and were used to help a practice administrator understand which type of insurance paid what amount during what period of time. Practice administrators used dashboards to estimate cash flow and know when to contact insurance companies for payments.

2.1.2 New Data Added for Medical Records

The term "electronic medical record" (EMR) has sometimes been used interchangeably with EHR because they both include data and systems/processes to support healthcare. The EMR was originally designed to add medical data to the practice management system. It replicated the patient's chart with notes written by the physician about the patient's condition and treatment. EMRs incorporated "medical" data and were used mostly for diagnosis and treatment (Garrett & Seidman, 2011).

Physician notes were frequently dictated and stored in the EMR as a series of large text files (think of those physician notes as .pdf documents) that were attached to the patient's record in the practice management system. These text files did not contain structured data that could be stored in separate fields on a computer and were not able to be easily searched and accessed with automated tools. This type of data is referred to as *unstructured* because it has unpredictable size, structure, and meaning (Baars & Kemper, 2008). Since the patient medical data were unstructured, they could use variable terms and formats and could convey nuanced information with narrative statements about a given encounter such as the time frame when symptoms were presented (i.e., yesterday or 6 months ago), the relative severity of symptoms, ideas about the possible etiology of the disease, and behavioral data directly related to the symptoms (i.e., lack of exercise, smoking, diet) (Bowman, 2013; Swinglehurst & Greenhalgh, 2015). The structure and content of the notes were often inconsistent among physicians and were very difficult to transfer between differing healthcare provider organizations – the data in an EMR doesn't travel easily from one organization to another (Garrett & Seidman, 2011; Kharrazi et al., 2018).

Unstructured data are difficult to use for analysis. For example, if a practitioner wants to know how many and which people have symptoms of depression, computer programs will have to search through many documents looking for specific keywords to find those data. And the computer will most likely not be able to create a count of these data but will instead have to simply point to the related keyword in the document and rely on a person to do the counting. The practitioner will have to then read the document to find the context of the information. If a practitioner wants to understand past patterns of a patient's behavior or history, each unstructured document will most likely have to be searched separately to find the pertinent information. For many practitioners, this work is too time-consuming to perform before a patient's visit.

2.2 Moving from Unstructured to Structured Medical Data

When practice management billing systems were repurposed to capture medical care-related data for healthcare rather than simply supporting billing and accounting processes, they required more precise coding of medically related data (de Lusignan, 2005). Templates were created to enter data, perform error checking, and provide flags for individuals using the system. The creation of the templates required participation from healthcare professionals to understand and provide structure to the complex process of medical diagnosis and treatment (Swinglehurst et al., 2012). The goal was to create an entire "health" record of a patient that could serve as a patient-centered continuum of care record, following the patient to differing healthcare providers so that all members of the healthcare team would have ready access to the latest information. These data had to be structured so that they could be transmitted more readily while also becoming predictable and consistent as it followed a patient.

The act of coding medical data for the purpose of medical care not only changed the purpose of the EMR but also changed the processes followed by physicians and other healthcare professionals. This meant that an uncertain diagnosis, or a set of potential diagnoses, might be treated as more certain than initially intended (Varpio et al., 2015). Creating a code and assigning it to a medical record could imply unwarranted (and unintended) assertions about diagnostic certainty (Swinglehurst & Greenhalgh, 2015). It was also possible that two different physicians might elect to code the same symptoms differently leading to inconsistent results.

As medical data became structured and were able to be transmitted (theoretically) between healthcare providers, the term EHR became more widely used. As of 2021, the US Office of the National Coordinator for Health Information Technology (ONC) created a new draft for the US Core Data for Interoperability (USCDI version 2) to clarify the data that should be part of a patient's health record (see Fig. 5.2 for the data elements recommended in this draft). The new USCDI adds two types of data (ONC, 2021c) to the data set defined in 2015:

- *Clinical notes*: Both structured and unstructured data may be included.
- *Provenance*: An audit trail of the data, showing where the data came from. This is especially important because the EHR is considered a legal document and the overall accuracy of all included data must be reviewed and signed off by a physician or appropriate practitioner (Cifuentes et al., 2015).

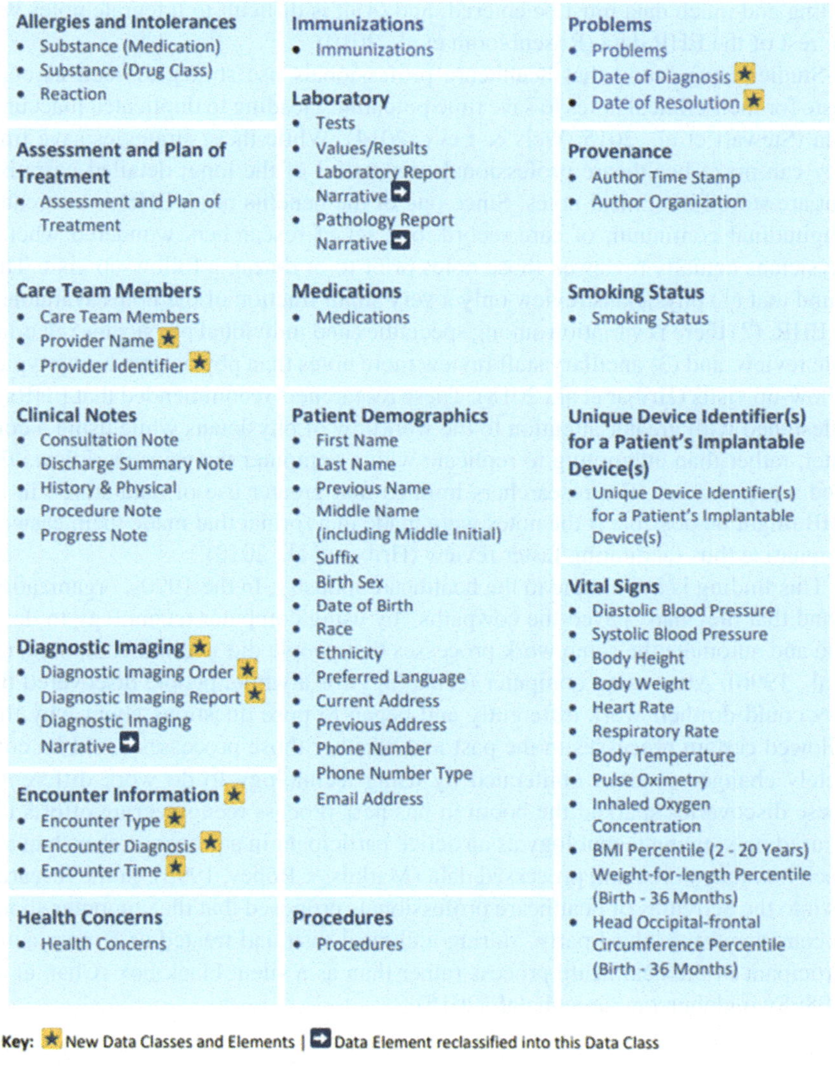

Allergies and Intolerances
Substance (Medication)
Substance (Drug Class)
Reaction
Assessment and Plan of Treatment
Assessment and Plan of Treatment
Care Team Members
Care Team Members
Provider Name
Provider Identifier
Clinical Notes
Consultation Note
Discharge Summary Note
History & Physical
Procedure Note
Progress Note
Diagnostic Imaging
Diagnostic Imaging Order
Diagnostic Imaging Report
Diagnostic Imaging Narrative
Encounter Information
Encounter Type
Encounter Diagnosis
Encounter Time
Health Concerns
Health Concerns
Immunizations
Immunizations
Laboratory
Tests
Values/Results
Laboratory Report Narrative
Pathology Report Narrative
Medications
Medications
Patient Demographics
First Name
Last Name
Previous Name
Middle Name (including Middle Initial)
Suffix
Birth Sex
Date of Birth
Race
Ethnicity
Preferred Language
Current Address
Previous Address
Phone Number
Phone Number Type
Email Address
Procedures
Procedures
Problems
Problems
Date of Diagnosis
Date of Resolution
Provenance
Author Time Stamp
Author Organization
Smoking Status
Smoking Status
Unique Device Identifier(s) for a Patient's Implantable Device(s)
Unique Device Identifier(s) for a Patient's Implantable Device(s)
Vital Signs
Diastolic Blood Pressure
Systolic Blood Pressure
Body Height
Body Weight
Heart Rate
Respiratory Rate
Body Temperature
Pulse Oximetry
Inhaled Oxygen Concentration
BMI Percentile (2 - 20 Years)
Weight-for-length Percentile (Birth - 36 Months)
Head Occipital-frontal Circumference Percentile (Birth - 36 Months)
Key: New Data Classes and Elements | Data Element reclassified into this Data Class

Fig. 5.2 US Core Data for Interoperability (USCDI v2). (ONC, 2021c)

2.2.1 Challenges Moving Clinical Notes to EHR

Clinical notes summarize interactions that occur between patients and healthcare professionals documenting the encounter. It was noted early in the implementation of EHRs that completing clinical documentation with an EHR is challenging because (1) early EHRs attempted to replicate the pre-EHR workflow for clinical notes which were usually notes generated through a process of dictation and transcription; (2) structured entry systems are constrained by the complexity of the user interface and differing contexts of healthcare; (3) documentation occurs in a chaotic setting and much data must be entered; and (4) it is difficult to integrate notes with the rest of the EHR data (Rosenbloom et al., 2010).

Studies have found that healthcare professionals use strategies such as copy/paste for their clinical notes to save time potentially leading to duplicated inaccurate data (Stewart et al., 2015; Weis & Levy, 2014). While these strategies save time, they can make healthcare professionals distrustful of the long, detailed narratives that are stored in clinical notes. Since one of the benefits of an EHR is to create a longitudinal continuum of care record, one set of researchers wondered whether physicians actually reviewed those notes prior to or during a follow-up visit. They found that (1) physicians review only a very small fraction of the notes available in an EHR, (2) there is variation among specialties and individual physicians regarding note review, and (3) ancillary staff review more notes than physicians during typical follow-up visits (Hribar et al., 2018). These researchers recommended that EHRs be redesigned with greater attention to the workflow of physicians while using a computer, rather than attempting to replicate with a computer the prior workflows that used a paper chart. The researchers implied that greater use of data stored in the EHR might be possible if the notes were made in a format that made them easier to summarize thus facilitating faster review (Hribar et al., 2018).

This finding is not unique to the healthcare industry. In the 1990s, organizations found that they had "paved the cowpaths" by using computer technology to duplicate and automate the same work processes that people did without computers (Yu et al., 1996). After using computer technology for a while, people discovered that they could do their work differently and began to pose questions about why they followed certain processes in the past and whether those processes could be completely changed or even obliterated by using technology to do work differently. These discoveries sparked the boom in business process reengineering efforts that focused on viewing technology as an active participant in a process rather than as a black box that stored and processed data (Markus & Robey, 1995). Some researchers into the activities of healthcare professionals proposed that the computer should be considered the "third party" during a clinical visit and treated as a more active participant in the healthcare process rather than as a silent black box (Chan et al., 2008; Swinglehurst & Greenhalgh, 2015).

2.2.2 Incorporating Behavioral Health Data into the EHR

Some EHRs target healthcare providers of physical health, some focus on behavioral health, and others combine both physical and behavioral health. The ONC defined the additional behavioral health data shown in Table 5.1 as important for inclusion in EHRs and federally required for transmission among healthcare providers (Matthews et al., 2016).

The data shown in Table 5.1 extend the original data set defined by the ONC and are frequently stored as unstructured data in an EHR.

A 2016 study investigated the extent of fragmentation of behavioral and physical health data in EHRs (Madden et al., 2016). The researchers studied one healthcare

Table 5.1 Behavioral health data required for inclusion in the EHR (ONC, 2016a)

Sociodemographic	Psychosocial	Health behaviors
Residential address for geocoding	Stress	Physical activity levels
Race/ethnicity	Depression	Tobacco use
Education	Intimate partner violence	Alcohol use
Overall financial resource strain		

system that served 300,000 people and included multiple healthcare providers all using the same EHR vendor. They focused on two conditions, depression and bipolar disorder, to analyze whether data related to those conditions would be recorded completely in the EHR. To accomplish this goal, they compared the data in payment claims data with data available in the medical/health records section of the EHR. They found that almost all service encounters related to the conditions were collected in the payment claims data, but a substantial majority of encounters that existed in the claims data were not documented in the medical/health records of the patients. These encounters occurred with behavioral health providers who recorded claims data but did not interface with the EHR system to record behavioral health data of the patients. Even though all providers were using the same EHR, the data were incomplete.

When a healthcare professional is treating a patient, incomplete data can be a problem, but the data can be recovered if the professional has the opportunity to ask the patient for the data again. Researchers are not so fortunate – if the data do not exist, then they cannot be recreated. Researchers are concerned that patients may seek behavioral care from practitioners who are separate from other healthcare professionals leading to fragmentation in patient care (Madden et al., 2016).

Some EHRs do not provide a way to enter behavioral health data and the resulting appropriate intervention protocols. A recent study (Bruni et al., 2021) evaluated the use of EHRs to document and track primary care physician actions in response to positive PHQ-9 screens. While the interface of the EHR collected data about PHQ-9 screening, it did not collect data about appropriate actions that should be taken based on the screening. From a data collection perspective, what was interesting is that the EHR interface did not incorporate the protocol for behavioral activation that the researchers believed necessary for informing physician actions. The EHR did not collect the necessary data for the researchers to conduct their study. Thus, before the study could be performed, the researchers worked with psychologists, pediatricians, and an EHR analyst to develop the interface needed to gather the necessary data about healthcare professional actions.

2.2.3 Challenges Incorporating Behavioral Health Data into the EHR

The two general areas of healthcare, physical and mental, have differing needs and reporting requirements, so it can be challenging to combine the two into a single EHR system. However, creating an effective and efficient clinical care team that works closely with patients as active participants requires that all stakeholders have access to the data necessary for effective decision-making.

The question of whether data should be captured and stored as structured or unstructured data is particularly salient for behavioral health data. Structured data are easy to transmit and share among multiple healthcare providers, while unstructured data are much more difficult to share. As stated in the previous section, a recent study found that clinical notes in unstructured, text format are reviewed infrequently by other providers in follow-up visits with patients (Hribar et al., 2018).

The sociodemographic data listed in Table 5.1 could be collected easily as structured data, while the psychosocial and health behavior categories are more problematic. Even something relatively straightforward like tobacco use could lead to many different questions. For example, entering that a patient smokes may lead to questions about how many cigarettes per day are smoked and for how long the patient has been smoking. It could lead to gathering data about when a person started smoking and how often the person has tried to stop smoking. From a psychological context, it could lend itself to further discussions about the relative dependency of the patient on smoking for comfort. Capturing these data as text produces richer information for treating a single patient but makes it very difficult to sort, summarize, or even find that information in the future. Capturing these data as text makes the data difficult to share and less likely that they will be reviewed by others, even if those others are using the same EHR with the same data.

The psychosocial data in Table 5.1 are also challenging to collect. Coding data, such as "stress" or "depression," requires that the people using the system have agreed upon a coding scheme. Structured data are collected in an EHR through completion of a series of templates where the healthcare professional selects items from drop-down boxes, checklists, and check boxes. These selections are created by knowledgeable designers, but they inevitably reflect an underlying model of analysis. For example, there are many ways to evaluate "depression" including the Center for Epidemiologic Studies Depression Scale, the Beck Depression Inventory, Patient Health Questionnaire (PHQ-9 or PHQ-2), and the PROMIS-8 scale. In order to record that data as a structured code in an EHR, it is necessary to select a preferred coding scheme, which will privilege one form of analysis and understanding over another (Matthews et al., 2016; Roberts, 2017). Even more difficult, these coding schemes should be standardized measures used by all practitioners for consistency across healthcare professionals in a discipline (Adler & Stead, 2015).

2.2.4 Integrating Data About the Social Determinants of Health in the EHR

Table 5.2 expands the lists of sociodemographic, psychosocial, and health behavior variables to add data suggested to be collected in the EHR during encounters with healthcare professionals. These data are not federally required to be included in the EHR data for transmission among healthcare providers (ONC, 2021b).

Table 5.2 Social determinants of health suggested for the EHR (Matthews et al., 2016)

Sociodemographic	Psychosocial	Health behaviors
Country of origin	Anxiety	Dietary pattern
Food insufficiency	Social connections/isolation	Health literacy
Housing insecurity	Conscientiousness	Sexual behavior
Employment	Optimism	
	Patient engagement	
	Self-efficacy	
	Stress in childhood	
	Sexual identity	

The social determinants of health listed in Table 5.2 affect health risks; hence, practitioner awareness of their presence for a given patient may impact the suggested treatment program. Incorporating data about social determinants of health not only can help healthcare professionals provide better targeted care but also can help with appropriate referrals (Gruß et al., 2021). Past research shows that incorporating these data into the EHR can help create automatic triggers for capturing additional important data and also notifying social service agencies (Gottlieb et al., 2015). Gottlieb et al. (2015) studied three different case studies of EHR inclusion of social determinant data to analyze how the data could be used to provide services more efficiently to patients. They found that when the data were captured in a structured format, reports could be generated that helped leadership in healthcare organizations make better decisions about which interventions provided better quality patient care. These structured data also improved efficiency in the clinic which produced cost savings. This was accomplished in one organization because the data could be used to create automated referrals for patients to other agencies. For example, one of the clinics frequently created utility shut-off protection letters stating that a patient had a chronic illness and that the patient's treatment depended on the utility. Each letter used to take 30 min to produce, but the data from the EHR cut that time to 30 s. "The provider can auto-populate the letter with the patient's demographic information and, with the patient's permission, note that the patient has a serious chronic condition" (Gottlieb et al., 2015, p. 216).

2.2.5 Challenges Integrating Data About the Social Determinants of Health into the EHR

Like the behavioral health data, the social determinants of health data are subtle, complex, and diverse. They are difficult to include in a standard template within an EHR system. Past research found that EHRs generally lack standard templates to document social determinants of health and practitioners frequently use areas allocated in the systems for unstructured notes as a workaround (Cifuentes et al., 2015). However, once data are stored in an unstructured format, it will be difficult to search, sort, and aggregate in the future. That means it will be challenging to provide important data for follow-up care, create reports that summarize service provided by a healthcare provider, or help analyze the efficacy of given interventions.

Roberts (2017) clarifies the tension that is produced between attempting to capture unstructured, nuanced text in structured data in an EHR,

> … however data are structured, the clinician can only consider the fixed set of patient characteristics and features allowed by the structured representation and has no way to stray beyond those parameters. Clinicians cannot easily describe the personal, social, and cultural circumstances of patients; the interplay between their disease, life, and treatment; or the particular way in which they experience their disease. (Roberts, 2017, p. 283)

Understanding this tension between rich description and structured coding is critical for both those who are designing EHRs and those who use the systems. Practitioners need to understand both what they gain and what they lose by structuring data so that they can better participate in the design process as true subject matter experts.

2.2.6 Integrating Patient-Generated Health Data into the EHR

Patient-generated health data (PGHD) are data that are created, recorded, and collected by patients or their caregivers. PGHD is distinct from data generated in a clinical setting because it is the patient who is responsible for gathering the data, validating the accuracy of the data, and deciding what data will be shared with healthcare professionals (Shapiro et al., 2012). PGHD can include data from home glucose monitors, personal blood pressure devices, smartphones, and wearable fitness devices like smart watches. While patients have previously shared general information verbally with healthcare professionals, PGHD provides the opportunity to formalize these digital data within the EHR. Rather than providing a single snapshot of data, PGHD can provide a more continuous look at measurements for a patient over time (Ancker et al., 2019).

PGHD can engage a patient more directly in his/her care and thus enhance the working relationship between the healthcare professional and the patient while at the same time potentially degrading the relationship if the patient substitutes PGHD for face-to-face visits with healthcare professionals (Reading & Merrill, 2018). While the data have been shown to be very helpful in managing chronic care in diagnoses of diabetes and certain types of cancer, PGHD has not yet been integrated often into the EHR because of the concern for the accuracy, consistency of context, completeness, and reliability of the data (Melstrom et al., 2021; Salvi et al., 2019).

A study examined the current use of PGHD within mental healthcare practices, focusing on the workflow, practitioner's perspectives, and how the data were interpreted and shared (Wu et al., 2020). This study reviewed data gathered from patient-reported outcomes while using smartphone apps that helped patients report their sleep quality and mood status. As with previous studies, the practitioners were concerned about the accuracy and reliability of the data. The practitioners found it difficult to incorporate the data into the workflow because there were no applications (apps) that easily integrated the PGHD into the EHR, so the data had to be evaluated manually. They also found it difficult to identify the most appropriate smartphone apps for patients to use. On the other hand, the practitioners found that using the app engaged patients more closely into their mental healthcare and created an environment where care continued beyond the face-to-face visit into an ongoing process.

Healthcare professionals work with their patients to manage many acute and chronic conditions. Patients will potentially work with many different professionals over time, so they need a continuum of care record that reflects the history of their treatment. EHRs were not intended to stand alone; they were intended to serve as key source data for a nationwide network of interconnected health data. The next section discusses the sharing and integration of health data.

3 Exchanging Data to Coordinate Care

A key benefit of storing health data in a digital format within an EHR is the ability to share it more readily in legally appropriate circumstances. Figure 5.3 is a general overview of sharing health-related data and information.

The left box on Fig. 5.3 is a summarized view of the standardized health data defined by the ONC as required for interoperable health information exchange. These data may be fragmented for a given patient, because they are stored in the EHRs of many different healthcare providers. The right box on Fig. 5.3 represents those people and organizations who generate that data, create information from it, and use that data for primary healthcare purposes and/or secondary research. Data are exchanged through three general methods as depicted by the large two-way arrow in the middle of Fig. 5.3: (1) a shared EHR that allows all professionals within a healthcare organization to access data as legally permitted, (2) a patient portal that allows a patient and/or caregivers to access data about a specific patient,

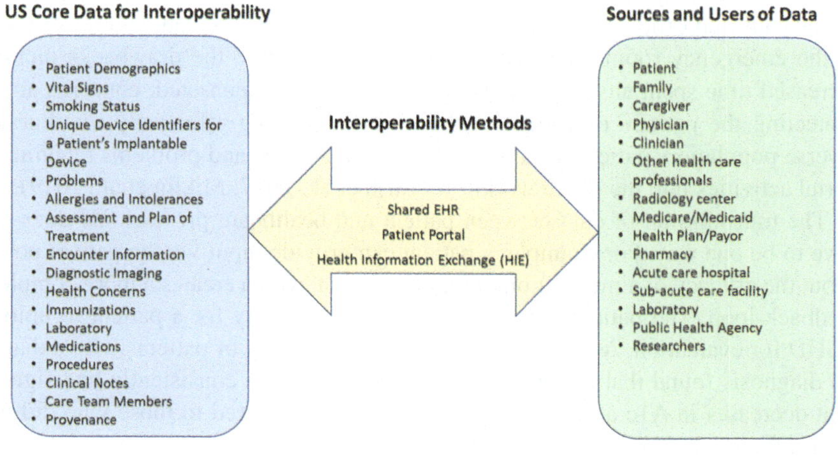

Fig. 5.3 Exchanging data among sources and users

and (3) a health information exchange (HIE), which is a platform for electronically exchanging data among independent healthcare providers. We discussed sharing data through an EHR in the previous section of this chapter, so this section will discuss the patient portal and HIE as methods for sharing data.

3.1 Sharing Data Through a Patient Portal

Data available through an EHR can be shared with patients through a patient portal. As part of the US government effort to promote the use of EHR as a strategy to improve health outcomes, ensure better population health, and provide cost efficiencies, patient portals are used to demonstrate provider-to-patient exchange of data (CMS, 2021). A patient portal is a secure website usually tied to a specific EHR from which patients can view their health-related data. Data available on a patient portal include medication lists, recent doctor visits, discharge summaries, lab results, and immunizations. Some patient portals allow a patient to securely message a doctor, request prescription refills, schedule appointments, download forms, and view additional educational materials (ONC, 2017).

Patients report that the benefits of using a portal include (1) accessing data more easily, especially viewing longitudinal records of test results, (2) communicating more quickly with a healthcare professional via messaging, (3) ordering prescription refills easily, (4) understanding medical conditions more thoroughly, and (5) increasing medication adherence (Delbanco et al., 2012; Portz et al., 2019). The drawbacks, from a patient's perspective, include (1) poorly designed user interfaces making it difficult to read or understand the text, (2) incomplete data, (3) inaccurate or inconsistent data, (4) barriers to access the portal through passwords, and (5) different patient portals for different healthcare providers using different interface formats (Cross et al., 2021; Dendere et al., 2019; Portz et al., 2019). From a healthcare provider's view, the benefits are decreases in no-show appointments, fewer low-risk phone calls and office visits, greater loyalty to a given health plan, and fewer visits to the emergency room (Avdagovska et al., 2020), while the drawbacks include increased time spent answering messages that is not compensated, concerns about protecting the privacy of patients, difficulties addressing effectively a culturally diverse population, patient avoidance of necessary visits, and problems integrating portal activities into the office workflow (Bush et al., 2017; Miklin et al., 2019).

The transmission of data between patient and healthcare professional does not have to be one way. For example, a patient can provide input via the patient portal about the efficacy of a medication or treatment plan, which creates a more complete feedback loop. The patient portal can also serve as a way for a patient to upload PGHD for evaluation. A retrospective observational study of patients with a diabetes diagnosis found that patients who uploaded their data consistently had significant decreases in A1c and body mass index when compared to those who did not upload their data (Ancker et al., 2019).

A recent study (Turvey et al., 2021) found that healthcare providers often deny patient access to treatment documentation for mental health issues. This study found that of the 80 organizations they surveyed, only 36% provided patient access to records for mental health through the patient portal. Of the providers who gave access to patients, they found that many patients asked more questions when they used the patient portal – some were distressed by the data in the notes, some engaged in self-destructive behavior, others were comforted, some exhibited greater adherence to medications, and a majority had increased trust in the practitioner (Turvey et al., 2021). While it is not required by law in the USA to share the internal notes written by a clinical psychologist with a patient, there are some who argue strongly that detailed notes should be included in the data shared through the patient portal to enhance open communication between practitioner and patient and also to encourage greater patient participation in the behavioral healthcare process (Mangino & Danis, 2020).

3.2 *Sharing Data Through a Health Information Exchange*

A health information exchange (HIE) is not a specific architecture or technology but instead is a concept defined by its capabilities and intended benefits. Applying these capabilities and benefits, an HIE is the integration and secure electronic transfer of individually identifiable clinical health information among disparate, independent health-related organizations intended to improve patient safety, the clinical management of chronic disease conditions, and clinical quality and efficiency (ONC, 2020).

Many use cases have been proposed for HIE including the need to have data available for treatment of patients in the emergency room when timely knowledge of patient allergies and medications may be critical to survival. A second use case is using the HIE to limit the number of unique, expensive tests that must be performed for a given patient since all healthcare providers would be able to share in the test results generated for a patient. Another use case for HIE is supporting patients transitioning between care settings. Poor information sharing at the time of hospital discharge can contribute to the disruption of patient care. However, effective use of HIE depends on how hospitals choose to use them; hospitals have discretion over what information they send, when they send it, and how it is structured (Adler-Milstein et al., 2021). Another use case for HIE is related to secondary research using data from the HIE. An HIE could be used as the source for data which could then be de-identified by the owners of that data before including the data for population-level research.

Rather than transmitting only raw data, an HIE frequently transmits summarized or pre-filtered information about a given patient. While it is possible to transmit entire EHR records for a patient, the goal of the HIE is to deliver information that is best suited to help with healthcare for a patient.

The acronym HIE can refer to the organization that provides communication interfaces, the vendor who supplies the technology for the interfaces, or it can refer to the actual type of platform that is used. Communities in the USA have been experimenting with the HIE concept for at least 25 years under various implementation names such as Community Health Information Network (CHIN) and Regional Health Information Organization (RHIO) (Fontaine et al., 2010).

As of 2021, the ONC recognizes three different HIE methods summarized in Table 5.3.

The information transmitted through a HIE is primarily the US Core Data for Interoperability (USCDI), and it does not usually include the non-required data on social determinants of health described in Table 5.2. It also does not usually include patient-generated health data (PGHD).

3.2.1 Barriers to Sharing Data Through a Health Information Exchange

Despite many years of experimentation and significant investment of federal US dollars through the US Health Information Technology for Economic and Clinical Health Act (HITECH), adoption and use of HIE have been painfully slow (Adler-Milstein et al., 2017; Sun, 2021). The differing rates of diffusion of HIE in other countries indicate that this is not only a problem in the USA; there is wide variation across countries in the amount of progress toward full information exchange (Payne et al., 2019). Many studies have analyzed the growth and adoption of HIE and have identified the categories of barriers shown below (Everson & Adler-Milstein, 2020; Everson & Butler, 2020; Heath & Porter, 2019; Mello et al., 2018; Shen et al., 2019; Sun, 2021):

- *Technical*: There are many different EHR vendors with different data storage methods and different formats that make it difficult to share beyond a single

Table 5.3 Health information exchange methods

Type	Common names	Description
Directed exchange	Direct, secure email	This method is a "push" method of sending information. The provider sending the information initiates the exchange. For example, directed exchange might be used to send records of COVID-19 immunization to a public health agency
Query-based exchange	State HIE, ACO HIE, national HIE, enterprise HIE	This method is a "pull" method of requesting information. The healthcare provider that wants to receive information initiates a request to the exchange and then receives the information in return. This could occur when a patient is in an emergency room and the physicians utilize a query-based exchange to access patient information such as allergies, medications, or recent tests
Consumer-mediated exchange	OpenNotes, past examples – Google Health, Microsoft HealthVault	This method is conceptualized as a way for patients to aggregate and control the use of health information among providers. The patient controls what data are exchanged and allows healthcare providers the ability to upload and access the data that are stored in a protected exchange

Adapted from Sun (2021) and ONC (2020)

vendor. In addition, some data are stored in a structured format, while other data are unstructured leading to unpredictable data that cannot be used to create integrated shared information. While there are standard protocols for data transmission and sharing (i.e., HL7 and FHIR), the context or meaning of the data must also be shared among those participating in an HIE. After gaining access to the information via the HIE, the receiving organization needs to decide what and how to integrate that information into its EHR. There are many different HIE and EHR vendors resulting in unique methods of integration that must be used for each vendor. Integrating data from the HIE into the EHR is frequently not part of the standard workflow for the receiving healthcare provider organization.

- *Financial*: EHR vendors charge a premium for the translation and integration of data into an HIE. Some regions have multiple HIE platforms available for the exchange of data requiring that an EHR vendor translates its data formats for varying numbers of different HIE platforms. Some EHR vendors charge for data conversion for each HIE. For many small healthcare providers, this cost of integration is prohibitive. In addition to the direct cost of providing data exchange functionality, healthcare providers are concerned that easy exchange of data may lead to a loss of revenue from patients who then have decreased switching costs between providers creating a more fluid and competitive environment.
- *Social/Cultural*: This category incorporates social/cultural issues on the parts of both the medical community and patients. The use of data outside of a given EHR system accessible from an HIE must be incorporated into the workflow of a given practice to make it useful. In addition, healthcare providers find it difficult to trust information from unfamiliar sources or medical technologies. Patients are concerned about the protection of their privacy; the reaction of others to information contained within healthcare data, especially mental health information, can significantly affect a patient's work and personal life. Patients must trust their healthcare professionals to have an effective patient-provider relationship, and the outside exchange of data gathered inside that relationship may go beyond what is anticipated by the patient.
- *Legal/Political*: The US federal Health Insurance Portability and Accountability Act (HIPAA) Privacy Rule declares that some healthcare data are protected health information (PHI) and requires written patient authorization for release of the data. While no authorization is required for the use of PHI for treatment, payment, or healthcare operations, it is critical that appropriate security measures be taken to protect the identity of the individual data. Fear of legal prosecution under HIPAA has delayed acceptance of HIE by some healthcare providers. Federal 42 CFR Part 2 rules restrict the disclosure of data regarding substance abuse, which constrains the ability of practitioners to exchange some behavioral health data.
- Current federal policy blocks creation of a unique patient identifier in the USA that is universal to all health records. This poses a significant political issue. HIE and EHR software must contain extensive matching algorithms to ensure that the health record for a specific patient from one healthcare provider matches to the same patient from another healthcare provider. Matching errors can lead to seri-

ous health consequences. For example, if "Jane Smith" in the emergency room does not have an allergy to penicillin, yet she is matched with a second "Jane Smith" who does have an allergy to penicillin, the physicians treating the first "Jane Smith" might believe that they are actually the same person and treat her as if she has an allergy to penicillin.

An ongoing challenge for HIE is that the exchange of information among healthcare providers may not be considered strategically beneficial to all participants (Everson et al., 2021). HIE may make it easier for patients to change healthcare providers, decreasing the loyalty to a particular group and increasing the fear of losing revenue for that group. HIE may make it easier for healthcare providers to switch EHR vendors, decreasing the reliance on a single EHR vendor and increasing the fear of the EHR vendor of losing revenue. EHR vendors may charge very high prices for data integration both to generate new revenue streams and to retain customers who would switch to a new vendor if data could be transferred more easily (Everson & Adler-Milstein, 2020; Everson et al., 2021).

3.2.2 Addressing the Barriers to Health Information Exchange Through Legislation

The US Congress passed the 21st Century Cures Act in 2016 with the intent to encourage greater sharing of data by preventing "information blocking." Information blocking is "a practice by a health IT developer of certified health IT, health information network, health information exchange, or healthcare provider that, except as required by law or specified by the Secretary of Health and Human Services (HHS) as a reasonable and necessary activity, is likely to interfere with access, exchange, or use of electronic health information (EHI)" (ONC, 2021a). There are many exceptions to information blocking in the Cures Act which could make it difficult to enforce, but it may, in the future, make it challenging for stakeholders in the realm of health information technology to purposefully withhold data and strangle the exchange of data.

In summary, the data stored in an EHR can be used to inform the process of healthcare by sharing it among patients, designated care givers, and healthcare providers. These data can be integrated in such a way as to create a continuum of care record that could accompany a patient on his/her journey to maintain good health. There are many barriers to the exchange of data including the type of data originally captured (structured vs. unstructured; clinically collected vs. patient collected), the context and meaning of the data, as well as the technical, financial, social/cultural, and legal/political roadblocks that prevent successful exchange.

We have focused so far in this chapter on using technology and digital data to coordinate primary care for a given patient. Some of the studies referenced used publicly available data from the US Centers for Medicare & Medicaid Services (CMS) that has only recently become available due to new requirements for reporting data from EHRs. The next section briefly explores how data captured for the primary care of a patient could also be used for research to provide insight into future care.

4 Using the Data

De-identified data from the EHR can be used to support research into new methods to produce cost-efficient, good quality healthcare. This secondary use of data (beyond the need for primary care of patients) can help inform future healthcare decision-making. These research activities require aggregating data for sets of patients, rather than focusing on summarizing and integrating data for a single patient. A few examples of secondary research using data from EHRs and other sources are provided in Table 5.4. These examples include supporting decision-making regarding providing better quality healthcare (e.g., identify suicidal behavior among psychiatrically hospitalized adolescents) and improving the business practice of healthcare (predict patient flows in facilities to ensure better staffing on a real-time basis).

Many of the studies focus on extracting data from unstructured clinical notes trying to pull diagnoses, treatments, and healthcare professional's sentiments about the relative extent of the symptoms under examination (Shickel et al., 2017). These studies first must create natural language processing algorithms that will correctly identify medical terminology before they can move into using the unstructured data for decision-making. After identifying the terms correctly, then text mining and sentiment analysis algorithms are tested on that data (Pulmano & Estuar, 2016). Some of the studies attempt to compare structured claim and diagnosis data with unstructured clinical notes to validate the results of using natural language processing algorithms (Kharrazi et al., 2018). Each step of the process requires painstaking work to ensure that the data extracted from unstructured notes is viable for input into predictive analytics.

These studies are starting to yield interesting results now that there is more de-identified data available from EHRs for use.

5 Conclusion

This chapter described the data that are captured in EHRs and used to support decision-making for current and future patients. The EHR is a set of apps that are written by people to automate the workflows to deliver healthcare. These apps are not set in concrete; they have the potential to change and can be adapted as new needs arise. These apps will continue to evolve as people use them and recognize that technology can both hinder and facilitate workflows. Future healthcare professionals will be called upon to enhance these systems so it would be helpful for you

Table 5.4 Sample analytic research using data from EHR and social media sources

Study citation	Description	Data source(s)
Zheng and Hu (2020)	Predict progression of Alzheimer's disease (AD) using longitudinal data	Uses AD neuroimaging data gathered from EHR data over multiple points in time integrating behavioral and physical health data (imaging)
Carson et al. (2019)	Identify suicidal behavior among psychiatrically hospitalized adolescents	Uses unstructured clinical notes in EHR to identify phases associated with suicide attempts and outcomes
Feller et al. (2020)	Explore whether social and behavioral determinants of health (SBDH) can be detected from unstructured clinical notes	Uses unstructured clinical notes in EHR data to identify key factors that compose SBDH
Sundararaman et al. (2018)	Predict readmission post-hospital discharge	Uses publicly available critical care database of congestive heart failure admissions that was gathered from acute care hospital EHR records
Bertsimas et al. (2021)	Predict patient flows, identify short-term vs. long-stay patients, predict discharge destination (sub-acute care facility use)	Uses past EHR data for prediction and current EHR data for daily hospital decision-making
Feng et al. (2017)	Develop a real-time perioperative complication risk assessment system. Calculates risk scores for each new patient	Uses real-time streaming EHR data
Mohammadi et al. (2018)	Predict no-show's to appointments to better understand appointment adherence in underserved populations	Uses EHR and appointment data
Kharrazi et al. (2018)	Explore and categorize the components of "geriatric syndrome"	Compares structured claims data and unstructured clinical notes
Pulmano and Estuar (2016)	Predict a diagnosis based on unstructured clinical notes. This text mining application could better automate the billing claims process	Uses EHR data, including claims and clinical notes, to predict the final diagnosis
Trotzek et al. (2018)	Detect depression at an early stage	Uses social media (Reddit) posts and comments from other Reddit posts over time
Thorstad and Wolff (2019)	Detect depression and other categories of mental illness (anxiety, ADHD, bipolar disorder)	Uses social media (Reddit and subreddit) posts and comments over time from discussion forums not associated with healthcare

to think about how technology could serve more effectively as your companion during a visit with a patient.

EHRs, their connected patient portals, and HIEs are written and maintained by technology professionals, and they need the support of healthcare professionals to create systems that will work. A healthcare professional is perceived by a technology professional as a subject matter expert – a person who is an authority on the workflow of healthcare and the data that can best support those workflows.

Technology can help you do your job more effectively but only if it is designed and implemented in a way that supports your work rather than detracts from it.

In summary, this chapter focuses on five key issues that could help you serve as a more effective subject matter expert:

1. Data from EHRs are used as the basis for patient healthcare and for studies analyzing healthcare practices. Accuracy and consistency of these data are critical to providing good quality healthcare and also for underlying meaningful research.
2. Data can be stored in either a structured or unstructured format. Structured data can be searched, summarized, and shared more easily than unstructured data. Structured data can be used to create information visualizations that help people see patterns. On the other hand, unstructured data can provide a richer description through detailed, nuanced narrative.
3. Data that are unstructured now but are being transformed into structured data may require healthcare professionals to agree upon a coding scheme. This coding scheme will become explicit in the EHR but may no longer be visible to those using it – it will simply become the accepted way of analyzing a given patient's condition. Choosing an effective coding scheme has long-term ramifications for those using the EHR.
4. Unstructured data are being used for population-level healthcare analyses. These data may be derived from an EHR and/or many different types of social media. These data should be viewed as potentially incomplete, inaccurate, or inconsistent, depending on the source of the data.
5. Sharing data among differing healthcare providers is challenging due to technical, financial, social/cultural, and legal/political issues. These barriers could potentially be overcome with good, coordinated design efforts performed by enthusiastic subject matter experts and competent technology professionals.

References

Adler, N. E., & Stead, W. W. (2015). Patients in context—EHR capture of social and behavioral determinants of health. *Obstetrical & Gynecological Survey, 70*(6), 388–390. https://doi.org/10.1097/01.ogx.0000465303.29687.97

Adler-Milstein, J., Embi, P. J., Middleton, B., Sarkar, I. N., & Smith, J. (2017). Crossing the health IT chasm: Considerations and policy recommendations to overcome current challenges and enable value-based care. *Journal of the American Medical Informatics Association, 24*(5), 1036–1043. https://doi.org/10.1093/jamia/ocx017

Adler-Milstein, J., Raphael, K., O'Malley, T. A., & Cross, D. A. (2021). Information sharing practices between US hospitals and skilled nursing facilities to support care transitions. *JAMA Network Open, 4*(1), e2033980. https://doi.org/10.1001/jamanetworkopen.2020.33980

American Medical Association (AMA). (2014). *Improving care: Priorities to improve electronic health record usability.* https://www.ama-assn.org/sites/ama-assn.org/files/corp/media-browser/member/about%2D%2Dama/ehr-priorities.pdf

Ancker, J., Mauer, E., Kalish, R., Vest, J., & Gossey, J. (2019). Early adopters of patient-generated health data upload in an electronic patient portal. *Applied Clinical Informatics, 10*(02), 254–260. https://doi.org/10.1055/s-0039-1683987

Avdagovska, M., Menon, D., & Stafinski, T. (2020). Capturing the impact of patient portals based on the quadruple aim and benefits evaluation frameworks: Scoping review. *Journal of Medical Internet Research, 22*(12), e24568. https://doi.org/10.2196/24568

Baars, H., & Kemper, H.-G. (2008). Management support with structured and unstructured data—An integrated business intelligence framework. *Information Systems Management, 25*(2), 132–148. https://doi.org/10.1080/10580530801941058

Bertsimas, D., Pauphilet, J., Stevens, J., & Tandon, M. (2021). Predicting inpatient flow at a major hospital using interpretable analytics. *Manufacturing & Service Operations Management*. https://doi.org/10.1287/msom.2021.0971

Bowman, SE. (2005). Coordination of SNOMED-CT and ICD-10: Getting the most out of electronic health record systems. *Perspectives in Health Information Management*, Spring 2005 (May 25, 2005).

Bowman, S. (2013). Impact of electronic health record systems on information integrity: Quality and safety implications. *Perspectives in Health Information Management, 10*(Fall). https://www.ncbi.nlm.nih.gov/pmc/articles/PMC3797550/

Bruni, T., Lalonde, L., Maragakis, A., Lee, J., Caserta, A., Kilbourne, A. M., Smith, S., Orringer, K., Quigley, J., McCaffery, H., & Lancaster, B. (2021). The use of electronic health record tools to improve evidence-based treatment of adolescent depression in primary care. *Academic Pediatrics*. https://doi.org/10.1016/j.acap.2021.05.022

Bush, R. A., Connelly, C. D., Pérez, A., Chan, N., Kuelbs, C., & Chiang, G. J. (2017). Physician perception of the role of the patient portal in pediatric health. *Journal of Ambulatory Care Management, 40*(3), 238–245. https://doi.org/10.1097/jac.0000000000000175

Carson, N. J., Mullin, B., Sanchez, M. J., Lu, F., Yang, K., Menezes, M., & Cook, B. L. (2019). Identification of suicidal behavior among psychiatrically hospitalized adolescents using natural language processing and machine learning of electronic health records. *PLoS One, 14*(2), e0211116. https://doi.org/10.1371/journal.pone.0211116

Centers for Medicare and Medicaid Services (CMS). (2021). *2021 program requirements*. https://www.cms.gov/regulations-guidance/promoting-interoperability/2021-program-requirements

Chan, W.-S., Stevenson, M., & McGlade, K. (2008). Do general practitioners change how they use the computer during consultations with a significant psychological component? *International Journal of Medical Informatics, 77*(8), 534–538. https://doi.org/10.1016/j.ijmedinf.2007.10.005

Cifuentes, M., Davis, M., Fernald, D., Gunn, R., Dickinson, P., & Cohen, D. J. (2015). Electronic health record challenges, workarounds, and solutions observed in practices integrating behavioral health and primary care. *The Journal of the American Board of Family Medicine, 28*(Supplement 1), S63–S72. https://doi.org/10.3122/jabfm.2015.s1.150133

Colligan, L., Potts, H. W., Finn, C. T., & Sinkin, R. A. (2015). Cognitive workload changes for nurses transitioning from a legacy system with paper documentation to a commercial electronic health record. *International journal of medical informatics, 84*(7), 469–476. https://doi.org/10.1016/j.ijmedinf.2015.03.003

Congressional Budget Office (CBO). (2008). *Evidence on the costs and benefits of health information technology Pub. No. 2976*. The Congress of the United States. http://www.cbo.gov/ftpdocs/91xx/doc9168/05-20-HealthIT.pdf

Cross, D. A., Levin, Z., & Raj, M. (2021). Patient portal use, perceptions of electronic health record value, and self-rated primary care quality among older adults: Cross-sectional survey. *Journal of Medical Internet Research, 23*(5), e22549. https://doi.org/10.2196/22549

de Lusignan, S. (2005). Codes, classifications, terminologies and nomenclatures: Definition, development and application in practice. *Journal of Innovation in Health Informatics, 13*(1), 65–69. https://doi.org/10.14236/jhi.v13il.580

Delbanco, T., Walker, J., Bell, S. K., Darer, J. D., Elmore, J. G., Farag, N., Feldman, H. J., Mejilla, R., Ngo, L., Ralston, J. D., Ross, S. E., Trivedi, N., Vodicka, E., & Leveille, S. G. (2012). Inviting patients to read their doctors' notes: A quasi-experimental study and a look ahead. *Annals of Internal Medicine, 157*(7), 461–470. https://doi.org/10.7326/0003-4819-157-7-201210020-00002

Dendere, R., Slade, C., Burton-Jones, A., Sullivan, C., Staib, A., & Janda, M. (2019). Patient portals facilitating engagement with inpatient electronic medical records: A systematic review. *Journal of Medical Internet Research, 21*(4), e12779. https://doi.org/10.2196/12779

Dimara, E., Franconeri, S., Plaisant, C., Bezerianos, A., & Dragicevic, P. (2020). A task-based taxonomy of cognitive biases for information visualization. *IEEE Transactions on Visualization and Computer Graphics, 26*(2), 1413–1432. https://doi.org/10.1109/tvcg.2018.2872577

Everson, J., & Adler-Milstein, J. (2020). Sharing information electronically with other hospitals is associated with increased sharing of patients. *Health services research, 55*(1), 128–135. https://doi.org/10.1111/1475-6773.13240

Everson, J., & Butler, E. (2020). Hospital adoption of multiple health information exchange approaches and information accessibility. *Journal of the American Medical Informatics Association, 27*(4), 577–583. https://doi.org/10.1093/jamia/ocaa003

Everson, J., Patel, V., & Adler-Milstein, J. (2021). Information blocking remains prevalent at the start of 21st century cures act: Results from a survey of health information exchange organizations. *Journal of the American Medical Informatics Association, 28*(4), 727–732. https://doi.org/10.1093/jamia/ocaa323

Feller, D. J., Bear Don't Walk, J. O., IV, Zucker, J., Yin, M. T., Gordon, P., & Elhadad, N. (2020). Detecting social and behavioral determinants of health with structured and free-text clinical data. *Applied Clinical Informatics, 11*(1), 172–181. https://doi.org/10.1055/s-0040-1702214

Feng, Z., Bhat, R. R., Yuan, X., Freeman, D., Baslanti, T., Bihorac, A., & Li, X. (2017). *Intelligent perioperative system: Towards real-time big data analytics in surgery risk assessment*. https://doi.org/10.1109/DASC-PICom-DataCom-CyberSchiTec.2017.201

Fontaine, P. R., Stephen, E., Zink, T., & Schilling, L. M. (2010). Systematic review of health information exchange in primary care practices. *Journal of the American Board of Family Medicine, 23*(5), 655–670. https://doi.org/10.3122/jabfm.2010.05.090192

Garrett, P., & Seidman, J. (2011, January 4). *EMR vs EHR – What is the difference?* HealthIT Buzz – The Latest on Health Information Technology from ONC. https://www.healthit.gov/buzz-blog/electronic-health-and-medical-records/emr-vs-ehr-difference

Goodwin, N. (2016). Understanding integrated care. *International Journal of Integrated Care, 16*(4). https://doi.org/10.5334/ijic.2530

Gottlieb, L. M., Tirozzi, K. J., Manchanda, R., Burns, A. R., & Sandel, M. T. (2015). Moving electronic medical records upstream: Incorporating social determinants of health. *American Journal of Preventive Medicine, 48*(2), 215–218. https://doi.org/10.1016/j.amepre.2014.07.009

Gruß, I., Bunce, A., Davis, J., Dambrun, K., Cottrell, E., & Gold, R. (2021). Initiating and implementing social determinants of health data collection in community health centers. *Population Health Management, 24*(1), 52–58. https://doi.org/10.1089/pop.2019.0205

Heath, M., & Porter, T. (2019). Sensemaking through a storytelling lens: Physician perspectives of health information exchange. *Qualitative Research in Organizations and Management: An International Journal, 14*(4), 428–443. https://doi.org/10.1108/qrom-05-2018-1648

HMSA. (2018). *Diagnosis Related Group (DRG)*. HMSA Resource Center. https://hmsa.com/portal/provider/zav_pel.fh.DIA.650.htm

Hoffer, J. V., Ramesh, V., & Topi, H. (2019). *Modern database management* (13th ed.). Pearson.

Homeland Security Association (HSA). (2020, March 18). *Snapshot: Combatting human trafficking with analytics*. Homeland Security-Science and Technology. https://www.dhs.gov/science-and-technology/news/2020/03/18/snapshot-combatting-human-trafficking-analytics

Hribar, M. R., Biermann, D., Goldstein, I. H., & Chiang, M. F. (2018). Clinical documentation in electronic health record systems: Analysis of patient record review during outpatient ophthalmology visits. *AMIA Annual Symposium Proceedings, 2018*, 584–591.

Kharrazi, H., Anzaldi, L. J., Hernandez, L., Davison, A., Boyd, C. M., Leff, B., Kimura, J., & Weiner, J. P. (2018). The value of unstructured electronic health record data in geriatric syndrome case identification. *Journal of the American Geriatrics Society, 66*(8), 1499–1507. https://doi.org/10.1111/jgs.15411

Kodner, D. L. (2009). All together now: A conceptual exploration of integrated care. *Healthcare Quarterly (Toronto, Ont.), 13 Spec No*, 6–15. https://doi.org/10.12927/hcq.2009.21091

Kohli, R., & Tan, S. S.-L. (2016). Electronic health records: How can IS researchers contribute to transforming healthcare? *MIS Q, 40*(3), 553–573. https://doi.org/10.25300/misq/2016/40.3.02

Lee, S. Y., & Kwon, Y. (2018). Twitter as a place where people meet to make suicide pacts. *Public Health, 159*, 21–26. https://doi.org/10.1016/j.puhe.2018.03.001

Lewis, R. Q., Rosen, R., Goodwin, N., & Dixon, J. (2010). *Where next for integrated care organisations in the English NHS*. The Nuffield Trust for Research and Policy Studies in Health Services. https://www.nuffieldtrust.org.uk/files/2017-01/where-next-integrated-care-english-nhs-web-final.pdf

Madden, J. M., Lakoma, M. D., Rusinak, D., Lu, C. Y., & Soumerai, S. B. (2016). Missing clinical and behavioral health data in a large electronic health record (EHR) system. *Journal of the American Medical Informatics Association, 23*(6), 1143–1149. https://doi.org/10.1093/jamia/ocw021

Maisto, M. (2016, June 1). U.S. adoption of electronic health records nears 100 percent. *E-Week IT Management*. https://www.eweek.com/it-management/u-s-adoption-of-electronic-health-records-nears-100-percent/

Mangino, D. R., & Danis, M. (2020). Sharing ethics consultation notes with patients through online portals. *AMA Journal of Ethics, 22*(9), E784–E791. https://doi.org/10.1001/amajethics.2020.784

Markus, M. L., & Robey, D. (1995). Business process reengineering and the role of the information systems professional. In V. Grover & W. Kettinger (Eds.), *Business process change: Concepts, methods, and technologies* (pp. 591–611). Idea Group, Inc.

Matthews, K. A., Adler, N. E., Forrest, C. B., & Stead, W. W. (2016). Collecting psychosocial "vital signs" in electronic health records: Why now? What are they? What's new for psychology? *American Psychologist, 71*(6), 497–504. https://doi.org/10.1037/a0040317

Mello, M. M., Adler-Milstein, J., Ding, K. L., & Savage, L. (2018). Legal barriers to the growth of health information exchange-boulders or pebbles? *The Milbank Quarterly, 96*(1), 110–143. https://doi.org/10.1111/1468-0009.12313

Melstrom, L. G., Rodin, A. S., Rossi, L. A., Fu, P., Jr., Fong, Y., & Sun, V. (2021). Patient generated health data and electronic health record integration in oncologic surgery: A call for artificial intelligence and machine learning. *Journal of Surgical Oncology, 123*(1), 52–60. https://doi.org/10.1002/jso.26232

Miklin, D. J., Vangara, S. S., Delamater, A. M., & Goodman, K. W. (2019). Understanding of and barriers to electronic health record patient portal access in a culturally diverse pediatric population. *JMIR Medical Informatics, 7*(2), e11570. https://doi.org/10.2196/11570

Mohammadi, I., Wu, H., Turkcan, A., Toscos, T., & Doebbeling, B. N. (2018). Data analytics and modeling for appointment no-show in community health centers. *Journal of Primary Care & Community Health, 9*, 215013271881169. https://doi.org/10.1177/2150132718811692

National Institute of Mental Health (NIMH). (2021, May 2021). *Suicide mental health information*. https://www.nimh.nih.gov/health/statistics/suicide

Office of the National Coordinator for Health Information Technology (ONC). (2015). *Cures Act final rule: Health care provider definition and cross-reference table*. Health.It.Gov https://www.healthit.gov/cures/sites/default/files/cures/2020-08/Health_Care_Provider_Definitions_v3.pdf

Office of the National Coordinator for Health Information Technology (ONC). (2016a). *Common clinical data set*. Health.It.Gov https://www.healthit.gov/sites/default/files/commonclinicaldataset_ml_11-4-15.pdf

Office of the National Coordinator for Health Information Technology (ONC). (2016b). *Health IT legislation and regulations*. Health.It.Gov. https://www.healthit.gov/policy-researchers-implementers/health-it-legislation-and-regulations

Office of the National Coordinator for Health Information Technology (ONC). (2017). *What is a patient portal?* Health.It.Gov. https://www.healthit.gov/faq/what-patient-portal

Office of the National Coordinator for Health Information Technology (ONC). (2020). *What is HIE?* Health.It.Gov. https://www.healthit.gov/topic/health-it-and-health-information-exchange-basics/what-hie

Office of the National Coordinator for Health Information Technology (ONC). (2021a). *Information blocking*. Health.It.Gov. https://www.healthit.gov/topic/information-blocking

Office of the National Coordinator for Health Information Technology (ONC). (2021b). *Representing housing insecurity*. Health.It.Gov. https://www.healthit.gov/isa/representing-housing-insecurity

Office of the National Coordinator for Health Information Technology (ONC). (2021c). *USCDI – United States core data for interoperability draft version 2*. Health.It.Gov. https://www.healthit.gov/isa/sites/isa/files/2021-01/Draft-USCDI-Version-2-January-2021-Final.pdf.

Payne, T. H., Lovis, C., Gutteridge, C., Pagliari, C., Natarajan, S., Yong, C., & Zhao, L.-P. (2019). Status of health information exchange: A comparison of six countries. *Journal of Global Health, 9*(2). https://doi.org/10.7189/jogh.09.020427

Portz, J. D., Bayliss, E. A., Bull, S., Boxer, R. S., Bekelman, D. B., Gleason, K., & Czaja, S. (2019). Using the technology acceptance model to explore user experience, intent to use, and use behavior of a patient portal among older adults with multiple chronic conditions: Descriptive qualitative study. *Journal of Medical Internet Research, 21*(4), e11604. https://doi.org/10.2196/11604

Pourmand, A., Roberson, J., Caggiula, A., Monsalve, N., Rahimi, M., & Torres-Llenza, V. (2018). Social media and suicide: A review of technology-based epidemiology and risk assessment. *Telemedicine and e-Health, 25*(10), 880–888. https://doi.org/10.1089/tmj.2018.0203

Pulmano, C. E., & Estuar, M. R. J. E. (2016). Towards developing an intelligent agent to assist in patient diagnosis using neural networks on unstructured patient clinical notes: Initial analysis and models. *Procedia Computer Science, 100*, 263–270. https://doi.org/10.1016/j.procs.2016.09.153

Reading, M. J., & Merrill, J. A. (2018). Converging and diverging needs between patients and providers who are collecting and using patient-generated health data: An integrative review. *Journal of the American Medical Informatics Association, 25*(6), 759–771. https://doi.org/10.1093/jamia/ocy006

Roberts, A. (2017). Language, structure, and reuse in the electronic health record. *AMA Journal of Ethics, 19*(3), 281–288. https://doi.org/10.1001/journalofethics.2017.19.3.stas1-1703

Rosenbloom, S. T., Stead, W. W., Denny, J. C., Giuse, D., Lorenzi, N. M., Brown, S. H., & Johnson, K. B. (2010). Generating clinical notes for electronic health record systems. *Applied Clinical Informatics, 01*(03), 232–243. https://doi.org/10.4338/aci-2010-03-ra-0019

Roy, A., Nikolitch, K., McGinn, R., Jinah, S., Klement, W., & Kaminsky, Z. A. (2020). A machine learning approach predicts future risk to suicidal ideation from social media data. *NPJ Digital Medicine, 3*(1). https://doi.org/10.1038/s41746-020-0287-6

Sabo, T. (2019, April 5). Countering human trafficking using text analytics and AI. *SAS Blogs*. https://blogs.sas.com/content/sascom/2019/04/05/countering-human-trafficking-using-text-analytics-and-ai/

Salvi, E., Bosoni, P., Tibollo, V., Kruijver, L., Calcaterra, V., Sacchi, L., Bellazzi, R., & Larizza, C. (2019). Patient-generated health data integration and advanced analytics for diabetes management: The AID-GM platform. *Sensors, 20*(1), 128. https://doi.org/10.3390/s20010128

Shapiro, M., Johnston, D., Wald, J., & Mon, D. (2012). *Patient-Generated Health Data*. ONC. https://www.nationalehealth.org/ckfinder/userfiles/files/PGHD%20White%20Paper_April%202012.pdf

Shen, N., Sequeira, L., Silver, M. P., Carter-Langford, A., Strauss, J., & Wiljer, D. (2019). Patient privacy perspectives on health information exchange in a mental health context: Qualitative study. *JMIR Mental Health, 6*(11), e13306. https://doi.org/10.2196/13306

Shickel, B., Tighe, P. J., Bihorac, A., & Rashidi, P. (2017). Deep EHR: A survey of recent advances in deep learning techniques for electronic health record (EHR) analysis. *IEEE Journal of Biomedical and Health Informatics, 22*(5), 1589–1604. https://doi.org/10.1109/jbhi.2017.2767063

Stephens, K. A., Van Eeghen, C., Mollis, B., Au, M., Brennhofer, S. A., Martin, M., Clifton, J., Witwer, E., Hansen, A., Monkman, J., Buchanan, G., & Kessler, R. (2020). Defining and measuring core processes and structures in integrated behavioral health in primary care: A cross-model framework. *Translational Behavioral Medicine, 10*(3), 527–538. https://doi.org/10.1093/tbm/ibz163

Stewart, E., Kahn, D., Lee, E., Simon, W., Duncan, M., Mosher, H., Harris, K., Bell, J., El-Farra, N., & Sharpe, B. (2015). Internal medicine progress note writing attitudes and practices in an electronic health record. *Journal of Hospital Medicine, 10*(8), 525–529. https://doi.org/10.1002/jhm.2379

Sun, Z. C. (2021). Mapping the landscape of health information exchange (HIE) networks in the United States. *Communications of the ACM, 49*, 483–514.

Sundararaman, A., Valady Ramanathan, S., & Thati, R. (2018). Novel approach to predict hospital readmissions using feature selection from unstructured data with class imbalance. *Big Data Research, 13*, 65–75. https://doi.org/10.1016/j.bdr.2018.05.004

Swinglehurst, D., & Greenhalgh, T. (2015). Caring for the patient, caring for the record: An ethnographic study of 'back office'work in upholding quality of care in general practice. *BMC Health Services Research, 15*(1), 177. https://doi.org/10.1186/s12913-015-0774-7

Swinglehurst, D., Greenhalgh, T., & Roberts, C. (2012). Computer templates in chronic disease management: Ethnographic case study in general practice. *BMJ Open, 2*(6), e001754. https://doi.org/10.1136/bmjopen-2012-001754

Thorstad, R., & Wolff, P. (2019). Predicting future mental illness from social media: A big-data approach. *Behavior Research Methods, 51*(4), 1586–1600. https://doi.org/10.3768/s13428-019-01235-z

Trotzek, M., Koitka, S., & Friedrich, C. M. (2018). Utilizing neural networks and linguistic metadata for early detection of depression indications in text sequences. *IEEE Transactions on Knowledge and Data Engineering, 32*(3), 588–601. https://doi.org/10.1109/tkde.2018.2885515

Turvey, C. L., Fuhrmeister, L. A., Klein, D. M., Moeckli, J., Howren, M. B., & Chasco, E. E. (2021). Patient and provider experience of electronic patient portals and secure messaging in mental health treatment. *Telemedicine and e-Health*. https://doi.org/10.1089/tmj.2020.0395

Varpio, L., Day, K., Elliot-Miller, P., King, J. W., Kuziemsky, C., Parush, A., Roffey, T., & Rashotte, J. (2015). The impact of adopting EHRs: How losing connectivity affects clinical reasoning. *Medical Education, 49*(5), 476–486. https://doi.org/10.1111/medu.12665

Ware, C. (2019). *Information visualization: Perception for design*. Morgan Kaufmann.

Weis, J. M., & Levy, P. C. (2014). Copy, paste, and cloned notes in electronic health records. *CHEST, 145*(3), 632–638. https://doi.org/10.1378/chest.13-0886

Wu, D. T. Y., Xin, C., Bindhu, S., Xu, C., Sachdeva, J., Brown, J. L., & Jung, H. (2020). Clinician perspectives and design implications in using patient-generated health data to improve mental health practices: Mixed methods study. *JMIR Formative Research, 4*(8), e18123. https://doi.org/10.2196/18123

Yu, E. S. K., Mylopoulos, J., & Lesperance, Y. (1996). AI models for business process reengineering. *IEEE Expert, 11*(4), 16–23. https://doi.org/10.1109/64.511773

Zheng, Y., & Hu, X. (2020). Healthcare predictive analytics for disease progression: A longitudinal data fusion approach. *Journal of Intelligent Information Systems, 55*(2), 351–369. https://doi.org/10.1007/s10844-020-00606-9

Chapter 6
How Will You Know Whether Your Efforts to Strengthen Patient Health Are Effective and Efficient? How Will You Convince Others?

Jeanne Wendel

1 Introduction to Health Program Evaluation

Clinicians and administrators use program evaluation studies to assess program performance, to identify strategies for improving program outcomes and efficiency, and to understand the program's fiscal impacts. These analyses are an essential component of efforts to strengthen patient health and eliminate inefficiencies currently embedded in the US healthcare system. Evaluation study results equip clinicians and program administrators to quantify impacts of their programs on patient health and to document evidence of these impacts. This chapter will discuss questions that must be addressed by teams designing these studies.

The term program evaluation is an umbrella term that describes several types of analyses of program operations, including estimation of program impacts on patient health, health-related behaviors, healthcare utilization, and (in some cases) the cost of providing care. Studies that estimate program impacts on patient health, health behaviors, and/or healthcare utilization are known as comparative effectiveness research (CER) studies.[1] Studies that estimate both health impacts and financial impacts are known as cost-effectiveness analysis (CEA) studies. Healthcare providers and payers utilize these studies to fine-tune program design; to support decisions to continue, expand, or discontinue programs; to inform provider contracting decisions; and to inform payer coverage and formulary decisions (Centers for Disease Control and Prevention [CDC], 2012).

[1] CER studies are also known as comparative clinical effectiveness research studies.

J. Wendel (✉)
Department of Economics, The University of Nevada, Reno, NV, USA
e-mail: wendel@unr.edu

L. C. James et al. (eds.), *Clinical Health Psychology in Military and Veteran Settings*, https://doi.org/10.1007/978-3-031-12063-3_6

Comparative effectiveness research (CER) studies address questions such as the following:

- Does the treatment generate physical health and/or mental health benefits for individuals who elect to participate?
- Does the treatment attract participation by the people who are most likely to benefit from the treatment?
- Can the treatment design be modified to increase participation and/or increase the health benefits enjoyed by participants?

Cost-effectiveness analysis (CEA) utilizes the same statistical methods to estimate both health impacts and financial impacts of operating specific treatments.[2] These studies report a ratio that measures the financial cost of achieving a specific health benefit (CDC, 2012, 2017).

Cost-effectiveness analysis (CEA) studies are utilized to support decisions to allocate resources across existing treatments, and they support decisions regarding health insurance coverage of new drugs and treatments. As provider and payer organizations make these decisions, they consider questions such as the following:

- How does the cost of achieving a specific health benefit via a particular treatment compare with the cost of utilizing alternate strategies to achieve the same benefit?
- How do the benefits generated by a particular treatment compare to the financial impacts of providing that treatment?
- Does the ratio of benefits to costs vary across subgroups of treatment participants (CDC, 2012)?

Answers to these questions may support payer decisions regarding coverage of new treatments. They also support provider organization decisions to allocate resources to specific treatments and assessments of an array of management issues such as (i) risks and benefits of participating in shared savings contracts and (ii) likely impacts of treatments on publicly posted quality measures and the probability of earning quality-based incentive payments.[3]

High-quality CER and CEA studies estimate causal impacts of treatments on patient health and on costs and revenues. Therefore, both types of studies require careful design to ensure that the study results will reflect causal relationships. Results that simply report correlations between treatments and outcomes do not

[2] Cost benefit analysis (CBA) studies also utilize estimates of both health and financial impacts. The two types of studies differ in the format used to compare the health and financial impacts. CEA studies, which are widely used to evaluate programs that generate health impacts, report the two sets of results using the format "net costs per unit of health benefit." Health benefits may be measured as "statistical lives saved," "statistical life years saved," or "quality-adjusted life years saved." CBA studies compute a monetary valuation of the health benefits and then report the ratio of the monetary value of health benefits to the program's net costs. For additional details, see Culyer, A.J. and K. Chalkidou, Economic Evaluation for Health Investments En Route to Universal Health Coverage: Cost-Benefit Analysis or Cost-Effectiveness Analysis? 2019. Value in Health 22: 99–103.

[3] See Chaps. 2 (The US Healthcare System: Components and Functional Areas) and 3 (Clinical Practice and Financial Management) for discussions of payment structures and risk management.

necessarily inform decision-makers about treatment impacts, because the correlations could, instead, reflect parallel trends in the treatment and outcome variables or the impact of a lurking variable not included in the analysis. The well-known economist Franklin Fisher illustrated this point with the following anecdote:

> There was once a cholera epidemic in Russia. The government, in an effort to stem the disease, sent doctors to the worst-affected areas. The peasants of [one] province ... discussed the situation and observed a very high correlation between the number of doctors in a given area and the incidence of cholera in that area (i.e. more doctors were observed in cholera areas than elsewhere). Relying on this hard fact, they rose and murdered their doctors. (Fisher, 1966)

Incentives to conduct CER and CEA studies stem from pressures to increase healthcare system efficiency. This focus on efficiency is rooted in the US Triple Aim health policy. The Triple Aim focuses on boosting healthcare quality and increasing access to healthcare while reducing the growth rate of healthcare expenditures. To achieve simultaneous progress on all three goals, healthcare payers and providers must develop and implement strategies to develop efficient and effective strategies for generating health benefits for patients (Tanenbaum, 2017). CER and CEA studies will be used to help clinicians asses the value of the care they deliver, identify opportunities for improvement, and demonstrate that value to payers (Beaudin-Seller et al., 2021; Figueroa et al., 2019). These studies will equip clinicians to address two questions: How do you know whether your efforts to strengthen patient health are successful and efficient? How will you convince others?

In this environment, clinicians face growing incentives to conduct program evaluation studies. Payers are utilizing two payment system strategies to incentivize providers to identify and implement efficient strategies for delivering care. Managed care organizations receive monthly capitated payments to provide specified care for all individuals enrolled in the managed care plan. These organizations have strong incentives to produce care efficiently while ensuring that the care meets quality standards. In addition, payers utilizing fee-for-service payments are increasingly including value-based payment incentives in the provider payment. For example, physician reimbursement for treating patients covered by Medicare may be subject to value-based rewards and penalties specified in the 2015 Medicare Access and CHIP Reauthorization Act (MACRA).[4] To the extent that integrated care strengthens performance on quality metrics while reducing overall healthcare expenditures, this delivery strategy can help physician practices maximize reimbursement for treating Medicare patients.

Some clinicians and entities contract with managed care companies and healthcare providers to offer cost-effective programs, such as integrated care, under shared savings contracts. Under these contracts, the program vendor's revenue hinges on generation of reductions in the managed care company's healthcare expenditures. These "savings" are "shared" between the program vendor and the managed care

[4] See Chap. 2 (The US Healthcare System: Components and Functional Areas) for a description of the MACRA value-based payment system.

company (Slater & Culkin, n.d.). CEA studies provide the information needed to assess whether it is wise to sign such a contract and - after a contract is signed - to determine year-end payments.

In addition to these monetary incentives to increase healthcare efficiency, healthcare providers increasingly face reputation incentives. Provider-level quality performance and payment data are now available to patients and payers. The CMS website *Care Compare* provides star ratings summarizing performance on quality of care and patient satisfaction for hospitals (including VA hospitals) and clinicians (including psychologists). In addition, states aiming to increase healthcare transparency are creating all-payer claims databases (APCDs) that store provider-level information that can support analyses to compare practice patterns across provider organizations (All-Payer Claims Database Council, 2021). Provider groups working in states that maintain APCDs can use these data to compare the quality and efficiency of their own practice patterns with the practice patterns of their peers.

Some clinicians deploying evidence-based programs may question the value of conducting CER and CEA studies to measure the impacts these programs in their clinics or practices. Despite the availability of published estimates[5] of the impacts of programs implemented in other locations, clinicians and practice administrators conduct site-specific CER and CEA studies because program impacts can differ across sites for several reasons. Site-specific variations in program impacts stem from differences in participant characteristics, differences in the program environment (payment and utilization incentives, insurance coverage, availability of complementary services such as transportation or day care), and subtle site-specific differences in program implementation details. Characteristics of eligible individuals may differ across sites if, for example, one site primarily treats patients covered by Medicaid while another site primarily treats individuals covered by private sector employer-sponsored insurance. Characteristics of the subset of patients who elect to participate in the program may differ across sites if, for example, one site successfully induces individuals with high BMI to participate in a wellness program, while most participants in the wellness program offered at another site are individuals who were already interested in exercise and healthy diets before the program was implemented (US Government Accountability Office, 2012).

Program evaluation study teams include individuals with diverse types of expertise. Clinician input is essential in the study design phase and in the assessment of the implications of the study results. The study team will also include individuals with detailed knowledge of data available in electronic medical records systems,

[5] Quantitative study results are denoted as "estimated impacts" rather than "computed impacts" because the data used in the study provides information about the specific set of patients who participated in the treatment or program. This set of patients is a random sample, in the sense that the set of patients who will participate next year will be different. They may be different people, or they may be the same people with new health issues and circumstances due to the passage of time. Quantitative analysis of the data uses statistical methods that account for variability within the sample of program participants, and the methods use this variability to generate the information needed to determine whether the program impacts are statistically significant.

along with individuals with knowledge of the program's implementation and management processes, and detailed understanding of substitutes and complements for the services offered by the program. The team will also include individuals with expertise in multivariate statistical techniques designed to distinguish between results that reflect correlations among variables and results that reflect causal relationships among variables. These individuals may be econometricians or biostatisticians. If they are not available within the healthcare provider or payer organization, clinicians and healthcare administrators can partner with university researchers who can provide the necessary econometric skills and treatment evaluation experience. In addition to providing essential skills, these researchers offer a neutral perspective, because they are not associated with treatment implementation and operation. Professors with this expertise may work in several types of university departments, including economics, statistics, and public health.

For CEA studies, the team will also include individuals with detailed knowledge of the payer and/or provider organization's fixed and variable costs and provider organization reimbursement rates and incentive structures. In addition, input may be needed from individuals with detailed understanding of the organization's budgeting processes. If the program is expected to generate costs or savings over a multiyear period, the study team will also include an individual with experience addressing issues posed by the time value of money.

Clinicians may be the team leaders for some CER and CEA studies. In other situations, clinicians may prefer to delegate this role to neutral entities or individuals who do not have vested interests in demonstrating the success of a specific treatment. Whether clinicians are team leaders or team members, they play significant roles in defining the study goals, specifying useful measures of treatment performance, ensuring that the individuals designing the analytical methods have clear and accurate understandings of treatment processes, and clarifying implications of the study results.

This chapter is not a manual specifying technical methods to complete a study. Instead, this chapter aims to equip clinical professionals and treatment managers to engage in meaningful and productive collaboration with econometricians and/or statisticians. Section 2 focuses on issues addressed by teams designing CER or CEA studies. Section 3 discusses additional issues considered by teams planning CEA studies. Section 4 addresses controversies about appropriate uses of CEA, to help study teams anticipate issues that could potentially arise when they report study results. Section 5 concludes the chapter. To streamline the discussion in this chapter, we will use the terms "program" and "treatment" interchangeably, to refer to the broad array of activities, initiatives, and programs that aim to strengthen patient or client health.

2 Tasks Required to Conduct a CER or CEA Study

While CER and CEA studies address several types of specific questions, the planning processes for all of these studies share a common structure. For both types of studies, the study designers must specify the key questions to be addressed in the study, metrics that will be used to evaluate the impacts of the treatment on participant health, the study sample, and the experimental design and statistical methods that will be used to generate reliable estimates of the treatment impacts (Adams & Neville, 2020). In addition, the study designers will assess the types of reports that will be used to convey the results to the study stakeholders. Clinicians play important roles as subject matter experts at each stage of this process.

2.1 Task # 1: Specify the Study Questions and the Date for Reporting Results to the Study Stakeholders

Specifying the questions to be addressed in the study is an essential first step that shapes subsequent decisions about the study's key evaluation metrics and the analytical strategy. In this subsection, we discuss three key questions that must be addressed to complete this task.

Who Are the Study Stakeholders? What Questions Are Important to These Entities? Completing a CER or CEA study requires staff time and financial resources. Careful study design is needed to ensure that the results of this effort will be useful to decision-makers. The first step is identification of the study stakeholders and specification of the questions that are salient for these individuals and entities. The CDC *Framework for Program Evaluation* (2017) highlights the importance of careful consideration of the questions that will be addressed by the study:

> …good evaluation does not merely gather accurate evidence and draw valid conclusions, but produces results that are used to make a difference. To maximize the chances evaluation results will be used, you need to [focus the evaluation] on questions that are most salient, relevant, and important. (CDC, 2017)

The task of specifying the study goal includes specification of relevant types of health impacts, subgroups for which impacts should be estimated, additional questions identified by the study stakeholders, and the duration of the study.

What Types of Health Impacts Are Important to the Study Stakeholders? Specification of relevant types of health impacts requires a careful trade-off. The definition must be broad enough to capture key treatment benefits, and it must be focused enough to avoid introducing statistical noise by including health events that may be also impacted by myriad other factors.

For example, an employee wellness program might include gym memberships and ergonomic consultations as strategies to reduce surgeries for musculoskeletal injuries. To estimate whether these strategies significantly reduce expenditures for musculoskeletal surgeries, it would be useful to exclude surgeries for patients with diagnoses indicating trauma, patients with recent surgeries, and patients referred to fitness facilities to complete rehabilitation programs. If data on such diagnoses are not available, analysts could alternately exclude patients with unusually long hospital stays. Similarly, for a wellness program focused on encouraging employees to comply with cancer screening recommendations, the relevant outcome metric might be expenditures for cancer treatments. In this case, analysts might control for prior employee tobacco use among program participants and nonparticipants.

What Other Issues Are Important to the Study Stakeholders? If the key study stakeholder is the program manager, that individual might be interested in both documenting program impacts and identifying opportunities for program improvement. This individual might be interested in program impacts on outcome variables, and she may also be interested in impacts on intermediate process measures. For a tobacco cessation program, for example, the manager might be interested in the program's impacts on the outcome of abstaining from tobacco use for 1 year. She might also be interested in intermediate process measures such as the proportion of eligible individuals who begin participating in the program, proportion of initial participants who complete the program, and the proportion who relapsed by year-end after abstaining for 6 months.

Should Impacts Be Estimated for Subgroups of Program Participants? In addition to estimates of program impacts on the full set of participants, stakeholders may request additional results such as estimates of program impacts by participant income category. Understanding the distributions of program participation and health benefits across subgroups of patients or clients may be important to support efforts to address equity issues or efforts to broaden the treatment's reach. Identifying subgroups for which impacts should be estimated may require consideration of shifting societal priorities and emphases and the degree to which these societal concerns are relevant to the current study. Subgroups may be delineated by a range of factors such as:

- Geographic proximity between the treatment's potential participants and treatment sites
- Socioeconomic characteristics of potential treatment participants such as education
- Demographic characteristics of potential treatment participants such as race and ethnicity
- Health risk levels of potential treatment participants defined by factors such as smoking status or the presence of specific diagnoses
- Proximity to areas affected by environmental risks such as wildfire smoke, mosquitoes carrying specific viruses, or exposures to pollution or toxins

Analyses of participation decisions by demographic or socioeconomic subgroups may help program managers adjust program design and communication strategies to optimize participation patterns. For example, evaluation of an employee wellness program indicated that employees with relatively high wages were more likely to participate in treatment events than employees with lower wages. The program vendor responded by indicating that this result highlighted an opportunity to improve the treatment design. Because employees with relatively high wages were disproportionately employed in office locations, while lower wage workers were more likely to work in non-office locations, the study result highlighted the importance of careful consideration of the locations and scheduling of program events (Mukhopadhyay & Wendel, 2013).

When Will the Study Team Report to the Study Stakeholders? From a program management perspective, it is reasonable for the treatment funder to be interested in the treatment's first-year results, to assess whether the treatment should be continued and/or modified.[6] However, specifying the report due date constrains the duration of the time available for program operation and data collection. This is an important issue for two reasons. First, if data for an ongoing treatment are to be gathered prospectively, the study duration will determine the potential number of treatment participants to be included in the study dataset. Second, the study duration will also determine the time available for observing health impacts.

The definition of a reasonable study duration depends on the types of impacts targeted by the treatment. For example, funders may be interested in first-year results, to make decisions about ongoing funding. This time frame is long enough to assess whether the program successfully helped women quit smoking while pregnant, but it would not be long enough to assess whether the program successfully helped these women maintain abstinence for a year following completion of the pregnancy. Employee wellness programs that aim to reduce employee healthcare expenditures by increasing compliance with cancer screening behaviors face a similar challenge. This strategy requires an initial investment to fund the increased cancer screenings. Thus the immediate effect of this strategy will be increased healthcare expenditures for the screenings, expenditures to determine whether patients with positive screening results actually have cancer, and expenditures to treat newly identified early cancers. However, the savings generated by treating these cancers "early" will not be realized for 6 or 7 years (Pyenson & Zenner, 2005).[7]

---

[6] The program funder is likely to be either the payer organization, the provider organization, or a grant-funding organization. See Chap. 2: The US Healthcare System: Components and Functional Areas.

[7] In addition, participation in cancer screening may increase short-term healthcare expenditures, if the screening leads to additional treatments to determine whether positive screening results accurately identify cancer cases or are simply false-positive results. Diagnostic and treatment efforts triggered by false positive can add substantial cost to a screening program. For one example, see Ong, M-S and K. D. Mandl. 2015. National Expenditure for False-Positive Mammograms and Breast Cancer Overdiagnoses Estimated at $4 Billion a Year, Health Affairs April 2015.

2.2 *Task # 2: Specify the Study Sample*

Study designers must specify whether the study will focus on analyzing the impact of the treatment on individuals who actually participated and engaged in the treatment or analyzing the impact of the treatment on all individuals who were eligible to participate in the treatment. Studies that report the impact of a treatment on individuals who participated in the treatment are said to estimate the impacts of the "treatment on the treated individuals" (TT). Studies that focus on the average impact of a treatment on the full set of individuals who were eligible to participate in the treatment are said to report the impact of "the intent to treat" (ITT). Both types of estimates are useful; however, they address different questions. TT estimates focus on the ability of the treatment to generate benefits for participants. ITT estimates of the treatment's impact capture the combined result of the program's recruitment efforts and the program's impact on participants. This type of result is relevant when the program funder pays a monthly fee for each eligible individual.[8] In this situation, the ITT permits comparison of the per capita expenditure and the per capita program impact.

For studies that report both TT and ITT impacts, the difference between TT and ITT estimates of treatment impacts yield insights about individual participation decisions. These decisions are known as "selection" decisions, and analysis of these decisions yields information about the program's ability to "target" individuals with high potential to benefit from the program. Two types of selection are possible:

Selection Type 1 People with low potential to benefit from the treatment might be more likely to participate than people who could potentially gain larger benefits by participating in the treatment. For example, "health-conscious" women may be more likely to be nonsmokers and are also more likely to initiate prenatal care during the first trimester than other women. If so, women who do not smoke would be more likely to obtain recommended prenatal care than women who are smokers. To the extent that assistance with smoking cessation is an important component of prenatal care, this would imply that women who are most likely to benefit from prenatal care (i.e., smokers) are also less likely to initiate prompt prenatal care. In this situation, the TT estimate of the impact of prenatal care would underestimate the impact that would occur if a random sample of eligible individuals obtained prenatal care. Individual selection decisions make it difficult for the treatment managers to achieve the goal of maximizing treatment benefits achieved with the resources allocated to the treatment. An increase in the proportion of eligible individuals who participate in the program would lead to an increase in the average estimated impact per participant.

---

[8] For more details on payment structures, see Chap. 2, "The US Healthcare System: Components and Functional Areas."

Selection Type 2 Alternately, women who smoke might proactively seek assistance with quitting during pregnancy. In this case, smokers would be more likely to obtain prenatal care than nonsmokers. The TT estimates of treatment impacts would overestimate the potential impact of expanded participation in a prenatal care program. In this situation individual selection decisions are congruent with treatment managers' efforts to maximize the benefits achieved with the resources allocated to the treatment. An increase in the proportion of eligible individuals who participate in the program would lead to a decrease in the average estimated impact per participant.

Consider an employee wellness program, for example. Selection impacts are likely to be important because per-person healthcare expenditures vary dramatically across individuals. Nationwide, the most expensive 5% of people spend 50% of the nation's healthcare dollars, while the least costly half of the population spends less than 3% of the nation's healthcare dollars[9] (Mitchell, 2019). Suppose a large employee group has a similar distribution of healthcare expenditures across the insured individuals. In this situation, an employee wellness treatment can only generate net savings if it successfully engages individuals who incur high healthcare expenditures along with individuals who are likely to enter that group in the future. In contrast, an employee wellness treatment that attracts participation by health-conscious individuals (who incur minimal healthcare expenditures) is not likely to generate net savings.

Selection patterns have implications for both study design and treatment design (Lewis et al., 2014). From a study design perspective, it is useful to understand the pattern of selection decisions. From a treatment design perspective, it is important to induce high levels of participation among individuals who are likely to benefit from the treatment. These efforts are known as "targeting" the program (U.S. Government Accountability Office, 2012).

2.3 *Task # 3: Specify Data Sources and Variables*

CER and CEA studies employ four types of variables: measures of program outcomes, measures of the degree and duration of program participation, variables that measure individual characteristics that may shape participation decisions, and variables that control for factors that affect program impacts such as individual health status prior to program participation. Analysts may also utilize information about confounding variables, such as major disruptions that could affect program delivery

[9]This data indicates that the 5% of people with the highest healthcare expenditures (per year) account for half of US personal healthcare expenditures. The next 45% of people account 47% of US personal healthcare expenditures. Thus, the most expensive half of US residents account for 97% of US personal healthcare expenditures. The remaining half of US residents account for 3% of US personal healthcare expenditures.

(such as government-imposed COVID lockdown restrictions, or evacuations triggered by major environmental disruptions including hurricanes or wildfires). As study designers consider the variables that will be utilized in the study, they typically confront two types of data questions: Will the study measure treatment impacts by focusing on outcome measures or process measures? Will the study utilize any proxy measures?

Will the Study Rely on Outcome Measures or Process Measures of Participant Health? Some treatment evaluation studies focus on outcome measures, such as reduced numbers of cardiac events, while other studies utilize process measures, such as participation in screenings for high blood pressure or attendance at weight management sessions. The distinction between process and outcome measures is generally clear; however, the classification of a metric as either "process" or "outcome" can be affected by the study goal. If the treatment goal is BMI reduction, then this variable would be an outcome measure. However, if the treatment focused on BMI reduction as a strategy to achieve the larger goal of reducing expenditures for cardiac events, then expenditures for cardiac events would be an outcome measure, and the BMI reduction variable would be an intermediate process variable.

Some argue that studies should focus on outcome measures, because they provide more useful and relevant information than process measures (Gross, 2012). However, some studies cannot focus on outcome measures due to time frame constraints or sample size constraints.

Time Frame Constraints Consider a study designed to estimate the financial impact of an employee wellness program. To inform the employer's decision to either continue or terminate the program, it was necessary to complete the study using 3 years of data. However, an actuarial study completed by Milliman concluded that cancer prevention treatments do not begin to reduce healthcare expenditures for 6 or 7 years after the screenings are performed (Pyenson & Zenner, 2005). Thus, outcome variables could not be used to inform the employer's contracting decision. However, process variables could provide preliminary information about program participation. This information could include analyses of changes in proportions of employees obtaining screenings (stratified by employee characteristics) or employee success in achieving BMI reductions or smoking cessation.

Sample Size Constraints Process variables may also offer an advantage over outcome variables for evaluating programs that aim to prevent high-cost outcomes that occur in only small proportions of individuals. Consider, for example, the sample size needed to be able to conclude that a 33% reduction in the incidence of an adverse outcome represents a statistically significant change. If 30% of patients initially experience the adverse outcome, the initial probability of the adverse outcome is $P = 0.30$. Suppose that only 20% of patients experienced the adverse outcome following implementation of an improvement program. This represents a 33% reduction in the incidence of the adverse outcome. If the number of patients studied was at least 143, the reduction would be statistically significant (at the 5% level, with $t >= 1.96$).

In contrast, suppose that only 3% of patients experienced the adverse outcome in the initial situation and only 2% experienced this outcome following implementation of the improvement treatment. This represents a 33% reduction in the incidence of the adverse outcome, but this change would not be statistically significant if the sample size were 143. In this case, the sample size needed to conclude that the change was statistically significant is 1875 (see Table 6.1).

For studies designed to prevent low-probability events, the key outcome is the incidence of the low-probability event. However, study designers may not be able to construct samples that are large enough to draw meaningful conclusions about this type of outcome measure. In this situation, it may be necessary to focus on process measures. However, process measures only provide insight about the treatment's impact on outcomes when estimates of the treatment's impact on a process measure are combined with published estimates of impacts of the process measure on outcomes achieved in other settings. For example, evaluation of a treatment designed to increase compliance with mammogram screening recommendations might provide evidence that the treatment increased the number of 50–59-year-old women with repeated screenings by 10,000. Study results cited by the US Preventive Services Task Force suggest that recommended screening for 10,000 women in this age category would reduce the number of breast cancer deaths by eight statistical deaths (Nelson et al., 2016). Hence, analysts would conclude that the treatment would likely reduce breast cancer deaths by approximately eight deaths.

This type of indirect estimate must be interpreted cautiously, however, because this estimation strategy does not account for possible differences in the risk factors associated with women who were screened in the program under evaluation and those who were screened in the studies that generated the published evidence. If the risk factors associated with the two sets of women differ, however, the number of

Table 6.1 Impact of the initial incidence of an adverse outcome on the sample size needed to conclude that a reduction is significant

	Percent of individuals who experience the adverse outcome			
	Incidence of adverse outcome			
	High		Low	
	Initial	After treatment participation	Initial	After treatment participation
	0.30	0.20	0.03	.002
Percent reduction in percent experiencing adverse outcome		0.33		0.33
Sample size needed to conclude that the reduction is statistically significant 5% level with $t >= 1.96$		143		1875

Computation by author

deaths averted by the treatment could be significantly higher or significantly lower than 8.

Will the Set of Independent Control Variables Include any Proxy Measures? In addition to variables measuring treatment participation and outcomes, the study dataset will include variables measuring key factors that could potentially mediate the relationship between treatment participation and outcomes. These variables are denoted as independent variables or control variables. They may identify subgroups for which the study sponsor requests separate estimation of treatment impacts. In addition, independent variables may capture individual characteristics that are hypothesized to affect either individual participation decisions or the probability that treatment participation will generate a significant impact on the individual.

However, direct measures of some important mediating variables are not always available. In these situations, it may be possible to construct proxy variables to capture key issues. For example, an evaluation of a diabetes management treatment utilized a proxy variable to measure the complexity of each participant's diabetes management task. The annual cost of each individual's diabetes-related prescriptions provided the proxy measure for the complexity variable (Wendel & Dumitras, 2005).

Detailed discussions between clinical personnel and the analysts are needed to define useful proxy measures. In addition, the analysts may estimate treatment impacts with and without inclusion of the proxy measure to assess the sensitivity of the study results to inclusion of the proxy measures in the analysis.

In other situations, it might be useful to include an independent variable to control for patient income because income might be a measure of challenges faced by the patient attempting to implement medical recommendations. Income is not generally included in medical record databases. In this situation, insurance type may be used as a proxy measure of income: individuals with low income may be eligible for Medicaid, while individuals covered by employer-sponsored insurance are likely to have higher income. Similarly, some analysts use coverage by Medicare as a proxy measure for age 65 or older. These proxy measures do not represent the key variables with complete accuracy: some low-income individuals are covered by employer-sponsored insurance, and some individuals younger than age 65 are covered by Medicare. However, these proxy measures are used as independent control variables because they provide reasonable representations of the indicated income and age categories.

2.4 *Task # 4: Specify the Analytical Strategy*

Designing a CER or CEA evaluation study to estimate a causal impact of the treatment on outcome variables requires either randomized experimental design or a multivariate econometric estimation strategy capable of yielding estimates that are likely to reflect causal relationships. Multivariate estimation techniques are used because they allow the analyst to control for an array of individual-level characteristics that potentially affect treatment participation and/or health outcomes.

Implementing a randomized experimental design for a prevention program or a clinical treatment that will be offered to a population of eligible individuals can be accomplished in several ways.

- The treatment may be implemented sequentially at different locations. Locations that have not yet implemented the treatment can serve as the control group if the eligible populations have similar characteristics at each location, the treatment implementation details are uniform at all locations, and the sequence of locations is randomly selected.
- If the treatment can initially accommodate only one-half of eligible individuals, every other caller could be enrolled in the treatment, while the remaining callers constitute the control group until treatment capacity can be expanded.
- If the study is conducted to test alternate strategies for implementing a treatment, eligible individuals may be randomly assigned to groups that will participate in alternate versions of the treatment.

Studies that use these types of randomization strategies are known as "field experiments," because the experimental design must accommodate requirements imposed by the treatment's purpose and methods and by ethical considerations raised by decisions to offer treatments or programs to selected groups of individuals.

The evaluation task is more challenging for programs that are mandatory for eligible individuals or entities. The analytical strategy used to estimate the impacts of one value-based purchasing program provides an example of issues faced by study designers in this situation (Shapoval, 2020). This study estimated whether a pay-for-performance incentive system successfully induced hospitals to reduce hospital-acquired conditions (HACs). This study utilized national data to estimate the impact of a value-based payment program administered by the federal Centers for Medicare & Medicaid Services. The Hospital-Acquired Condition Reduction Program (HACRP) was designed to incentivize hospitals to develop and implement strategies to reduce the incidence of hospital-acquired conditions for Medicare patients. The study used hospital-level performance scores reported by all hospitals included in the incentive program. The program was announced in August 2013, and the first penalties were applied in 2015. Because there is a lag between the year for which hospitals report data and the year in which penalties were used to reduce Medicare reimbursements for the penalized hospitals, the 2015 penalties reflected performance that predated the announcement of the program.

To test the hypothesis that the incentive program generated reductions in HACs, the researcher constructed a dataset that included HACRP penalty information for the years 2015, 2017, and 2019. The worst-performing 25% of hospitals were penalized in 2015, with a one percent reduction in payments earned by treating Medicare patients. For the first round of analysis, these hospitals were viewed as the "treatment" group, because they received the "treatment" of a monetary penalty and public posting of hospital-level data documenting this penalty based on activities that occurred before the incentive program was announced. The remaining hospitals were viewed as the "control" group, because they were not immediately impacted by the penalty. This presented the researcher with "before" and "after" observations for members of treatment and control groups. The fact that the initial penalties were based on actions that predated the program announcement mitigated concerns about potential selection effects. Multivariate regression indicated that the disparity between the worst performers (i.e., hospitals penalized in 2015 due to poor performance prior to announcement of the HACRP program) and the top performers (i.e., hospitals that were not likely to ever be affected by HACRP due to strong performance prior to 2015) decreased significantly by 2017, and it decreased further by 2019.

Results using this framework (of before and after observations of hospitals in the treatment and control groups) are generally viewed as likely to reflect a causal relationship. However, this type of analysis would normally be accompanied by analysis of HAC trends occurring in the two groups of hospitals for several years prior to the program announcement. Because the available data were not sufficient to support analysis of these trends, the researcher focused, instead, on additional analyses to assess whether the reduction in the gap between the worst performers and the top performers reflected a meaningful relationship or simply regression to the mean.[10]

One characteristic of causal relationships is a dose-response relationship, in which hospitals facing a greater "dose" would exhibit a larger response. The researcher tested whether a dose-response relationship was present by constructing a "threat" variable. The 25% of hospitals that were the worst performers received immediate penalties in 2015. At the same time, all hospitals received the threat that they could fall into this category in 2017, if low-performing hospitals improved their HAC scores. The threat was greatest for hospitals with scores close to the 25th percentile threshold, and it was attenuated for hospitals with scores further from this value. Multivariate analysis of the "threat" variable indicated that the data does exhibit a dose-response relationship.

One hospital administrator commented on this finding, by stating that his hospital faces incentives and pressures to improve on a broad array of metrics. If the hospital discovers that performance on one specific metric is above average, it reallocates staff time and effort to work on metrics that posed more immediate concerns.

While the researcher reported additional exploratory analyses, she cannot rule out the possibility that the results could simply reflect the phenomenon of "regression to the mean." Because the results are consistent with both hypotheses, the study results must be viewed as preliminary. If the study had been conducted to inform resource allocation decisions, the study conclusion would have provided a careful explanation of the limitations imposed by available data, and the administrator or program manager would review the results with caution until additional years of data become available.

[10] The term "regression to the mean" refers to the fact that the results could potentially be consistent with random movements from one category to other categories.

2.5 Task # 5: Specify the Types of Reports to Inform the Stakeholders About the Study Results

CER and CEA studies require thoughtful consideration of the econometric and statistical results, to draw conclusions, identify questions for further examination in the study data or in future work, and explore implications of the study results for program management strategies (Adams & Neville, 2020). Interactions among the clinicians, analysts, and program managers are useful at this point, to ensure insightful examination of these issues.

Based on the number and types of stakeholders and stakeholder requests, it may be useful to generate two types of reports, to explain (i) estimates of program impacts on all participants and on subgroups of participants and (ii) results of analyses of intermediate process measures and other issues that suggest opportunities for quality improvement.

3 Additional Tasks Required for CEA Studies

Individuals designing a CEA study will address all of the questions required for CER, for the health impact component of the CEA study. In addition, the study designers will address four questions specific to the financial impact analysis. Two of these questions add additional components to Task 1, while the other two add additional components to Task 5.

3.1 Additional Steps Required to Specify the Study Goal in Task 1

Whose Financial Impacts Will Be Estimated? CER and CEA studies estimate health benefits enjoyed by treatment participants. However, the financial impacts generated by these treatments may affect a larger set of individuals and entities. Therefore, an important issue that must be addressed during the study design phase for a CEA study is what individuals and what types of entities will be included in the financial analysis. Will the study consider financial impacts on entities that provide healthcare for the treatment participants, entities that pay for this healthcare, the participants and their families, and/or other entities such as the participants' employers? While a narrowly focused CEA that estimates financial impacts on the relevant payer and provider offers the obvious advantage of streamlining the analytical task, a more comprehensive CEA that considered financial impacts to other individuals and entities, such as patients and their families and employers, could address an important question: Were costs shifted from one entity to another, or from one entity to patients and families?[11]

The answer to this question is typically shaped by the study purpose. If the study purpose is to support decisions about allocating resources within a provider organization, then the study will focus on estimating financial impacts on that entity. If an employer funds a CEA study to provide information about the financial impacts of a wellness program, then the financial analysis will focus on financial impacts on that employer. If a payer funds a CEA study to inform decisions about a shared savings contract with a provider, the study will focus on financial impacts on the payer.

The question is more complex when a CEA study is designed to inform a public payer's decision about covering a new treatment or treatment. CEA studies designed to inform public policy decisions may include analyses of impacts on patients and social service providers, along with estimates of financial impacts on providers and payers.

This "societal perspective" is receiving increasing attention. The Analytical Perspectives report for the 2003 federal budget discusses the importance of this perspective for federal agency CEA studies (Executive Office of the President of the United States, 2003). In a section titled "Which Costs Should Be Counted?", the report states:

> If one were only concerned about impacts on the Federal budget, then the only regulatory costs that would be counted would be those incurred (or saved) by a federal agency. To reflect the full effect of a regulation, all costs to society—whether Federal, State, or private costs—should be counted when cost-effectiveness ratios are computed.

Shafrin et al. (2018) expand this discussion, describing three perspectives for conducting a CEA study. In this typology, a CEA study of a medical treatment framed by the *Traditional Payer Perspective* would include estimates of medical costs to treat the patient, adverse medical events, and patient-reported outcomes that impact the patient's quality of life. A CEA study framed by the *Traditional Societal Perspective* would include those impacts plus productivity losses and non-medical costs such as transportation and cost of the patient's time. A study framed by the *Broad Societal Perspective* would add impacts on caregivers, the option value of treatment, the insurance value to non-patients, and the value of hope.

The Second Panel on Cost-Effectiveness in Health and Medicine recommended, in 2016, that cost-effectiveness analyses utilize both the societal perspective and the more focused strategy of analyzing financial impacts relevant to the entity sponsoring the study. This panel also recommended summarizing the range of potential program impacts by including a structured table that lists health and non-health

---

[11] Important cost shifts also occur for wellness or prevention programs that require an initial expenditure and generate a flow of savings in future years. For example, an employer may invest in a wellness program designed to prevent future cardiac conditions. If the firm's employees are typically age 50 or older, the savings may not occur until these individuals retire and enroll in Medicare. In this situation, the employer makes the initial investment, and Medicare reaps the subsequent reward.

impacts of the program. This table is denoted as an "impact inventory" (Neumann & Sanders, 2017). In subsequent discussion, some analysts question the feasibility and usefulness of recommending that all CEA studies should collect the information needed to support the analyses required by a societal perspective. These analysts focus on the recommendation that CEA studies should be designed to address questions posed by the study stakeholder(s).

What Types of Financial Impacts Will Be Estimated? Studies utilizing the traditional payer perspective may (a) focus on the treatment's impacts on explicit costs incurred by healthcare providers or payers, (b) focus on the treatment's impacts on both costs and revenues, or (c) expand the analysis to address impacts on implicit costs along with the impacts on explicit costs and revenues. (The term "implicit costs" refers to costs, such as patient wait time, that do not involve monetary transactions.) The decision to include (or exclude) implicit costs may be particularly important for studies that include analyses of impacts on informal care provided by families or studies of programs that affect the duration of time patients will be unable to work (Paterson, 2014).

Cost impacts are the central financial issue for CEA studies that are funded to support shared savings contracts, and they are also the central financial issue when a treatment is expected to impact cost, with no impact on revenue. This could occur, for example, if a fixed budget clinic evaluates a treatment, to provide input into resource allocation decisions.

Impacts on both costs and revenues may be relevant for a healthcare provider facing quality-based incentive payments such as the MACRA[12] incentive system that affects payments for services provided to patients covered by traditional FFS Medicare. For example, a private sector primary care practice (PCP) might hire a team of psychologists to provide integrated care. If the integrated care treatment strengthens medication adherence and wellness behaviors among patients with type 2 diabetes, the treatment would generate two types of health impacts for these patients: increased numbers of screening visits and reduced numbers of visits to treat preventable conditions. Each of these health impacts would affect clinic costs and clinic revenues.[13] In addition, the health impacts could potentially boost patient revenue by increasing the clinic's quality-based incentive payments.

The revenue impacts of such treatments depend on payment structures and quality-based incentive structures, which vary across payers and providers. Conducting a CEA study, which analyzes both cost and revenue impacts, requires detailed information about the incentive structure offered by each payer that contracts with this PCP and proportions of patients and visits covered by each of these

[12] See Chap. 2, "The US Healthcare System: Components and Functional Areas," for a description of the MACRA incentive system.

[13] Improved patient health could also reduce the clinic's revenue if it leads to a reduction in the total number of patient visits at this clinic. This would occur if the reduction in visits requested by current patients was not offset by visits from new patients.

payers. In this situation, the study team will include professionals with expertise in billing and accounting, along with those needed to conduct a CER study.

Many CER and CEA studies focus on costs and revenues from the perspective of a single payer or a single provider. Expanding the study to encompass both a payer and a contracting provider raises an additional complication: payments made by the payer to reimburse the provider appear as costs to the payer and revenue to the provider. The cost of care that triggered the reimbursement appears as a cost incurred by the provider. Whether the provider's revenue completely offsets the cost of providing that care depends on the terms of the contract between the payer and the provider.

4 Additional Steps Required to Specify the Reporting Format in Task 5

CEA studies are widely used, to evaluate healthcare programs and treatments and to evaluate regulations and programs in other areas such as environmental regulations. However, the details of CEA study design and reporting can be controversial. Anticipating and addressing concerns about the use of CEA in the study report can facilitate communications with study stakeholders. In addition to reporting study results to stakeholders within the organization that requested the study, study results may be submitted for publication. Some organizations will value the credibility established by published study results, while others will view the results as proprietary.

Metrics for Measuring Impacts on Health and Mortality Several metrics are used to measure the benefits generated by healthcare providers, including statistical lives saved, statistical life years saved, and quality-adjusted life years saved. The metric "statistical lives saved" is equal to the number of deaths averted. The metric "statistical life years saved" is useful for assessing the impacts of treatments that are expected to extend life for a period of time such as 1 year or 5 years.

The metric quality-adjusted life years saved (QALY) was developed to measure improvements in health status as well as extensions in years of life expectancy. QALYs are frequently used to account for the fact that healthcare services may reduce pain or increase ability to conduct activities of daily living (ADLs) or instrumental activities of daily living (IADLs). If a treatment strengthens the ability of individuals to conduct ADLs, without affecting life expectancy, this improvement generates an increase in QALY scores.

Statistical lives saved can be converted to statistical life years saved, to create a common metric. To make this conversion, analysts compute the average age of individuals who lives may be saved. To illustrate, suppose the relevant population is all employed US residents. US data indicate that the median age of these workers is 43 years (https://www.bls.gov/cps/cpsaat18b.htm). Average life expectancy in the

USA is 78 years (Arias et al., 2021); hence, the average remaining life expectancy of US workers is 35 years. One statistical life saved would therefore represent 35 statistical life years saved in this population.

One year of life with perfect health is measured as one QALY. Thus, the number of QALYs saved is the same as statistical life years saved if the entire population is in perfect health until death occurs. For individuals with chronic conditions or disabilities that create difficulties conducting ADLs or IADLs, the number of QALYs is less than the number of statistical life years. (Technically, QALYs are also statistical constructs, but it is not stated explicitly because the term QALY is assumed to imply this.) The weights used to compute QALYs for years of life with less-than-perfect health are derived from surveys designed to elicit public preferences regarding the myriad ways that chronic conditions or disabilities can create difficulties with ADLs or IADLs, or create pain or mental disturbances (NICE glossary, n.d.).

Reporting Format Issue 1: Will the Health and Financial Impacts Be Reported as a Ratio? CEA studies generate estimates of the impacts of programs on participant health benefits and on costs and revenues of payers, providers, patients, and others. These results are typically reported as a ratio of costs to benefits, known as the *cost-effectiveness ratio.*[14] For example, the study results might indicate that $12 million dollars would be spent and statistical two deaths would be averted. This could be reported as $6 million dollars spent per statistical life saved.

Reporting Format Issue 2: Will the Ratio Be Compared to a Threshold? If a payer were considering several programs, it could maximize the number of lives saved with its budget, by funding programs with the lowest ratio of dollars to statistical lives saved. The payer's decision problem is more complex when it expects to receive an ongoing stream of proposals and expects to make decisions to fund (or reject) proposals as they are received. This type of organization may want to ensure that all decision-makers use consistent standards and that system resources are allocated to the set of treatments that maximize benefits to patients. In this situation, organizations may set a threshold and fund projects that generate health benefits at relatively low cost while rejecting projects that generate health benefits at higher levels of cost.

Why Use a Threshold? To examine the logic underlying the threshold-based decision strategy, consider a hypothetical organization that will allocate $60 million to implement new programs. To simplify the discussion, we assume that the cost of implementing each program is $20 million and all of the people whose lives may be saved are the same age. In this hypothetical scenario illustrated in Table 6.2, the number of statistical lives saved by each program ranges from one to ten, as detailed below:

[14] Some sources use the acronym CER to refer to the cost-effectiveness ratio. We do not use this acronym in this chapter, because we have already used CER to refer to comparative effectiveness research. Sources that use the acronym CER to refer to the cost-effectiveness ratio are typically focused on CEA studies and are not considering CER studies.

Table 6.2 Hypothetical example: CER

Treatment	Cost	Statistical lives saved	Cost per statistical life saved = Cost-effectiveness ratio (CER)
A	$20 million	10	$2 million
B	$20 million	6	$3.3 million
C	$20 million	4	$5 million
D	$20 million	2	$10 million
E	$20 million	1	$20 million

The organization would begin by funding treatment A, which would save ten statistical lives. It would also fund treatments B and C. Together, programs A, B, and C would cost $60 million, and they would save 20 lives. Thus, the organization would spend $3 million per life saved. This strategy of funding the three treatments with relatively low CERs would maximize the number of lives saved given that the organization is willing to spend $60 million for this purpose. If the organization substituted treatment D for treatment C, for example, the cost would remain at $60 million, but the total number of statistical lives saved would decrease from 20 to 18.

Implementation of the strategy of allocating resources to treatments with low cost-effectiveness ratios is straightforward if all of the treatments are known at one moment in time. Decision-makers face a more difficult decision if information about treatments becomes available as they are proposed throughout the year. These decision-makers realize that new treatments will be proposed during each budget year, and it will be necessary to either implement or reject each of these treatments as they are proposed. Suppose this decision-maker wants to fund treatments with relatively low cost-effectiveness ratios while accommodating the need to make funding decisions sporadically as treatments are proposed during the upcoming year. He could use data from recent years to set a decision threshold. If the information summarized in the table above represented treatments proposed in recent years, that threshold would be equal to $5 million. Any treatment proposed with a cost-effectiveness ratio less than or equal to $5 million would be funded. Treatments with higher cost-effectiveness ratios would not be funded.[15]

[15] The cost-effectiveness ratio of health benefits to net costs should include benefits and costs that occur over a multiyear period. For example, an expensive drug might require an initial investment that would be rewarded by a reduction in expenditures for costly treatments in future years. The CEA study should measure impacts for enough years to measure both initial and future impacts.

4.1 What Types of Agencies Compare the Cost-Effectiveness Ratio to a Threshold?

CEA is widely used to guide treatment funding decisions in healthcare and in an array of government agencies, in the USA, and in other countries. We will briefly summarize information about regulatory agencies that compare cost-effectiveness ratios to a threshold. We then discuss relevant policies of US healthcare entities.

Agencies That Compare Cost-Effectiveness Ratios to a Threshold Health benefits are generated by an array of federal programs outside the healthcare system, such as the Department of Transportation (responsible for vehicle safety standards and projects to improve highway safety), the Environmental Protection Agency (sets chemical exposure standards), and the Occupational Safety and Health Administration (which sets workplace safety and exposure standards). These agencies make controversial decisions that save lives and extend lives while also imposing costs on individuals who own small businesses, invest retirement funds in stocks, buy vehicles, and/or pay taxes. Analysts argue that it is important to implement regulations and treatments that save lives at relatively low cost while eschewing regulations and treatments that save lives at relatively high cost. For example, the Organization for Economic Cooperation and Development (OECD, 2008) focuses on CEA as a tool to guide regulatory decisions, and federal budget analysts argue that the CEA threshold decision strategy can help the federal government increase transparency and consistency of federal agency decisions that affect health and safety risks. The EPA computes cost-effectiveness ratios for proposed regulations and compares these ratios to a threshold, which is currently approximately $10 million per statistical life saved. This threshold was set in the 2000 *Guidelines for Preparing Economic Analyses*, and it is updated to reflect increases in the Consumer Price Index (US Environmental Protection Agency [EPA], 2021).

The British National Institute for Health and Care Excellence (NICE) uses a similar strategy to assess drugs and treatments and to recommend to the British National Health Service (NHS) whether each intervention is a cost-effective use of NHS resources (Sculpher et al., 2001). NHS has an annual budget each year. Therefore, offering a new drug or procedure that does not generate net savings has a clear opportunity cost: the funds expended on the new drug or procedure will not be available to provide established treatments to patients. In the NICE system, treatments that cost more than $45,000 per QALY are less likely to be recommended than treatments that generate QALYs at lower cost (Dillon, 2015). The British strategy is not unique. Similar systems are used in other EU countries, Australia, and Canada. For example, the Canadian Agency for Drugs and Technologies in Health assesses both clinical effectiveness and cost-effectiveness of new drugs and provides nonbinding recommendations to drug plans operated by Canadian provinces other than Quebec (Tikkanen et al., 2020).

CEA and Threshold Policies in HealthCare Entities in the USA In the USA, policies regarding the use of CEA in healthcare are mixed. The Centers for Medicare & Medicaid Services (CMS) does not use CEA to assess new drugs and procedures. This policy applies directly to CMS approval decisions for individuals enrolled in the traditional FFS component of Medicare. Medicare Advantage Plans[16] may elect to provide additional coverage that is not specified by CMS. The CMS decision to approve the drug Provenge illustrates the difference between decisions made on behalf of individuals enrolled in traditional FFS Medicare and decisions made on behalf of individuals enrolled in Medicare Advantage Plans (Medicare Coverage Database, 2011). Provenge was approved by the FDA in 2010, and it was approved by CMS for patients enrolled in traditional FFS Medicare with asymptomatic or minimally symptomatic metastatic prostate cancer that was resistant to other treatment[17] (National Cancer Institute, n.d.). However, the CMS decision letter specifically stated that local contractors offering Medicare Advantage Plans could make their own decisions regarding coverage for patients with less advanced cancers, when these patients are enrolled in clinical trials (Mendelson & Carino, 2011). Thus, the CMS decision against covering Provenge for patients with less advanced cancers did not block coverage through managed care plans for patients enrolled in clinical trials.

In contrast with the CMS decision, the British NICE concluded, in January 2015, that the cost-effectiveness ratio for Provenge was too low to recommend this treatment. The NICE decision noted that Provenge is an immunotherapy that stimulates the patient's own immune cells to identify and attack prostate cancer cells (National Institute for Health and Care Excellence, 2015). It was the first drug of this type to be approved by the FDA. To the extent that coverage decisions affect pharmaceutical research initiatives, the difference between the CMS and NICE decisions represents a difference in policies regarding both pharmaceutical innovation and health insurance coverage.

The Affordable Care Act (ACA) expressly prohibited the use of CEA in research funded by the new Patient-Centered Outcomes Research Institute (PCORI). The PCORI was created in the ACA to generate the evidence needed to reduce waste without harming patient outcomes (Patashnik, 2020). The ACA specified that PCORI-funded analyses would focus on clinical effectiveness, without analyzing cost-effectiveness:

> The Patient Centered Outcomes Research Institute … shall not develop or employ a dollars per quality adjusted life year… as a threshold to establish what type of health care is cost

---

[16] See Chap. 2, "The US Healthcare System: Components and Functional Areas," for a discussion of payment systems.

[17] The CMS decision stated: "Nationally Covered Indications The Centers for Medicare and Medicaid Services (CMS) proposes that the evidence is adequate to conclude that the use of autologous cellular immunotherapy treatment – Sipuleucel-T; PROVENGE® improves health outcomes for Medicare beneficiaries with asymptomatic or minimally symptomatic metastatic castrate-resistant (hormone refractory) prostate cancer, and thus is reasonable and necessary for this on-label indication under 1862(a)(1)(A) of the Social Security Act."

> effective or recommended. The Secretary shall not utilize such an adjusted life year … as a threshold to determine coverage, reimbursement, or incentive programs under title XVIII. (The PPACA) (Neumann & Weinstein, 2010)

However, when Congress reauthorized PCORI at the end of 2019, for another 10 years, it softened the prohibition against the use of PCORI funding for cost-effectiveness analysis. The 2019 bill authorized PCORI to fund research that would address a broad range of outcomes:

> Research shall be designed, as appropriate, to take into account and capture the full range of clinical and patient-centered outcomes relevant to … patients, clinicians, purchasers and policy-makers in making informed health decisions. In addition to the relative health outcomes and clinical effectiveness, clinical and patient-centered outcomes shall include the potential burdens and economic impacts of the utilization of medical treatments … on different stakeholders and decision-makers…. These potential burdens and economic impacts include medical out-of-pocket costs, including health plan benefit and formulary design, non-medical costs to the patient and family, including caregiving, effects on future costs of care, workplace productivity and absenteeism, and healthcare utilization. (CITE: P 1423. Extension of appropriations to the patient centered outcomes research trust fund; Subsection (d)(2) of such section 1181 is amended by adding: (F) Consideration of full range of outcomes data)

Despite the impact of this expansion in the types of outcomes that may be considered in PCORI-funded research, Congress continues to constrain PCORI from funding studies designed to compare a cost-effectiveness ratio with a threshold. The PCORI website states:

> … even with this expanded provision, our authorizing law still does not allow developing or employing a dollars-per-quality adjusted life year as a threshold to establish what type of health care is cost-effective or recommended…. (New Provision Bolsters Relevance, Usefulness of PCORI's Work Sept 22, 2020. http://www.pcori.org//blog-topic/research)

In contrast, other public and private entities are utilizing CEA to support health and healthcare decisions (Neumann & Sanders, 2017), including the CDC Advisory Committee for Immunization Practices (CDC, 2021), the American College of Cardiology and the American Heart Association (Anderson et al., 2014), and the Institute for Clinical and Economic Review (ICER, n.d.; Neumann & Cohen, 2018). In 2017, the VA began utilizing ICER cost-effectiveness evaluations for prescription drugs. Glassman et al. (2020) summarize the results of this collaboration:

> Overall, the VA-IOCER collaboration has been highly beneficial to VA on several fronts, most notably to help VA better understand the relative value of new drugs and in providing more concrete pricing benchmarks for medications that are often extremely costly upon release. (p. 5)

In comparing CMS and VHA policies on the use of CEA, it is useful to note that the VHA has a fixed annual budget set by Congress, while CMS deficits are financed through general fund dollars.

The fact that agencies outside the healthcare industry have established thresholds provides a useful context for considering cost-effectiveness ratios computed for healthcare interventions. The EPA strategy for setting the threshold focuses on actual decisions made by individuals when they face trade-offs between risk and money. Individuals face this decision when they weigh the costs and benefits of buying a smaller, cheaper, and less safe vehicle against the costs and benefits of a larger, heavier, and safer vehicle. Individuals also face this decision when they consider employment in jobs that provide a base rate of pay and additional payment in the form of "hazard pay" for individuals facing elevated on-the-job risk (Catolico, 2020). The EPA website posts a review of published studies on decisions in which people reduce risk by paying higher prices (or accepting lower wages). The EPA's explanation of its logic focuses on trade-offs individuals make between dollars and risk in our daily lives:

> The EPA does not place a dollar value on individual lives. Rather, when conducting a benefit-cost analysis of new environmental policies, the Agency uses estimates of how much people are willing to pay for small reductions in their risks of dying from adverse health conditions that may be caused by environmental pollution.
>
> This is best explained by way of an example. Suppose each person in a sample of 100,000 people were asked how much he or she would be willing to pay for a reduction in their individual risk of dying of 1 in 100,000, or 0.001%, over the next year. Since this reduction in risk would mean that we would expect one fewer death among the sample of 100,000 people over the next year on average, this is sometimes described as "one statistical life saved." Now suppose that the average response to this hypothetical question was $100. Then the total dollar amount that the group would be willing to pay to save one statistical life in a year would be $100 per person × 100,000 people, or $10 million. This is what is meant by the "value of a statistical life." Importantly, this is not an estimate of how much money any single individual or group would be willing to pay to prevent the certain death of any particular person.
>
> What does it mean to place value on life? (EPA, 2020)

Based on these studies, the EPA concludes that the American public is willing to pay approximately $10 million per statistical life saved. This conclusion does not state that any individual would be willing to exchange his life for this amount of money. Instead, this conclusion indicates that a large population has demonstrated willingness to spend a total of $10 million to avoid one statistical death, or $286,000 to avoid losing on statistical life year. This number exceeds the NICE threshold by a substantial margin.

Anticipate Concerns About CEA Methods and Address These Concerns in the Study Report

The concept of allocating government funds to treatments that generate benefits at relatively low cost is widely accepted as an essential component of efforts to increase healthcare efficiency. However, some aspects of this concept are controversial. It may be useful for study designers to anticipate concerns articulated by individuals and groups opposing the use of CEA and CEA thresholds.

- *There may be substantive gaps in the information available to support the CEA study.*

Information is not always available to support evidence-based estimates of costs and benefits of new treatments. This issue is particularly salient when long-term costs and benefits are important and when individual behavioral responses are important. To address this concern, CER and CEA reports should provide detailed information about limitations imposed by the available data.

- *Reliance on the QALY metric could disadvantage disabled individuals.*

The use of the QALY metric raises concerns about comparisons of treatments that would extend life for individuals in perfect health versus treatments that would extend life for individuals with chronic conditions or disabilities. One extra year of life would generate more QALYs for individuals in otherwise perfect health than for individuals with chronic conditions or disabilities. Some analysts and policy-makers view this problem as sufficient reason to ban the use of CEA for insurance coverage decisions. Analysts can address this concern by reporting two CEA ratios, with one ratio using the QALY metric and the second ratio using statistical life years saved.

- *The manner of death may be important.*

Some analysts argue that people may generally dread death due to cancer more than sudden death due to an accident. NICE addresses this concern by setting a separate threshold for treatments that extend life for cancer patients.

- *Maximizing the total number of statistical lives saved is a simplistic goal. It ignores the question of whether there is an equitable distribution of statistical lives saved across groups delineated by geographic, socioeconomic, race/ethnicity, age, and health status characteristics.*

Some opponents of using CEA argue that the threshold decision strategy is likely to focus attention on healthcare system efficiency while diverting attention from equity issues. These analysts argue that equity concerns require careful consideration of the impacts of CEA decision strategies across subgroups of people differentiated by geography, socioeconomic status, race/ethnicity, age, differences in health status, and other characteristics (Neumann & Sanders, 2017).

- *Using a CEA threshold to make health insurance coverage decisions is a smokescreen to disguise rationing or limiting care. Restricting access to costly care could harm current patients and impede medical innovations that might benefit future patients.*

Some critics of using CEA thresholds as a tool to guide health insurance coverage decisions fear that comparing CEA ratios to a threshold is likely to limit healthcare expenditures. Advocates of the use of CEA counter this argument by stating that resource allocation decisions cannot be avoided and CEA increases the transparency of the trade-offs facing decision-makers (Neumann & Sanders, 2017).

Analysts also note that some expensive drugs are cost effective. In this situation, the CEA approach offers a logical approach to drug assessment. For example, some cancer drugs are expensive. Compared with money spent to avert statistical deaths in non-healthcare situations, however, some expensive healthcare treatments are bargains (Lakdawalla et al., 2010; Philipson et al., 2012; Lichtenberg, 2013). For example, Lakdawalla et al. (2010) conclude life expectancy for patients diagnosed with cancer during the years 1988–2000 increased by 4 years. Despite the much discussed high prices for cancer drugs, they also conclude that expenditures per statistical life year saved were substantially lower than the EPA threshold. They conclude that healthcare producers received less than 20% of the net gain, while patients enjoyed the majority of this gain. These results indicate that CEA offers a more nuanced assessment strategy than the "cost containment" approach for improving healthcare system efficiency (Murphy & Topel, 2006).

- *The term "statistical life" is confusing.*

The term "statistical life" does not facilitate communication about the fact that people routinely make decisions that involve trade-offs between money and risk. The EPA has announced intention to clarify its focus on risk reduction by changing from setting a threshold based on Value of Statistical Life (VSL) to setting a new type of threshold measuring the Value of Mortality Risk (VMR). The EPA explains the logic underlying this change as follows:

> For decades economists have been studying how people make tradeoffs between their own income and risks to their health and safety. These tradeoffs can reveal how people value, in dollar terms, small changes in risk. For example, purchasing automobile safety options reveals information on what people are willing to pay to reduce their risk of dying in a car accident. Purchasing smoke detectors reveals information on what people are willing to pay to reduce their risk of dying in a fire. (EPA-e: How will the EPA Estimate the Value of Mortality Risk (VMR))

In conclusion, clinicians participating in planning CEA studies and reporting CEA study results should be aware of controversies regarding CEA. Despite these controversies, however, this analytical strategy is widely used. It may be useful to note that much of the controversy focuses on the question of whether cost-effectiveness ratios should be compared to thresholds, to support public agency resource allocation decisions. When CEA results are not compared to thresholds, they may be used to help decision-makers develop a broad understanding of benefits generated by various alternative strategies. In addition, they may be used to support pharmaceutical price negotiations. Finally, CEA study results can place trade-offs between alternate healthcare treatments within the larger context of trade-offs between alternate regulatory policies that affect health such as environmental, highway safety, or product safety regulations.

5 Conclusion

Clinicians recommend treatments for individual patients, yet they are increasingly expected to consider population health issues when they make these recommendations. For example, the CMS clinician payment incentives include healthcare expenditures as a metric for measuring the value of the clinician's work. In this environment, clinicians are incentivized to develop and implement strategies to work more efficiently, and they are expected to consider impacts of individual treatment decisions on total healthcare expenditures. Therefore, clinicians are likely to be increasingly involved in CER and CEA studies as members of study teams and as "consumers" of other study results. As members of study teams, clinicians will contribute to study design, interpretation of the statistical results, and communication of the study conclusions.

References

Adams, J., & Neville, S. (2020). Program evaluation for health professionals: What it is, what it isn't and how to do it. *International Journal of Quantitative Methods, 19*, 1–11. https://doi.org/10.1177/1609406920964345

All-Payer Claims Database Council. (2021). *Interactive state report map.* Retrieved July 9, 2021, from https://www.apcdcouncil.org/state/map

Anderson, J. L., Heidenreich, P. A., Barnett, P. G., Creager, M. A., Fonarow, G. C., Gibbons, R. J., Halperin, J. L., Hlatky, M. A., Jacohs, A. K., Mark, D. B., Masoudi, F. A., Peterson, E. D., & Shaw, L. J. (2014). ACC/AHA statement on cost/value methodology in clinical practice guidelines and performance measures: A report of the American College of Cardiology/American Heart Association task force on performance measures and task force on practice guidelines. *Journal of the American College of Cardiology, 63*(21), 2304–2322. https://doi.org/10.1016/j.jacc.2014.03.016

Arias, E., Tejada-Vera, B., & Ahman, F. (2021). *Provisional life expectancy estimates for January through June, 2020* (Vital Statistics Rapid Release Report No. 010). Centers for Disease Control and Prevention. https://www.cdc.gov/nchs/data/vsrr/VSRR10-508.pdf

Beaudin-Seller, B., Miller, G., & Fendrick, M. (2021, November 1). Enhancing value by evaluating health care services. *Health Affairs Blog*. https://doi.org/10.1377/hblog20211028.15012.

Catolico, E. (2020, August 28). *Deal to avoid Detroit teachers 'safety' strike would offer COVID-19 testing, hazard pay.* Chalkbeat Detroit. https://detroit.chalkbeat.org/2020/8/28/21405179/deal-to-avoid-detroit-teachers-safety-strike-would-offer-covid-19-testing-hazard-pay

Centers for Disease Control and Prevention. (2012). *Introduction to program evaluation for public health programs: A self-study guide* [Report]. https://www.cdc.gov/eval/guide/introduction/index.htm

Centers for Disease Control and Prevention. (2017). Framework for program evaluation in public health [Recommendations and reports]. *Morbidity and Mortality Weekly Report, 48,* No. RR-11. https://www.cdc.gov/mmwr/PDF/rr/rr4811.pdf

Centers for Disease Control and Prevention. (2021). *Advisory committee for immunization practices (ACIP): Evidence to recommendations framework.* https://www.cdc.gov/vaccines/acip/recs/grade/downloads/acip-evidence-recs-framework.pdf

Dillon, A. (2015, February 19). *Carrying NICE over the threshold.* NICE. https://www.nice.org.uk/news/blog/carrying-nice-over-the-threshold

Executive Office of the President of the United States. (2003). *Fiscal year 2003 budget of the U.S. government: Section 24, ranking regulatory investments in public health.* Office of Management and Budget. https://obamawhitehouse.archives.gov/sites/default/files/omb/assets/omb/inforeg/spec24.pdf

Figueroa, J., Horneffer, K., & Jha, A. (2019). Disappointment in the Value-based era – Time for a fresh approach? *JAMA* October 9. https://doi.org/10.1001/jama.2019.15918

Fisher, F. M. (1966). *The identification problem in econometrics*. McGraw-Hill Book Company. https://doi.org/10.2307/1236642

Glassman, P., Pearson, S., Zacher, J., Rind, D., & Valentino, M. (2020, June 15). VA and ICER at three years: Critics' concerns answered. *Health Affairs Blog.* https://www.healthaffairs.org/do/10.1377/hblog20200611.662048/full/

Gross, P. (2012). Editorial process versus outcome measures—the end of the debate. *Medical Care, 50*(3), 200–202. https://doi.org/10.1097/MLR.0b013e31824a59fb

Institute for Clinical and Economic Review. (n.d.). *Value assessment framework*. https://icer.org/our-approach/methods-process/value-assessment-framework/

Lakdawalla, D. N., Sun, E. C., Jena, A. B., Reyes, C. M., Goldman, D. P., & Philipson, T. J. (2010). An economic evaluation of the war on cancer. *Journal of Health Economics, 29*(3), 333–346. https://doi.org/10.1016/j.jhealeco.2010.02.006

Lewis, A., Khanna, V., & Montrose, S. (2014, November 25). Workplace wellness produces not savings. *Health Affairs Blog*. https://www.healthaffairs.org/do/10.1377/hblog20141125.042926/full/

Lichtenberg, F. R. (2013). Has medical innovation reduced cancer mortality? *CESifo Economic Studies, 60*(1), 135–177. https://doi.org/10.1093/cesifo/ift014

Medicare Coverage Database. (2011). *National coverage determination (NCD) for autologous cellular immunotherapy treatment (110.22)*. Centers for Medicare & Medicaid Services. https://www.cms.gov/medicare-coverage-database/details/ncd-details.aspx?NCDId=344&ncdver=1&bc=AAAAIAAAAAAA&

Mendelson, D., & Carino, T. (2011, April 4). Look carefully: Medicare's Provenge national coverage decision. *Health Affairs Blog*. https://www.healthaffairs.org/do/10.1377/hblog20110404.010073/full/

Mitchell, E. M. (2019). *Concentration of health expenditures and selected characteristics of high spenders, U.S. civilian noninstitutionalized population, 2016*. [MEPS/AHRQ Statistical Brief #521]. https://meps.ahrq.gov/data_files/publications/st521/stat521.shtml

Mukhopadhyay, S., & Wendel, J. (2013). Evaluating an employee wellness program. *International Journal of Health Care Finance and Economic, 13*(3–4), 173–199. https://doi.org/10.1007/s10754-013-9127-4

Murphy, K. M., & Topel, R. H. (2006). The value of health and longevity. *Journal of Political Economy, 114*(5), 871–904. https://doi.org/10.1086/508033

National Cancer Institute. (n.d.). *Definition: Castrate-resistant prostate cancer.*. National Institute of Health. https://www.cancer.gov/publications/dictionaries/cancer-terms/def/castrate-resistant-prostate-cancer

National Institute for Health and Care Excellence. (2015). *Final appraisal determination—Sipuleucel-T for treating asymptomatic or minimally symptomatic metastatic hormone-relapsed prostate cancer.* https://www.nice.org.uk/guidance/ta332/documents/prostate-cancer-metastatic-hormone-relapsed-sipuleucelt-1st-line-id573-final-appraisal-determination-document2

Nelson, H. D., Rochelle, F., Cantor, A., Pappas, M., Daeges, M., & Humphrey, L. (2016). Effectiveness of breast cancer screening: Systematic review and meta-analysis to update the 2009 U.S. Preventative Services Task Force recommendation. *Annals of Internal Medicine, 164*(4), 244–255. https://doi.org/10.7326/M15-0969

Neumann, P. J., & Cohen, J. T. (2018, March 12). America's "NICE"? *Health Affairs Blog*. https://www.healthaffairs.org/do/10.1377/hblog20180306.837580/full/

Neumann, P. J., & Sanders, G. D. (2017). Cost-effectiveness analysis 2.0. *New England Journal of Medicine, 376*(3), 203–205. https://doi.org/10.1056/NEJMp1612619

Neumann, P. J., & Weinstein, M. C. (2010). Legislating against use of cost-effectiveness information. *New England Journal of Medicine, 363*(16), 1495–1497. https://doi.org/10.1056/NEJMp1007168

NICE glossary. *National Institute for Health and Care Excellence*. (n.d.). https://www.nice.org.uk/glossary?letter=q

Organization for Economic Co-operation and Development. (2008). *Introductory handbook for regulatory impact analysis, version 1*. https://www.oecd.org/gov/regulatory-policy/44789472.pdf

Patashnik, E. M. (2020). Comparatively ineffective? PCORI and the uphill battle to make evidence count in US medicine. *Journal of Health Politics, Policy, and Law, 45*(5), 787–800. https://doi.org/10.1215/03616878-8543262

Paterson, M. A. (2014). *Healthcare finance and financial management: Essentials for advanced practice nurses and interdisciplinary care teams* (2nd ed.). DEStech Publications, Inc.

Philipson, T., Eber, M., Lakdawalla, D. N., Corral, M., Conti, R., & Goldman, D. P. (2012). An analysis of whether higher health care spending in the United States versus Europe is 'worth it' in the case of cancer. *Health Affairs (Millwood), 31*(4), 667–675. https://doi.org/10.1377/hlthaff.2011.1298

Pyenson, B., & Zenner, P. A. (2005). *Cancer screening: Payer cost/benefit through employee benefits programs*. Milliman, Inc.

Sculpher, M., Drummond, M., & O'Brien, B. (2001). Effectiveness, efficiency, and NICE: A NICE start but evidence costs money. *The British Medical Journal, 322*, 943–944. https://doi.org/10.1136/bmj.322.7292.943

Shafrin, J., Skornicki, M., Brauer, M., Villeneuve, J., Lees, M., Hertel, N., Penrod, J. R., & Jansen, J. (2018). An exploratory case study of the impact of expanding cost-effectiveness analysis for second-line nivolumab for patients with squamous non-small cell lung cancer in Canada: Does it make a difference? *Health Policy, 122*(6), 607–613. https://doi.org/10.1016/j.healthpol.2018.04.008

Shapoval, O. (2020). *Incentives and firm behavior: Evidence from the hospital-acquired condition reduction program* [Seminar]. University of Nevada, Reno. https://www.unr.edu/business/departments-and-disciplines/economics/seminars/2020-econ-seminars

Slater, J., & Culkin, J. J. (n.d.). *What you need to know about shared savings financial targets*. Axene Health Partners. https://axenehp.com/need-know-shared-savings-financial-targets/

Tanenbaum, S. J. (2017). Can payment reform be social reform? The lure and liabilities of the "Triple Aim". *Journal of Health Politics, Policy and Law, 42*(1), 53–71. https://doi.org/10.1215/03616878-3702770

Tikkanen, R., Osbon, R., Mossialos, E., Djordjevic, A., & Wharton, G. A. (2020). *International health care system profiles – Canada*. The Commonwealth Fund. https://www.commonwealthfund.org/international-health-policy-center/countries/canada

U.S. Environmental Protection Agency. (2020). *Mortality risk valuation*. https://www.epa.gov/environmental-economics/mortality-risk-valuation#means

U.S. Environmental Protection Agency. (2021). *Guidelines for preparing economic analyses*. https://www.epa.gov/environmental-economics/guidelines-preparing-economic-analyses

U.S. Government Accountability Office. (2012). *Preventive health activities: Available information on federal spending, cost savings, and international comparisons has limitations*. https://www.gao.gov/products/gao-13-49

Wendel, J., & Dumitras, D. (2005). Treatment effects model for assessing disease management: Measuring outcomes and strengthening program management. *Disease Management, 8*(3), 155–168. https://doi.org/10.1089/dis.2005.8.155

Chapter 7
Business Strategies and Disruption in Vision Care

John Appert

1 Introduction

Disruptive innovations have occurred in many industries, including health care. For example, Apple's music product (iTunes), disrupted the music industry, record stores, and payments to musicians when it allowed individuals to purchase songs and save them as electronic files. These innovations usually leverage new technology to provide services to potential customers that were neglected by the incumbent firms. These innovations can challenge both incumbent firms and regulators to adapt quickly while ensuring that consumer protections are sufficient to protect those with an information disadvantage. While this innovation poses challenges, it also provides an opportunity for those who are ready to take advantage of the change, and who understand the strategies used by stakeholders to protect their interests.

Health care providers, including psychologists working in integrated care, are affected by an ongoing stream of health care innovations, sparked by concerns about continued increases in health care expenditures, technological innovations, or unmet needs of individuals who are under-served or over-served by the current health care system. Innovations affecting psychologists include telehealth, substitution of social workers, substitution of masters-degree psychologists for PhD psychologists, and a plethora of online and cell-phone apps designed to help patients manage mental health conditions and behaviors contributing to chronic medical conditions. Additional pressures for change specific to the Veterans Health Administration include declining numbers of veterans and shifts in the locations of veterans. Finally, innovations, such as telehealth services and retail clinics offering convenient and relatively inexpensive treatments for minor illnesses and injuries, could weaken relationships between primary care practices and their patients. This could affect

J. Appert (✉)
Department of Economics, University of Nevada, Reno, Nevada, USA
e-mail: jappert@nevada.unr.edu

L. C. James et al. (eds.), *Clinical Health Psychology in Military and Veteran Settings*, https://doi.org/10.1007/978-3-031-12063-3_7

psychologists working in integrated care, to the extent that this delivery model presupposes strong ties between primary care physicians and their patients. The ongoing stream of innovations includes two types of innovations: those that strengthen the ability of the industry to function in the traditional manner, and those that disrupt the traditional industry. The degree to which psychologists are affected by disruptive innovations will depend on their strategic responses to the innovations.

This chapter provides a conceptual framework for understanding the types of innovations, the potentially positive impacts of disruptive innovations on some groups of consumers or patients, implications of these innovations for consumer protection, and the mix of positive and negative potential impacts of these innovations on health care professionals. The chapter begins by defining disruptive innovations and discussing a few examples in Sect. II. Section III focuses on a case study of a disruptive innovation that occurred within the health care industry but does not involve psychologists. This allows psychologists to focus on the business aspects of the challenges posed by the innovation and possible professional responses. The first part of Section III describes the innovation. The second part of Section III outlines a series of steps professionals can use to analyze a potentially disruptive innovation, and it illustrates the steps by analyzing the innovation highlighted in the case study. To facilitate comparisons between innovations in the health care industry and innovations in other industries, we use the words "products," "goods," and "services" interchangeably.

2 Disruptive Innovation

Two types of innovation drive growth in an economy (Schumpeter, 1942). The first type of innovation is a form of learning by doing. As a firm grows, it may innovate to reduce cost and displace rival companies. For example, aircraft manufacturers continually upgrade engine designs, creating engines that are more reliable and less expensive. The large size of firms that manufacture aircraft and their investments in innovation create a virtuous cycle: the firms improve steadily as they grow (Rosenberg, 1982). The challenge for successful incumbent firms is that the incentive to do this type of innovation is muted by the fact that the company is already successful. In this situation, change is risky.

The second type of innovation described by Schumpeter is creative destruction. In this model, innovators from outside the industry combine existing technologies, develop new technologies, or they use a combination of the two strategies to disrupt the incumbent firms. While an incumbent may have access to industry-specific technologies that are not widely available, there are other technologies that are well known and can be used across industries. Innovators may apply technology developed in one industry to disrupt a second industry. For example, Uber leveraged smartphone technology to disrupt the taxi industry.

The term "disruptive innovation" describes a specific type of industry disruption (Christenson et al., 2015). In a mature industry, incumbent firms tend to focus their efforts on supporting their most profitable customers. (Christensen et al., 2015) This focus on the most profitable customers usually means that some customers are under-served by incumbent firms, while others are over-served. Under-served customers may not buy any product from the industry because they would prefer to buy a streamlined product with a low price, but the industry does not offer this option. Over-served customers are currently buying products, but they would switch to an inexpensive streamlined product if it were available. In disruptive innovation, an outside group redesigns the production of a good to fulfill the demand of the under-served group for an inexpensive streamlined product. Initially, this innovator does not compete with the incumbent firms for its existing customers. The innovator will begin to compete with these firms, however, if existing customers begin switching to the inexpensive streamlined product or if the innovator begins to improve its product to appeal to existing customers, and eventually disrupt the incumbent's position.

This framework is helpful for thinking about innovation and the likely impacts of disruption. Analyzing how this dynamic plays out in other industries can also give some insight into the challenges psychologists could face in the future in their practice. First, it is important to understand what disruptive innovation is not. It is not innovation that serves the mainstream customers of the incumbent firms. Instead, disruptive innovations begin by targeting under-served customers and then improve the product to appeal to mainstream customers, eventually disrupting the mainstream market. While Uber did spark significant changes in the market for "rides for hire," it was not a disruptive innovation as it targeted the mainstream taxi customer from the beginning. Amazon was a disruptive innovator in the mid-1990s, as it targeted an under-served market of readers who wanted a wider selection than could be found in brick-and-mortar stores like Barnes and Noble. This is clear from the title of the first book sold on Amazon.com: "Fluid Concepts and Creative Analogies: Computer Models of the Fundamental Mechanisms of Thought" (Garber, 2012).

2.1 Examples of Disruptive Innovation

Amazon.com did more than just disrupt the businesses of large chain bookstores. Over time, it disrupted the businesses of book distributors, authors, and publishers. It then leveraged their business processes to take on big box retail in general. The impact of disruption extends to all members of the supply chain for a good or service, in some cases in very negative ways. For example, one book retailer, Borders Books, was eventually forced to declare bankruptcy in the face of the disruption brought by Amazon.com. However, Amazon.com also facilitated the success of authors and independent entrepreneurs through the launch of Kindle publishing and Fulfillment by Amazon. While the disruption brought by Amazon hurt some firms, it was leveraged by others to create new businesses and serve new customers. Disruptive innovation can either hurt or harm those involved in a mature industry, depending on how each stakeholder reacts to the disruption.

Retail health clinics provide an example of a potentially disruptive innovation in the health care industry. When the first retail clinic opened inside a retail store, the clinic offered a streamlined set of primary care services and did not have a system for billing insurance (Kaissi, 2016). Nurse practitioners or physician assistants provided a streamlined set of services; prices for specific services were posted and they were lower than prices charged by physician practices; services were offered during extended hours on weekends as well as weekdays on a drop-in basis only; and the clinics worked to ensure that wait-times did not exceed 15 min. The clinics were expected to appeal to uninsured individuals, who were under-served by physicians offering a broad array of traditional health care services in a physician office. As the retail clinic business grew, however, insured people also used the clinics, and the retail clinics acquired systems for billing insurance. Surveys indicated that insured individuals obtained care at retail clinics for minor illnesses and injuries because they preferred the convenience and low price offered by retail clinics (Cassel, 2018). Studies indicated that the quality of care provided by retail clinics was comparable to physician-provided care, for the types of services offered in retail clinics (Cassel, 2018). This innovation was potentially disruptive, but it did not generate major impacts on other components of the health care system, such as the volume of patients arriving at hospital emergency departments or urgent care facilities (Kaissi, 2016). One explanation focuses on the fact that some hospitals partnered with retail clinics, and they developed business strategies to utilize the clinics in ways that supported the hospital's business model (Kaissi, 2016). An additional explanation highlighted the fact that the substantial growth of retail clinics occurred as passage of the 2010 Patient Protection and Affordable Care Act (PPACA, 2010) triggered increased demand for primary care services (Kaissi, 2016). To the extent that patients who switched to retail clinics had been over-served by primary care physicians (because they were relatively healthy adults with only minor illnesses or injuries), the increase in retail clinic utilization helped primary care physicians focus on treating patients with more complex conditions.

2.2 *Impacts of Disruption on Skilled Individuals Working in the Incumbent Firms*

People who oppose innovations that automate production processes are known as "Luddites," after a textile worker named Ned Ludd who smashed a piece of textile equipment prior to the well-known Luddite incident. The Luddite incident is often framed as a revolt of unskilled labor against automation: however, the events that triggered the revolt were actually more complicated. Those who participated in the Luddite demonstrations were skilled members of the weaver's guild, a professional group which was similar to a modern labor union. In 1811, a group of English workers, the Luddites, assembled outside Nottingham, England and began to break automated weaving machines (known as "frames") (Beckett, 2012).

Why did the protests happen and why were skilled laborers being displaced at that time? At the beginning of the industrial revolution the primary constraint in the textile process was spinning cotton, wool, or other materials into thread. Through most of human history, this process was highly labor-intensive compared to weaving, and there were frequent shortages of thread supplied to weavers in eighteenth century England. In 1768, Richard Arkwright removed constraints to thread production when he perfected an automated spinning process to produce reliable supplies of thread that was both stronger and less expensive than thread produced with the previous methods (Postrel, 2020).

Within a few years, materials for creating textiles were plentiful, the textile industry grew rapidly, and shortages of skilled weavers became the chief constraint faced by producers of cloth. These weavers enjoyed several decades of high wages, until a second innovation (which was partly motivated by these high wages) reduced demand for them as well (Postrel, 2020).

The availability of stronger thread made it possible to automate parts of the weaving process (Postrel, 2020). The new automated weaving machines were initially used to produce relatively low-quality textiles. Thus, the innovation focused on changing production methods to serve a previously under-served customer base that preferred to buy inexpensive low-quality cloth. While skilled weavers were still needed to produce higher-quality textiles, use of the new machines reduced the immediate demand for weavers, and the Luddites correctly perceived that more affluent customers would eventually switch from buying hand-woven textiles to buying textiles woven with automated processes. One can imagine the distress this automation would cause, after skilled workers spent long years in apprenticeships to obtain high-paying employment, only to see technology make the occupation obsolete (Postrel, 2020).

This sequence of events recurs frequently throughout history, and accelerated sharply with the start of the industrial revolution:

1. Firms produced a popular product and sold it to consumers. Some individuals involved in the production process were able to earn high wages.
2. People completed extensive training to qualify for employment in these high-wage occupations.
3. Other people noted the high wages and high prices, and they began working to develop new methods of production to offer new types of goods to consumers at lower prices.
4. The new production methods (or the new products) reduced demand for the highly skilled workers who had been enjoying high wages.

2.3 Regulatory Issues Raised by Disruptive Innovations

In contrast to the impact of innovation on skilled workers, the impact of innovation on consumers is generally positive. During his Nobel Lecture, Paul Romer (2018) argued that most of the increase in living standards over the last 200 years can be attributed to the development of new technologies, new processes, and new scientific knowledge. However, while the benefits to society may be positive overall, subsets of people involved in a disrupted industry are negatively impacted by these changes. These groups use an array of strategies to try to mitigate damage. In particular, skilled labor may lobby for increased regulations, such as licensing laws, to minimize the risk that their jobs will be threatened by the new type of competition.

Consumer protection regulations, such as licensure requirements, play a particularly important role in the health care industry. Patients (customers) cannot usually judge the quality of care up front. Generally, this problem is mitigated by licensing and regulation. Therefore, innovators must address regulatory restrictions in addition to the task of creating a service that is valued by people who were under-served by incumbent providers. Regulators may have concerns about developing new types of consumer protection regulation to accommodate disruptive innovation. They have a primary responsibility to protect consumers. When the existing regulatory system was designed, lawmakers and regulators conceptualized "consumer preferences" and "consumer protection" in the context of the traditional health care system. When a disruptive innovation occurs, it typically offers new types of quality and convenience that were not provided by the incumbent providers. Protecting consumers in the evolving industry may require new definitions of "consumer protection" and new strategies for achieving that goal. It may also require weighing trade-offs between subsets of consumers because the innovation may allow some previously under-served individuals to gain access to the market, while the change in quality characteristics may pose a new risk for other consumers. In addition, regulatory agencies have typically worked with provider organizations for many years and may be reluctant to adjust regulations in ways that are likely to facilitate rapid disruption of the incumbent providers.

3 Case Study: EyeQue

New technology for providing vision care and prescription glasses illustrates issues posed by disruptive innovations and possible strategic responses. There are elements of vision care that require significant skill and judgement on the part of a medical professional, while other elements of vision case are more straightforward. Innovations like EyeQue allow providers to separate the two types of care, devoting more resources to the more complex cases, while possibly providing oversight and review on the more straightforward services needed by patients. If psychologists keep this mental model in mind as they approach their own care, they may identify strategies for leveraging the new technology to strengthen patient care while avoiding the pitfalls for providers that disruptive innovation can cause. In short, disruptive innovation in health care can offer benefits to providers who understand the dynamics of these changes and explore strategies for leveraging them to improve care or reduce health care expenditures.

3.1 The EyeQue Innovation

In 2015, two researchers at MIT, Tibor Laczay and John Serri, patented technology that would allow an individual with a smartphone and an inexpensive attachment to obtain the measurements required for eye glass prescriptions.[1] This technology was initially developed to serve adults without insurance or vision care plans. The researchers formed the company, EyeQue, to sell kits based on this technology to consumers (EyeQue, 2021a). In July 2021, the newest model could be purchased online for $69, and shared with friends and family members. Each user must open an online account; however, there is no charge for these accounts as of July 2021. In contrast, a visit to a medical provider for vision care was estimated to cost $171–$200 dollars for one individual.[2] These fees do not include the cost of frames and lenses, potentially several hundred dollars, which are often sold by the optometrist as well. David Gewirtz, writing for Zdnet.com during 2021, describes his experience using the EyeQue tool and procuring frames and lenses outside of the traditional path. He spent the $45 for the EyeQue kit in 2020, and then spent $21.95 to buy frames and prescription lenses from an online provider called EyeBuyDirect (Gewirtz, 2021).

EyeQue is attempting to disrupt part of the vision care market by allowing people to update or obtain the equivalent of an eyeglass prescription by using the technology it licensed from MIT. How does the process work? First, a customer buys an attachment for her smart phone from a retailer. As of this writing, the attachment was on sale at several retailers, includingAmazon.com. When the customer receives the attachment, she opens an account with EyeQue and downloads the app. The app requires the user to take the test three times and then generates what EyeQue refers to as "EyeGlass Numbers." These are the same measurements generated for a prescription, but EyeQue cannot legally refer to them using that term due to the fact that they are not generated by a licensed optometrist or ophthalmologist.

For example, under Nevada law, the following activities are included in the list of "acts constituting practice in optometry," which can only be conducted by licensed optometrists or under the supervision of an optometrist (NRS, 2021). These activities include measuring refractive errors. Similar activities are also described under the practice of ophthalmology. These activities include measuring refractive error, and they specify that eyeglass lenses and frames can only be dispensed when the patient has a valid prescription written by an optometrist or physician.

NRS 636.025: Acts constituting practice in optometry

> (b) Adapting, or prescribing or dispensing, without prescription by a practitioner of optometry or medicine licensed in this State, any ophthalmic lens, frame or mounting, or any part thereof, for correction, relief or remedy of any abnormal condition or insufficiency of the eye or any appendage or visual process.

[1] The attachment uses the smartphone's computer capabilities to perform a refraction test at home.

[2] This estimate was prepared by Fair Health, a nonprofit organization that aggregates payment data from health care claims (Nvisioncenters.com, 2021).

> (c) The examination, evaluation, diagnosis and treatment of the human eye and its appendages, the measurement of the powers or range of human vision by any means, including, without limitation, the use of an autorefractor or other automated testing device, unless performed under the direct responsibility of a licensed optometrist as authorized in NRS 636.346, the determination of the accommodative and refractive states of the eye or the scope of its function in general, … .

Generating the eyeglass numbers is only part of the information you need to buy a pair of glasses. Another key element is getting an accurate measure of pupillary distance, the distance between your pupils. This measurement is important as it determines where the lenses/frames need to sit to place the focal point of a corrective lens in the correct spot. The EyeQue kit includes a pair of white plastic frames with several markings on it to aid in accurately measuring this distance. A customer can put the frames on and take a picture of herself wearing the glasses. The EyeQue app uses the photo to capture the pupillary distance and frame measurements required to make a pair of glasses that fits, with the lens focus centered correctly over the pupil.[3] These are all steps that are traditionally carried out by a technician or an optometrist in the traditional vision care model.

While smartphone technology is able to detect vision problems, calculate the needed lens power for correction, and measure facial features was necessary for a disruptor like EyeQue, it is not sufficient for their business model to be successful. There are also stacks of other technologies and business processes that are required for a business model like this to work. The EyeQue business model also depends on the availability of online eyeglass retailers to address state laws requiring valid prescriptions prior to in-state sales of eyeglasses.

The EyeQue business model is only viable because customers can now purchase prescription glasses online from companies such as Zenni Optical, Glasses USA, and EyeBuy Direct. This is possible because businesses outside the health care industry have developed processes to support online sales over the last 20 years.

EyeQue and companies like it can provide a cheaper way to get the measurements for a corrective lens because other technologies and business processes enabled by the Internet support this business model. However, the EyeQue business model raises two important concerns. First, an eye exam generally entails more than just determining the appropriate corrective lenses for a patient. An eye exam also screens for other conditions such as macular degeneration, cataracts, and glaucoma. Patients who want to buy eyeglasses from brick-and-mortar stores must still obtain prescriptions from optometrist and ophthalmologists. One argument for maintaining this requirement focuses on the value of bundling the service that is often salient to individuals (eyeglasses) with the screenings that may be important for maintaining eye health, but are less salient to patients. The combination of benefits and harms generated by the EyeQue business model generates an important question: Does the benefit of increased access to corrective eyeglasses (generated by the low

[3] EyeGlass Numbers can be used, along with the measure of pupillary distance, to purchase eyeglasses, but they cannot be used to purchase contact lenses. The EyeQue system is not calibrated to provide the necessary information for purchasing contact lenses (EyeQue Support, 2021a, b, c).

cost of using EyeQue to obtain a vision test) offset the potential harm that could be caused if fewer people obtain annual eye exams screening for eye health issues? Second, regulators considering modifying the current consumer protection regulatory strategy could also be concerned about the quality of the eye glass numbers versus a prescription written by a trained optometrist. Some doctors have expressed these concerns. An optometrist, Dr. Heiting, summarized the two concerns (GeWirtz, 2020):

> I took a quick peek at the promo video for the device. It looks like it could work to determine a glasses prescription for single vision lenses (including astigmatism correction), but not a prescription for progressive lenses for someone with presbyopia.
>
> ...
>
> Finally, consumers should be made aware that this is not a substitute for a comprehensive eye exam, as it does not evaluate the health of the eyes or test eye pressure to rule out glaucoma. *https://www.zdnet.com/article/eye-exams-at-home-a-safe-way-to-update-your-eyeglass-rx-in-the-age-of-covid/*

Later, in the same article, Dr. Mesheca Bunyan, an opthalmologist in Maryland, said the following:

> I do think that technology such as EyeQue can work. The technology appears to be innovative and has the ability to offer a clear prescription if someone is unable to see their eye doctor.
>
> My thought is that it still can't replace a comprehensive eye exam which includes the refraction, the portion of the test that gives the eyeglass prescription.
>
> Optometrists have the ability to fine tune the prescription in ways that a piece of technology cannot. For example, there are instances in which a patient's prescription may be high in astigmatism and we might decrease it based on what the patient might be able to tolerate. Technology can't determine this. *https://www.zdnet.com/article/eye-exams-at-home-a-safe-way-to-update-your-eyeglass-rx-in-the-age-of-covid/*

These concerns could have important implications when we think about the impact of the EyeQue product on existing players in the vision care market. The fact that appointments with ophthalmologists and optometrists are still needed to check for other conditions impacts the effective cost for a consumer choosing between getting an eyeglass prescription while at their annual or biannual visit to their eye doctor or using EyeQue. This is particularly true for consumers who are willing to request their prescription at the end of an appointment and then use the same online eyeglass retailers that consumers using EyeQue use. For these consumers, there is the additional cost of EyeQue plus the added time and inconvenience of purchasing eyeglasses separately. This is an important thing to keep in mind as we review the potential impacts of the EyeQue product on the eyeglass market. Even if EyeQue provides a less expensive option for obtaining the information needed to purchase eyeglasses, customers might prefer to visit an optometrist because the optometrist can package several services at potentially a lower total cost, especially for consumers planning to purchase inexpensive eyeglasses online. Additionally, there is a risk factor with online sales: the glasses might not fit the customer's face correctly. If the glasses are purchased at a brick-and-mortar location, a technician fits the frames to the customer's face at the point of purchase.

3.2 Steps to Analyze Potential Impacts of a Disruptive Innovation (Illustrated for the EyeQue Case)

When professionals notice potentially disruptive innovations, they may assess the viability of the new firm and consider strategic responses. In this subsection, we use four steps to assess EyeQue's potential to disrupt optometry and ophthalmology services and to consider strategic responses. In the first step, we gather baseline information about the components of the vision care industry. In the second step, we examine payment structures that are likely to affect relationships among those components. In the third step, we consider the regulatory environment that could help – or hinder – the innovator's efforts. In the final step, we consider possible strategic responses to the innovation.

3.2.1 Components of the Vision Care Industry and Relationships Among Those Components

The US vision care industry has four major components: professionals offering diagnostic services and writing eyeglass prescriptions, firms manufacturing eyeglasses, firms distributing and selling eyeglasses, and vision care plans that form networks of optometrists and ophthalmologists and negotiate discounted prices for their services. Each component of this sequence of entities that create vision care for consumers has characteristics that can elevate prices paid by consumers. An innovator that can bypass points of inefficiency can potentially disrupt the industry. However, regulations designed to protect consumers and current guidelines for maintaining eye health pose challenges for potential disrupters.

Vision Care

The demand for vision care in the United States is high. Refractive errors that can usually be corrected with glasses or contact lenses impact approximately 30% of people over age 40 (Kempen et al., 2004). These services are traditionally provided by either optometrists or ophthalmologists, both highly trained professionals. An ophthalmologist is a medical doctor who can provide eye exams as well as perform surgery or treat conditions like glaucoma. As a medical doctor, she has completed medical school, residency, and an internship. An optometrist completes a four-year professional program after her undergraduate training. She can also provide eye exams, monitor certain medical conditions, and prescribe eyeglasses and contacts. She does not perform surgery.

Both professions were organized early in the twentieth century. In 1898, the Association of Opticians was formed (now known as the American Optometric Association), and by 1910, formal classes for the study of optometry were being offered at Columbia University (Bryan, 1981). The practice rapidly professionalized and the first Doctor of Optometry degrees were issued by the Pennsylvania College of Optometry in 1923. By 1928, the first state regulation limiting licensing to those with Doctor of Optometry degrees was established in New York. Similar developments occurred in professional training for ophthalmologists. The first ophthalmology specialty board exams were administered in 1916. Roles of the two professions continue to evolve. In 1986, Ronald Reagan signed a Medicare parity law that expanded the ability for optometrists to be reimbursed for vision care (Garland, 1987).

These professional organizations continue to provide leadership for eye-health providers and for consumers aiming to maintain eye health. A December 2020 letter written by the President of the American Optometric Association, which is posted on the organization website (Reynolds, 2020), states the organization's position on the EyeQue innovation:

> With regard to your question–whether the EyeQue Vision Monitoring kit is a good substitute for a trained professional, we can confidently say that, from a patient health and safety perspective, there is simply no replacement for an in-person comprehensive eye exam.
>
> https://www.aoa.org/about-the-aoa/press-room/statements/aoa-response-to-cnet-eyeque-review?sso=y

The position of the American Academy of Ophthalmology is more nuanced (see Box 7.1). This organization posted a list of mobile apps that might be useful for patients, along with a statement of disclaimer (Mukamal, 2021). EyeQue is one of the apps included in this list. The statement indicates that EyeQue does not replace an eye exam, but it can be used to obtain the information needed to buy eyeglasses.

Once licensed, some optometrists have attempted to maximize revenue by encouraging patients to purchase their glasses at the optometrist's office. These optometrists may withhold the written copy of the prescription until the patient specifically requests it or refuse to provide a written copy even when it is requested (Rottenberg, 1962).

Box 7.1: The American Academy of Ophthalmology on Eye Health Apps
Eye Health Screening Apps May Signal Need for Eye Exam

Reena Mukamal, Feb. 17, 2021.

Between visits to the eye doctor, some patients are turning to eye health apps. These apps don't replace a comprehensive eye exam by an ophthalmologist. But they may help you manage ongoing eye conditions and alert you when a doctor's input is needed.

Disclaimer: *These apps and technologies are presented for your information only. They are not the only such tools, but are merely representative of the types of tools that are available. These apps are not endorsed by the Academy, as the Academy never endorses products, companies or organizations. Ask your eye care team, including your ophthalmologist, to help identify apps and technologies that might best address your needs.*

VisionCheck 2 (EyeQue, $65 for the device and two-year subscription to the app)

This at-home vision test bundle includes a device that works in conjunction with your smartphone and an app. The device tests your vision, one eye at a time. You can measure the lens power needed to correct your nearsightedness, farsightedness, and astigmatism as well as any near-vision additional power you might need. The app generates eyeglass numbers that can be used to order glasses online. This bundle does not replace routine eye exams and does not screen for conditions like glaucoma, cataracts, and macular degeneration.

Source: Mukamal, R. (2021). Eye Health Screening Apps May Signal Need for Eye Exam. American Academy of Ophthalmology. https://www.aao.org/eye-health/tips-prevention/eye-health-app-covid-coronavirus-home-exam

The Federal Trade Commission responded to concerns about these strategies with the " Eyeglass Rule" in 1978. Under this rule, optometrists are required to provide a written prescription to each patient at the end of each appointment for no additional cost, whether the patient requests the prescription or not. In addition, optometrists may not condition an examination on a commitment to purchase any goods from the optometrist (FTC, 2020). This rule has been updated several times since 1978, and the FTC issued warning letters as recently as 2020 for violations of the EyeGlass rule (FTC, 2020).

Health care regulations are primarily controlled at the state level. Some of these regulations have been utilized to restrict competition among optometrists. State-level regulations on optometry have restricted the employment of optometrists by larger chain businesses, as well as the location and number of optometry offices in an area. Some of these restrictions made it unlawful for an optometrist to work for a non-optometrist or restrict the use of offices that are not dedicated entirely to optometry[4] (Haas-Wilson, 1986). This second restriction could increase the costs to entry for new optometrists, thereby limiting supply. Both of these restrictions are consistent with the hypothesis that regulation is often sought by an industry for its own benefit, particularly when one considers that state optometry boards are typically appointed by the governor from a list of optometrists who have practiced in that state for a minimum number of years (Haas-Wilson, 1986; Stigler, 1971).

[4] For an additional example, see L. Benham (1972) The Effect of Advertising on the Price of Eyeglasses, 15 J. L. & Econ. 337, and Kobayashi, B. and T. Muris (2013) I Can See Clearly Now: Lee Benham, Eyeglasses, and The Empirical Analysis Of Advertising And The Effects Of Professional Regulation, Competition Policy International, Vol. 9, No. 1, pp. 156–162, Spring 2013 George Mason University Law and Economics Research Paper Series.

Eyeglass Manufacturers and Distributors

The second and third components of the vision care industry are the eyeglasses manufacturers and distributors. The cost of manufacturing eyeglasses decreases as a firm produces a larger number of glasses. When this cost structure exists, large firms can charge lower prices than smaller firms. In this situation, the industry is likely to be dominated by a small number of large firms. The dominant position of the large firms can persist for many years, until a technological disruption occurs that allows new competitors to enter the market by using new production methods or offering new types of products.

In 1961, Leonardo Del Vecchio established Luxottica, an eyeglasses design and manufacturing firm (Luxotticaa, 2021). By 1974, it began wholesale distribution in Italy, and by the early 1980s, had expanded internationally. The firm continued to expand rapidly and today it manufactures 80% of the eyeglasses in the United States and 30% of eyeglasses worldwide. Today Luxottica manufactures prescription glasses and sunglasses, runs a vision benefits company with 52 million US members, provides optometrist services through Doctors at Luxottica, and owns retail outlets such as Sunglass Hut and the prescription eyeglass retailer LensCrafters. In 2017, Luxottica merged with the $49 billion French eyeglass firm Essilor, further consolidating the industry (Luxottica, 2021).

Payment Structures*: Vision Care Plan and Health Savings Accounts*

The fourth component of the industry includes entities and systems that help consumers pay for eye exams and glasses. Many health care insurers do not include eye exams and eyeglasses as covered benefits. These services are not covered by traditional Medicare, Medigap plans, (MedicareInteractive.org, 2021; Worstell, 2020), and adult vision care is not one of the essential benefits that must be covered in plans offered on the Health Insurance Exchanges (healthcare.gov, 2021). Instead, some employers offer managed vision care plans. The first of these, California Vision Services, was founded in 1955 by a group of optometrists in Oakland, California. By the mid-1970s, the practice had grown and changed its name to Vision Service Plan (VSP). Today, Davis Vision, EyeMed (owned by Luxottica), and VSP are some of the largest providers (IbisWorld, 2019). The typical vision care plan functions as a prepaid service. Customers purchase a plan with an annual premium. The vision care plan contracts with a network of licensed providers and negotiates price reductions for its members. By reducing consumer incentives to utilize price-saving strategies for obtaining the information needed to buy eyeglasses, however, vision care plans pose a challenge for EyeQue's efforts to disrupt the industry.

Contracts between vision care plans and the in-network optometrists may also contain a requirement that raises regulatory concerns. These contracts typically include clauses known as "Most Favored Nation" clauses. These clauses specify that the optometrist must offer her "best price" to the vision care plan. If the optometrist provides a service to any customer for a price below the negotiated price with the vision care plan, she must offer the same low price to the vision care plan. This requirement sounds good at first glance: this policy mandates that price discounts offered to a small set of individuals must be shared with all individuals covered by vision care plans. However, these clauses create a strong disincentive for an optometrist to offer price discounts to members of other vision care plans or individuals who are not covered by a vision care plan. For example, a provider could offer discounts to customers who are willing to be flexible on timing, and fill-in when a provider has a gap in her schedule. These discounts could be similar to discounts offered by airlines to "stand by" passengers. This would benefit the provider in that she utilizes otherwise-lost capacity, and a customer with scheduling flexibility who receives a price reduction for accepting a last-minute appointment. If the provider must also provide this reduced pricing to all members of a care plan, she may decide to accept the lost capacity. In this case, both the provider and the customer with some flexibility in time are worse off. This logic could also discourage an ophthalmologist from offering a discounted price to low-income individuals who are not covered by vision care plans.

Most Favored Nation clauses are widely used in business contracts; however, economists and regulators are concerned that these agreements can result in reduced price competition (Gurkaynak et al., 2015). Most Favored Nations clauses are not necessarily anticompetitive, but they can raise antitrust concerns in some circumstances. The federal Department of Justice filed an antitrust lawsuit against VSP in 1994, alleging that the Most Favored Nation clauses in its contracts with optometrists would discourage optometrists from offering discounts. The suit was settled by an agreement that prevented VSP from using this clause for five years (U.S. Department of Justice, 2020). Additionally, VSP was prohibited from taking any action that would discourage any doctor from participating in any other vision care plan's programs or charging lower fees than what she had contracted with the VSP to any other clients (U.S. Department of Justice, 1996). Since that time, the Justice Department has filed a handful of similar suits against dental plans and other health care plans (U.S. Department of Justice, 2020).

For individuals not covered by vision care plans, the EyeQue website notes that an individual with a Health Savings Account (HSA) may be able to use funds in that account to purchase the EyeQue kit. This is an advantageous purchasing strategy because some employers contribute funds to HSA accounts and money deposited in an HSA is not subject to federal income tax. The number of HSA accounts has grown from $6.3 million in 2011 to $30.2 million at the end of 2020 (Devenir Research, 2021). Compared with traditional insurance coverage, HSAs create incentives for individuals to be price-conscious when utilizing health care services. Under IRS regulations, funds in HSA accounts can also be used to pay for comprehensive eye exams and eyeglasses (Evans, 2021).

3.2.2 Regulatory Environment for Consumer Protection

Licensing laws protect consumers from improperly trained or incompetent providers (Rottenberg, 1962). Most consumers cannot assess the competence of a vision care provider on their own; hence these requirements are imposed to enforce a minimum level of training and knowledge (Haas-Wilson, 1986). In general, the regulatory system is created by a state legislature and then administered by a licensure board comprising members of the professional group being regulated. The legislature mandates that services may only be provided by licensed individuals, and the boards specify requirements for training and professionalism.

Health care licensing regulations address the asymmetry between information available to patients about the quality of care offered by individual health care providers, and information known to the providers themselves. An individual optometrist may know how skilled she is and the quality of service she provides. Her peers in an area may also know her skill level. However, there is limited opportunity for any individual patient to gain this knowledge. In the absence of any countervailing force to address this uncertainty, providers (with low skills or low scruples) could sell low-quality care at a low cost driving their competitors out of business. These countervailing forces vary by industry, from brand names, to retail chains, to third-party rating groups (Akerlof, 1970). In industries like law, health care, and vision care, these countervailing forces are generally licensing and educational requirements. In health care, licensing regulations play a central role in consumer protection.

While the arguments for licensing typically focus on protecting consumers; however, it is notable that the arguments for strong licensing requirements are also made by practitioners themselves. These arguments may be motivated by concern for standards; however, practitioners may also try to use stringent licensure requirements as a strategy to limit the number of new practitioners entering the field. If these efforts are successful, the existing practitioners may be able to charge higher prices (Rottenberg, 1962).

State licensure laws can also be used to block disruptive innovators such as EyeQue.

The position that licensure requirements are important is not controversial; however, there is ongoing controversy about the stringency of those requirements. If an industry successfully uses licensing to cap the number of entrants into a profession, consumers may be harmed by higher prices and inadequate access. In addition, individuals who have the skill and work ethic to enter the profession may be blocked by the costs of becoming licensed, including fees, training time, and/or tuition costs for training.[5] When a potentially disruptive innovation is introduced, lawmakers and regulators will be asked to weigh costs and benefits of specific licensure

[5]Adam Smith (1776) discussed this issue in The Wealth of Nations arguing that it is unjust to prevent a capable person from engaging in any field she wishes as long as she harms no one. "The patrimony of a poor man lies in the strength and dexterity of his hands; and to hinder him from employing this strength and dexterity in what manner he thinks proper without injury to his neighbor is a plain violation of this most sacred property."

requirements, and they will be asked to balance the need for quality against the harm caused by inadequate access and high prices.

3.2.3 Strategic Responses by the Incumbent Providers

How would we expect an optometry business to respond to the EyeQue innovation? We begin this analysis by considering an optometrist who produces two services: (i) vision exam that could generate a prescription for eyeglasses, and (ii) exams that screen for conditions such as glaucoma, macular degeneration, or cataracts. Ophthalmologists also produce these two services, along with an array of additional medical services.

One strategy an eye health professional could adopt is to refocus her time and efforts on providing services that require higher levels of skill. Pursuing this strategy could allow her to maintain her revenues even in the face of technological disruption, if there is sufficient demand for the higher-skill services. The US Bureau of Labor Statistics (BLS) projects continued growth of demand for optometrists' services through 2019, which will be partly spurred by the aging baby boomer generation (BLS, 2021). One analysis of the supply of optometrists' services reports a current surplus of optometrists that is decreasing as demand grows. This analysis also reports that sales of eyeglasses constitute a decreasing share of optometrists' income due to competition from retail chains and online retailers (VM, 2017).

The current oversupply of optometrists, along with the limited range of medical services offered by optometrists, suggests that these professionals will have difficulty maintaining current levels of revenue if substantial numbers of consumers switch to obtaining eyeglass prescription information from innovators such as EyeQue. In contrast, ophthalmologists provide a wider array of services beyond eyeglass prescriptions. They are more likely to be able to implement the strategy of shifting their time and efforts to produce services that require higher levels of skill. The difference in the market positions of these two professions is consistent with the difference in the public statements about EyeQue made by the two professional organizations (and noted above).

Optometrists and ophthalmologists pursing this "shifting" strategy may also look for new types of bundling opportunities. If individuals begin using devices like the EyeQue attachment to obtain the information needed to buy eyeglasses, the current practice of bundling the vision test with eye care screening tests could become obsolete. Eye care professionals might begin thinking about alternate bundling strategies. For example, an optometrist could potentially co-locate his office adjacent to a primary care practice. The two practices could contract with insurers to bundle the eye care screening with annual wellness visits or annual checkups.

The alternate strategy is to leverage the technology provided by EyeQue to increase patient engagement and to reduce the cost (to patients) of obtaining the information needed to buy eyeglasses. The EyeQue website suggests areas in which the EyeQue technology could be applied to strengthen the patient-doctor relationship (EyeQue, 2021c):

> Expand your practice and improve your relationship with patients by embracing leading-edge technology.
>
> - Attract more patients and create loyalty by being the coolest doc on the block.
> - Transform the annual visit to an ongoing conversation with regular at-home monitoring, alerts, and notifications.
> - Improve patient outcomes and monitor prescription stability in at-risk patients. https://www.eyeque.com/partner/

Eye Netra is a separate company offering "refraction testing powered by a cell phone.". This company's business model focuses on the concept that the device is a tool optometrists and ophthalmologists can use to (i) provide vision testing in a variety of settings (the battery can support 2 days of testing), and (2) strengthen the customer experience (Eye Netra, 2021):

> A provider using EyeNetra mobile tools empowers his or her patients to take a more active role in their eye care; fostering trust in the patient-provider relationship and vastly improving the customer experience. https://eyenetra.com/product-netra.html

3.2.4 EyeQue Market Experience

If EyeQue is able to supplant the traditional eye exam and eye prescription process for eyeglasses, purchases of "prescription" eyeglasses are expected to increase, as customers who currently rely on reading glasses would switch to "prescription" eyeglasses that correct vision errors in more detail. Further, the number of prescriptions provided by optometrists will decrease, and optometrists will shift more of their production to higher skilled services. Do we see these shifts, and if not, why?

The total size of the eyewear market can be difficult to estimate. However, according to Statista.com (2021), between 33% and 36% of Americans over 18 purchased glasses from a doctor's office in 2018. Additionally, Statista estimates that Luxottica had approximately $2.5 billion in sales in 2018 in the United States alone. We can also assume that some of those who cannot afford prescription eyeglasses buy reading glasses instead. That market was approximately $14 billion per year in 2018 (Insight, 2020). EyeQue began offering its devices to consumers in 2015, and its revenue is estimated at $6–$8 million per year (Owler.com, 2021). After 6 years of operation, EyeQue does not appear to be disrupting the vision care market. What could explain this lack of traction?

EyeQue may have difficulty disrupting the vision care market due to three challenges. First, optometrist and ophthalmologist traditionally bundled vision tests with other eye health services, and by regulatory issues. The fact consumers can obtain vision tests during recommended annual eye health exams suggests that the primary customer base for EyeQue will be individuals who do not have vision insurance. Second, individuals with vision insurance may not have strong incentives to seek low prices for vision tests and eyeglasses. Third, one company (Luxottica) provides optometry services and also manufactures and distributes eyeglasses. This company has market power in the manufacturing and distribution components of the vision care industry. Hypothetically, this company could work to thwart

EyeQue's effort to disrupt the market. Alternately, Luxottica could design its own disruptive innovation or it could acquire or partner with EyeQue.

Fourth, state regulations mandating that in-state eyeglass sales must be accompanied by prescriptions written by medical professionals may lead to raise questions in consumers' minds about the credibility of the EyeQue technology. The FDA does not require an approval process for this type of device. Without approval or certification from a reputable organization, products like EyeQue face the problem of asymmetric information: the company has access to data about the product's quality, but consumers cannot easily verify the product's quality for themselves. In this situation, the initial growth rate of a new product may be slow as the product gains a reputation for quality and reliability.

4 Other Examples of Disruptive Innovation in Health Care

A cardiologist, Eric Topol, has been speaking of the potential benefits of numerous low-cost smartphone-enabled testing devices, for both health care providers and their patients (Versel, 2013). For example, the FDA approved a device that allows consumers to perform electrocardiograms (ECG) at home (ACC, 2019). These systems allow inexpensive and frequent testing for patients and generate new types of data to inform interactions between patients and health care providers. Consumers can purchase the device at Walmart or through Amazon.com. The ECG device allows individuals to monitor heart conditions and provide the results to their physicians.

In a second example, Congress created a new category of over-the-counter (OTC) hearing aids in 2017 for use by adults with mild to moderate hearing loss. Traditionally, hearing aids could only be purchased with a prescription written by a licensed medical professional. Hearing aids are costly, and they are not typically covered by insurance. While many people over age 65 have some degree of hearing loss, most of these people do not purchase hearing aids. Consumers will be able to purchase the new OTC without prescriptions (NIDCD, 2021).

Congress mandated that the Federal Trade Commission (FTC) and Federal Drug Administration (FDA) will write consumer protection regulations to govern the new market. The logic of the new hearing aid category focuses on the fact that the majority of adults with mild to moderate hearing loss (such that they have difficulty hearing conversations in noisy places) need sound amplification and noise cancellation. Consumer electronics companies, such as Samsung and Bose, argued that they have expertise and experience producing headphone that provide these two services. Further, retail prices for these headphones are substantially lower than prices of hearing aids.

The market will open when the new regulations are complete. Writing these regulations required conceptualizing new types of consumer protection issues. Traditionally, consumer protection regulations focused on ensuring that consumers obtained health care from licensed professionals, and low-quality products were not available for sale. The new OTC headphones raise new issues such as: (i) Will headphone manufacturers be required to submit test results before advertising that the devices will help adults with age-related hearing loss; (ii) How will individuals know (before buying headphones) whether they would benefit from prescription hearing aids instead of the OTC devices? (iii) During audiologist visits, for hearing tests, individuals also received screenings for hearing-related medical conditions. If people can buy OTC devices to help them hear conversations in restaurants, will they experience adverse impacts from reductions in visits to audiologists?

The OTC hearing aids raise questions that parallel the questions raised by the EyeQue example. In both cases, licensed professionals bundled hearing or vision testing with routine screenings for related medical conditions. This system is useful for individuals who can afford the visits, but it may exclude others from obtaining the hearing aids or eyeglasses, because they cannot afford to obtain prescriptions written by these professionals under the current system. Bundling two goods, such as vision tests and eye-health screenings can provide convenience for consumers when it is covered by insurance, but it also raises the price of obtaining prescriptions for hearing aids or eyeglasses. Bundling can also raise antitrust concerns if it is mandatory.

5 Conclusions

Psychologists face an ongoing stream of innovations that are likely to affect their practices. These innovations include telemedicine, mental health apps, willingness of payers to substitute master's degree psychologists and social workers for PhD psychologists, consumers obtaining primary care in retail clinics (separate from primary care offices offering integrated care), teledoc services offered to enrollees by insurance companies (which could also weaken ties between patients and primary care providers), and the pressures for change faced by the Veterans Health Administration.

Clinicians considering potential impacts of innovations can:

1. Identify frameworks that help organize general information.
2. Identify a useful sequence of steps to structure detailed analyses.
3. Look at similar challenges faced by other professionals to conceptualize possible strategic responses.

In this chapter, we use the case of EyeQue to illustrate these steps. The EyeQue case is useful for psychologists for two reasons. Because this innovation occurred in vision care, rather than psychology, it may be easier for psychologists to focus on the strategic business issues rather than the content of the innovation itself. Second, many of the issues faced by vision care providers are similar to issues that psychologists are likely to face.

The dynamic illustrated by the EyeQue case is described by Christensen (1997) in his book "The Innovator's Dilemma." Christensen describes innovations that originate outside an industry and start by serving customers that were overlooked by the incumbent firms. For example, when Japanese firms entered the car market, they initially competed by selling low-end compact cars that were more fuel efficient than cars previously available in the market. Later, when Toyota had become a more established car brand, it began producing cars that appealed to higher-end customers and Korean car companies like Kia began to disrupt the low-end car market. This leads to a challenging situation for an established company as it is incentivized to compete for the higher end customers. However, this strategy leaves the door open for disruption from new competitors.[6]

In the health care space, this dynamic is more complicated. There are established eyeglass manufacturers and vision care providers that have incentives to continue competing at the higher end of the market. Regulators have the challenge of protecting consumers while expanding lower-cost treatments to individuals with straightforward conditions. Insurance plans blunt incentives for customers to shop for low prices, while asymmetric information makes it difficult for consumers to assess quality. External innovators will try to gain a foothold by offering products and services that are designed to appeal to individuals who are not currently served by the existing market. These innovators are likely to improve their product over time, to appeal to mainstream customers. Medical providers will face a dilemma: should they compete with these innovations, or shift their focus to providing services that require higher levels of skill?

Managing these dynamics will be a significant challenge for stakeholders in the vision care space over the next several years. Forward-looking vision care providers can explore strategies for leveraging this disruptive technology to provide better care to more patients. In fact, a company EyeNetra that uses the same technology as EyeQue is pursuing this path, focusing on partnering with optometrists to use these lower cost tools to improve the health care partnership between clinician and patient.

Regulators could work with providers to establish criteria for identifying patients that present straightforward vision issues that can be treated using the new low-cost technology, and make that technology more widely available to those patients. At the same time, regulators and health care providers will evaluate processes to identify those with more complicated problems that need more specialized treatments offered by licensed providers. At the national level, regulators and professional organizations may consider guidelines and tools to review or certify apps and related devices to help resolve the asymmetric information problem as it applies to innovative new apps.

Well-designed regulatory frameworks and app assessment guidelines could facilitate the development of affordable care for low-risk people, while allowing licensed health care providers to focus on people with complex health issues. Alternately, health care providers might use the new tools to strengthen patient relationships and patient engagement.

---

[6]Clay Christensen, Jerome Grossman, and Jason Hwang applied these ideas to the health care industry in a subsequent book: The Innovator's Prescription: A Disruptive Solution for Health Care. McGraw Hill. 2009.

Disruptive innovation and tools like EyeQue can provide a framework for health care providers in other fields to not only avoid the negative impacts of disruptive innovation on their practice, but also to leverage these innovations as a tool in.

their own practices. There are several lessons to learn both from the economic theory, and the example of EyeQue. First, disruptive innovation is likely to occur in the areas that are not served by current provider practices. Second, this type of disruptive innovation often focuses on areas where repeatable/algorithm-type decision-making occurs. Third, forward-looking health care providers can likely leverage this disruption to improve their own services, increase their resource allocation to higher-skilled tasks, and improve availability for their patients. In short, a forward-looking psychologist does not need to fear disruptive innovation. Instead, she can leverage it to improve her own practice and her service to the community.

Evaluating your clients can give you some insight into both who your practice is optimized to support and who are likely to be under-served potential customers. Perhaps customers without certain types of insurance coverage or other constraints on their life (work schedules, childcare, etc.) are under-served by your practice. Disruptive innovation is likely to target these groups in an effort to bring them affordable care. There may be a temptation to ignore these groups and focus on your primary client base. This can be risky though as disruptive innovators will leverage what they learn serving those groups to eventually disrupt your core business.

Second, it is important to review what types of services you provide and which services require higher-level decision-making versus more routine decision-making. Perhaps certain services you provide to your patients are fairly routine and some of them could be automated or sent to a lower skilled provider (for example a nutritionist). Where lower skilled, more rote decision-making overlaps with under-served populations there is risk for disruptive innovation.

Finally, if you can find areas in your practice where there are under-served patients and the potential to automate some of the simpler decision-making, you likely have also found an opportunity to expand your own practice. Reducing the resources allocated to these tasks can allow you to serve more patients at lower cost. Identifying such areas, that are ripe for disruptive innovation, can open doors to innovation within your own practice, to improve patient outcomes and potentially increase the number of clients you can serve. To protect the interests of patients, it may be necessary to work with licensing and regulatory bodies. Evaluation of necessary supportive technologies is also important. For example, the extent to which potential benefits of the innovation can be realized is conditioned on connectivity, computer literacy, and sufficient hardware support. Consider, for example, a veteran experiencing depression while living in a rural area that does not have Internet service. This individual would face substantive barriers blocking access to many of the online sites offering services to help manage depression. Clinicians may need carefully assess the fit between potentially useful innovations and each patient's capacity to use the innovation.

References

Akerlof, G. A. (1970). The market for "lemons": Quality uncertainty and the market mechanism. *The Quarterly Journal of Economics, 84*(3), 488–500. https://doi.org/10.2307/1879431

American College of Cardiology (2019, May 16). *FDA approves first six-lead personal ECG device.* https://www.acc.org/latest-in-cardiology/articles/2019/05/16/13/02/fda-approves-first-six-lead- personal-ecg-device

Beckett, J. (2012). *Luddites.* The Nottinghamshire Heritage Gateway. http://www.nottsheritagegateway.org.uk/people/luddites.htm

Bryan, S. (1981). *Pioneering specialists: A history of the American Academy of Ophthalmology and Otolaryngology.* American Academy of Ophthalmology. https://www.aao.org/about/history

Cassel, C. K. (2018). Can retail clinics transform health care? *JAMA, 319*(18), 1855–1856. https://doi.org/10.1001/jama.2018.2172

Christensen, C. M. (1997). *The innovator's dilemma.* Harvard Business Review Press.

Christensen, C. M., Raynor, M. E., & McDonald, R. (2015). *What is disruptive innovation?* Harvard Business Review. https://hbr.org/2015/12/what-is-disruptive-innovation

Devenir Research. (2021). *2020 year-end HSA research report.*. https://www.devenir.com/wp-content/uploads/2020-Year-End-Devenir-HSA-Research-Report-Executive-Summary.pdf

Evans, L. (2021). *What can I spend my HSA on?* All About Vision https://www.allaboutvision.com/vision-insurance/items-you-can-spend-with-hsa/

Eye Netra. (2021). *EyeNetra products.* Retrieved July 9, 2021, from https://eyenetra.com/product-netra.html

EyeQue. (2021a). *EyeQue homepage.* Retrieved July 9, 2021, from https://www.eyeque.com

EyeQue. (2021b). *Can I use eyeglass numbers to order contacts?* Retrieved July 9, 2021, from https://eyeque.zendesk.com/hc/en-us/articles/115008474228-Can-I-use-EyeGlass-Numbers-to-order-contacts-

EyeQue. (2021c). *Partner with EyeQue to make clear vision a reality around the world.* Retrieved January 18, 2021, from https://www.eyeque.com/partner/

Federal Trade Commission. (2020). *Eyeglass rule.* Retrieved January 1, 2018, from https://www.ftc.gov/enforcement/rules/rulemaking-regulatory-reform-proceedings/eyeglass-rule

Garber, M. (2012). Here is the first book ever sold on Amazon. *The Atlantic.* October 31. https://www.theatlantic.com/technology/archive/2012/10/here-is-the-first-book-ever-ordered-on-amazon/264344/.

Garland, N. (1987). Optometric parity legislation under Medicare. *Journal of the American Optometric Association, 58*(6), 518–519.

Gewirtz, D. (2020, October 8). *Eye exams at home: A safe way to update your eyeglass Rx in the age of covid-19.* Retrieved January 9, 2021, from https://www.zdnet.com/article/eye-exams-at-home-a-safe-way-to-update-your-eyeglass-rx-in-the-age-of-covid/

Gewirtz, D. (2021, January 4). *How to get a new prescription, new glasses, and see better from home (all for under $100).* Retrieved January 9, 2021, from https://www.zdnet.com/article/how-to-get-a-new-prescription-new-glasses-and-see-better-from-home- all-for-under-100/

Gurkaynak, G., Guner, A., Diniz, S., & Filson, J. (2015). Most-favored-nation clauses in commercial contracts: Legal and economic analysis and proposal for a guideline. *The European Journal of Law and Economics, 42*(1), 129–155. https://doi.org/10.1007/s10657-015-9515-y

Haas-Wilson, D. (1986). The effect of commercial practice restrictions: The case of optometry. *The Journal of Law and Economics, 29*(1), 165–186. https://doi.org/10.1086/467114

Healthcare.gov. (2021). *What marketplace health insurance plans cover.* Retrieved July 9, 2021, from https://www.healthcare.gov/coverage/what-marketplace-plans-cover/

IbisWorld. (2019, December 31). *Biggest companies in the vision insurance industry in the U.S. vision insurance industry in the US- market research report.* https://www.ibisworld.com/united-states/market-research-reports/vision-insurance-industry/

Kaissi, A. (2016). Health care retail clinics: Current perspectives. *Innovation and Entrepreneurship in Health, 47.* https://doi.org/10.2147/ieh.s88610

Kempen, J., Mitchell, P., Lee, K., Tielsch, J., Broman, A., Taylor, H., Ikram, M., Congdon, N., & O'Colmain, B. (2004). The prevalence of refractive errors among adults in the United States, Western Europe, and Australia. *Archives of Ophthalmology, 122*(4), 495–505. https://doi.org/10.1001/archopht.122.4.495

Luxottica. (2021). *Our history-Luxottica home page.* http://www.luxottica.com/en/about-us/our-history.

MedicareInteractive.org. (2021). *Medicare and vision care.* Retrieved July 5, 2021, from https://www.medicareinteractive.org/get-answers/medicare-covered-services/limited-medicare-coverage-vision-and-dental/medicare-and-vision-care. Accessed July 5, 2021.

Mukamal, R. (2021, February 17). *Eye health screening apps may signal need for eye exam.* American Academy of Ophthalmology. https://www.aao.org/eye-health/tips-prevention/eye-health-app-covid-coronavirus-home-exam

National Institute on Deafness and Other Communication Disorders (NIDCD). (2021). *Over the counter hearing aids.* Retrieved July 5, 2021, from https://www.nidcd.nih.gov/health/over-counter-hearing-aids

Nevada Revised Statutes (NRS). (2021). *Acts constituting practice in optometry.* Retrieved July 9, 2021, from https://www.leg.state.nv.us/nrs/nrs-636.html#NRS636Sec025

Owler.com. (2021). *EyeQue statistics.* Retrieved January 18, 2021, from https://www.owler.com/company/eye-que

Patient Protection and Affordable Care Act. Public Law No: 111–148: H.R. 3590. (PPACA). (2010). https://www.govinfo.gov/content/pkg/PLAW-111publ148/pdf/PLAW-111publ148.pdf

Postrel, V. (2020). *The fabric of civilization*. Basic Books.

Reynolds, W. (2020, December 17). *AOA response to CNET EyeQue review.* American Optometric Association. https://www.aoa.org/about-the-aoa/press-room/statements/aoa-response-to-cnet-eyeque-review?sso=y

Romer, P. M. (2018). *On the possibility of progress.* Lecture presented at Prize Lecture in Economics Sciences at Stockholm University. https://www.nobelprize.org/prizes/economic-sciences/2018/romer/lecture/.

Rosenberg, N. (1982). *Inside the BlackBox: Technology and economics*. Cambridge University Press.

Rottenberg, S. (1962). *The economics of occupational licensing*. Princeton University Press.

Schumpeter, J. (1942). *Capitalism, socialism, and democracy*. Harper and Brothers.

Smith, A. (1776). *An inquiry into the nature and causes of the wealth of nations.*

Statista.com. (2021). *Share of Americans who bought glasses /contact lenses at a doctor's office in the past 12 months in 2018, by age.* https://www.statista.com/statistics/228537/people-who-bought-glasses-contact-lenses-at-a-doctors-office-usa/

Stigler, G. T. (1971). The theory of economic regulation. *The Bell Journal of Economics and Management Science, 2*(1), 3–21.

U.S. Bureau of Labor Statistics. (2021, April 9). *Occupational outlook handbook.* https://www.bls.gov/ooh/healthcare/optometrists.htm#:~:text=4%25,Employment%20of%20optometrists%20is%20projected%20to%20grow%204%20percent%20from,lead%20to%20demand%20for%20optometrists

U.S. Department of Justice. (1996). Revised final judgment. United States of America vs. Vision Service Plan. https://www.justice.gov/atr/case/us-v-vision-service-plan

U.S. Department of Justice. (2020). *Summary of antitrust division health care cases (Since August 25, 1983).* Retrieved July 9, 2021, from https://www.justice.gov/atr/page/file/1077686/download

Versel, N. (2013, January 25). *Topol goes prime time with his message about smartphones, smart monitors.* Mobi Health News. https://www.mobihealthnews.com/20032/topol-goes-prime- time-with-his-message-about-smartphones-smart-monitors

Vision Monday (VM). (2017, November 13). *The future of optometry – Supply*. https://www.visionmonday.com/eyecare/optometry/article/the-future-of-optometry-supply/

Worstell, C. (2020, December 16). *Does medigap cover dental and vision care*? MedicareSupplement.com. Retrieved July 9, 2021, from https://www.medicaresupplement.com/coverage/medigap-cover-dentalvision/#:~:text=According%20to%20Medicare.gov%2C%20%E2%80%9C,or%20private%2Dduty%20nursing.%E2%80%9D

Chapter 8
Advancements in Health Care Communication

Alan Yang and Steve Lebedoff

1 Introduction

Information technology (IT) is changing the way patients and health care providers communicate with each other. Surveys have shown that over a third of American adults self-diagnose when they encounter a health problem and over 70% of American adults utilize the Internet as a resource for medical information (Hochberg et al., 2020). Surveys from 2021 report over 280 million smartphone users in the United States, which is 85% of the 2020 U.S. population (https://www.census.gov/quickfacts/fact/table/US/PST045219). Growth of the number of available digital health apps has paralleled recent exponential growth of cell phone and Internet usage (Smith, 2021). For health care professionals and their patients, these advancements provide opportunities to achieve new types of health care flexibility and convenience.

The medical provider is no longer the sole, authoritative source for health care information for most consumers. The onus is now on health care providers to keep pace with this innovation by offering patients a care experience customized to them through effective data management that allows for customized care experiences enabled through delivery of timely, relevant patient information. This chapter will address how to manage the technology and communication channels that are changing the health care system.

Proactive psychologists using new communication technologies will face strategic questions about patient data and its flow through the various actors within a

A. Yang (✉)
Department of Information Systems, University of Nevada, Reno, NV, USA
e-mail: alany@unr.edu

S. Lebedoff
PPN Health Access, Reno, NV, USA
e-mail: steve@ppnhealthaccess.com

L. C. James et al. (eds.), *Clinical Health Psychology in Military and Veteran Settings*, https://doi.org/10.1007/978-3-031-12063-3_8

health care system. How the data are stored, which individuals have access to specific types of data, and when the data are accessed are all important considerations for creating a competitive data-driven health care service. The field of clinical psychology is not immune to these changes. Phenomena once considered novel are now commonplace: patients entering behavioral data into their mobile phones, psychologists conversing with patients remotely, and psychological assessments conducted with the support of artificial intelligence. Understanding and adapting to these new phenomena will require careful analyses of the actors, the technology, and the data involved in these innovations.

This chapter will discuss developments in the field of health care communication that have begun to change the industry, as well as several issues that must be addressed as providers develop strategies for integrating these innovations into their workflows. This chapter includes five sections. Section 1 is this introduction. Section 2 will discuss three technologies that are changing the way patients communicate with providers: self-diagnostic tools, mobile health, and telehealth. Section 3 will address the five channels of communication that are managed in a technologically integrated health care environment along with five scenarios involving patients, providers, and technology. Section 4 is the conclusion.

2 Types of Technology

2.1 Self-Diagnostic Tools

Delivery of health information is not a one-way line of communication from provider to patient. As connectivity becomes more ubiquitous, health care providers are no longer the sole sources of health advice available to patients. Patients are now able to access information independently based on what has been communicated to them from their health records. Thanks to the many resources made available through information technology, patients can now independently search for information on their health conditions and read reports from other patients and medical professionals. In conducting these searches, patients can identify additional medical options that their health care providers may not have mentioned. Clinicians aware of these self-diagnostic tools and their capabilities can strengthen communications with patients, gather information about patient concerns and ensure that quality of care remains consistent.

Self-diagnostic tools began with basic symptom-checking of common conditions such as influenza or the common cold, but have now expanded to expert systems that encompass a myriad of conditions, including conditions such as ear infections, chronic conditions such as diabetes, and mental health conditions such as depression (Amisha et al., 2019). These innovations are driven by advances in artificial intelligence. As more data is supplied to these diagnostic tools, the predictions become more accurate within the context of the data pool (Fan et al., 2020; Jiang et al., 2017). The success of these tools has given rise to a new movement in health care consumerism: the educated and empowered patient or e-patient.

E-patients are health consumers who participate fully in their own medical care. They gather information about their health conditions from their health care providers and then use the Internet and other digital tools to obtain additional information. The term encompasses those who seek guidance for their own ailments, and the friends and family members who go online on their behalf. In the past, patients were more likely to seek external sources of information if the condition being treated was severe, such as cancer (Beisecker & Beisecker, 1990; Lambert & Loiselle, 2007). While the propensity for patients to seek external information is still higher for severe conditions, it is not uncommon now for patients to seek additional information sources for relatively minor conditions such as a seasonal allergy (Jacobs et al., 2017). This emergence of the informed consumer follows phenomena observed in other industries such as online retail (Major, 2019). The information asymmetry between patients and providers tends to be greater in health care than in other contexts due to the typical gap in expertise between patients and health care providers. However, the trend toward a more informed patient, facilitated by the vast amounts of information available online and the tools to simplify that information, may transform the health care industry the same way it has transformed others. In practice, online diagnostic tools are data-driven expert systems that rely on consistent feedback to improve future predictions.

Analysts discussing this potential impact of online information are not suggesting that patients will self-diagnose and self-treat serious conditions without consulting medical professionals. Instead, they suggest that patients may use the online self-diagnostic tools to assess whether it would be useful to seek professional help, or to address minor issues.[1]

A common flowchart for these diagnosis tools from the user's perspective is presented in Fig. 8.1. The flow chart walks through the progression of a patient as she accesses an online diagnostic system. The flowchart is separated by actors, actions that the patient would take are indicated by the nodes in the upper lane, while actions that the system would take are in the bottom lane. The patient begins by entering demographic data and selecting symptoms from lists. The diagnostic

[1]The book, *The Innovator's Prescription*, distinguishes between conditions treated with rules-based health care and conditions treated with intuitive care. Conditions treated with rules-based care are diagnosed using a straightforward test or readily observed symptoms, and treatment is guided by straightforward algorithmic treatment recommendations. Conditions requiring intuitive care are more difficult to diagnose, and they may require treatment regimens that are tailored to meet patient-specific requirements. The authors of *The Innovator's Prescription* argue that disruptive technologies may be useful for conditions that require rules-based diagnosis and treatment, but they are less likely to be useful for conditions requiring intuitive care. (Christensen, C, Grossman, J., and Hwang, J. (2009) The Innovator's Prescription. McGraw-Hill Education.

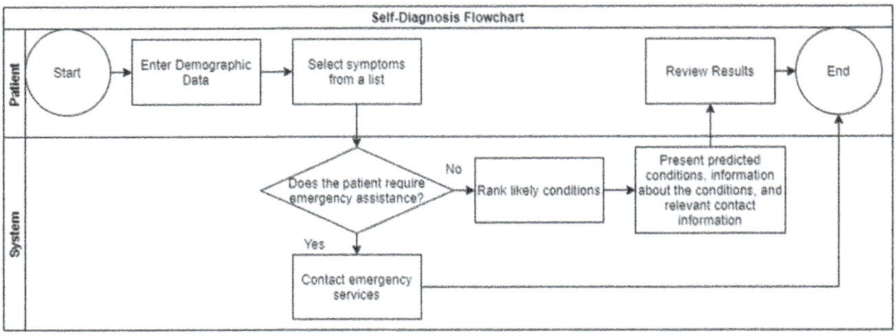

Fig. 8.1 Flowchart for an online diagnostic system

Gender: Male

Age: 51

Reported Symptoms: Headache, cough, fever between 100.4 to 102 f

Possible conditions

Influenza	**Moderate Match**	***More Information***
Bac. Pneumonia	**Moderate Match**	***More Information***
Common Cold	**Fair Match**	***More Information***
Coronavirus	**Fair Match**	***More Information***

Fig. 8.2 Template of typical physical health symptom checker results

system uses this information to make a determination, indicated by the diamond shape, on the question of whether the patient requires immediate emergency assistance. An example would be whether the patient reports an immediate difficulty breathing, a sensation nearing unconsciousness, or a direct indication that she requires immediate support. If the patient requires immediate care, the system recommends that the patient seek emergency care. If not, the system ranks possible diagnoses indicated by the patient's self-reported symptoms to provide a set of possible diagnoses, along with their calculated probabilities based on the symptoms reported. This type of system is patient-driven, with no human actor on the other end besides an expert system that uses the patient's data to generate a series of predictions.

Example results of these self-diagnostic tools are presented in Figs. 8.2 and 8.3. These reporting screens are shown to the patient at the end of the data entry and symptom evaluation process. Often the data the patient has entered are presented back to the patient for review. The likelihood of potential conditions is also reported. Most of these diagnostic tools provide an option for patients to access more information about any of the reported conditions. This feature guides the patient toward

Based on your responses, your depression test score was:

Moderate Depression (11/20)

Your responses indicate that you may be at risk of harming yourself or someone else. If you are in need of immediate assistance, please call the National Suicide Prevention Hotline to speak to a trained counselor.

More information about your results

Revise your answers

Take another test–

Fig. 8.3 Template of typical mental health symptom checker results

further research and may lead them to take proactive measures to address potential conditions.

Figures 8.2 and 8.3 provide illustrative examples of the types of results provided by self-diagnostic tools available online. Table 8.1 provides a summary of currently available tools along with links to the websites.

These systems use the information entered by the patient to generate a set of potential diagnoses. Most of these tools also provide resources for patients to learn more about the conditions, and possibly contact medical professionals virtually. If geolocational systems are involved, then these diagnostic assistants can recommend nearby health care providers and provide contact information directly through the interface.

While patient self-diagnosis tools can potentially guide patient decisions to seek care and may boost patient engagement in managing self-care behaviors, they also pose risks and dangers. Patient-driven information-seeking runs all the risks of any type of unsupervised browsing of the Internet (Liu et al., 2019). Self-diagnosis tools

Table 8.1 Self-assessment tools available online

Name	Description	Website
Mental Health Test	A collection of tests including depression, PTSD, addiction, and work health provided by the organization Mental Health America	https://screening.mhanational.org/screening-tools/
Symptomate	A general health checkup that determines the likelihood of health conditions based on user-input symptoms	https://symptomate.com/diagnosis/#0-66
WebMD Symptom Checker	A health checkup with additional functionality, including visual indicators for symptom locations and follow-up resources for health care assistance	https://symptoms.webmd.com/
Mental Health assessments from Psycom	A collection of self-assessment and screening tools for conditions, including depression, grief, ADHD, autism, bipolar disorder, addition, and stress	https://www.psycom.net/quizzes

can generate misleading predictions due to either weaknesses in the artificial intelligence embedded in specific self-diagnosis tools, or inaccurate information provided by patients. If patients act on these conditions and self-medicate for an incorrectly diagnosed condition, then the potential for harm increases due to exacerbation of a condition or the development of a new condition. Additionally, not all patients will exhibit information-seeking behavior equally. Factors such as patient educational status, access to the Internet, and trust in online health information can affect the search for information and how likely patients are to act upon advice from a source other than a health care provider (Morgan & Trauth, 2013; Peek et al., 2014).

Providers aware of the existence of these systems can communicate with patients to determine whether they are utilizing these resources as an additional source of information on their conditions. Providers can further limit the potential harm by recommending supported tools they are familiar with, and by asking patients to share the results from these self-diagnostic tests. By opening this channel of communication, providers can gain insight into patient concerns about their symptoms. With proper supervision, online diagnostic tools and the wider Internet at large can serve as a source of supporting information. Providers can advise patients to be critical about information obtained from these tools and to consult with a professional before following a course of treatment not directly prescribed by their clinician.

2.2 *Mobile Health*

Mobile health encompasses any device that can be carried or worn to decrease the temporal and spatial constraints associated with traditional health care (Steinhubl et al., 2015; Varshney, 2014). The goal of mobile health is to improve the health, comfort, and wellness of patients through information technology. Mobile health devices can be smartphone applications, wearable devices, or devices that are surgically implanted into a patient's body. Mobile health applications are the most popular form of mobile health intervention in use today due to the ubiquity of smartphones and the low overhead compared to dedicated devices. Therefore, this section will focus on implementation of mobile health apps as this is the most prevalent form of mobile health. The guidelines and considerations discussed in this section are also relevant to wearable and implanted mobile health technologies.

Commercial mobile health apps (such as apps provided on the Android or Apple application markets) and devices (such as FitBit or Apple Watch) are now capable of storing and transmitting information through a network. Over two-thirds of hospitals in North America integrate some form of mobile health in patient care, including mobile applications integrated with hospital electronic health records (EHRs) and applications designed to support maintenance activities such as medication adherence (Dick et al., 2020; Llorens-Vernet & Miró, 2020). In the field of clinical psychology, government applications, such as the Post Traumatic Stress Disorder (PTSD) Coach, Insomnia Coach, and VetChange, are providing additional resources

Table 8.2 Mobile applications from the US Department of Veterans' Affairs

Application name	Website
PTSD Coach	https://mobile.va.gov/app/ptsd-coach
Insomnia Coach	https://mobile.va.gov/app/insomnia-coach
Exposure Ed	https://mobile.va.gov/app/exposure-ed
Live Whole Health	https://mobile.va.gov/app/live-whole-health
Mindfulness Coach	https://mobile.va.gov/app/mindfulness-coach
Stay-Quit Coach	https://mobile.va.gov/app/stay-quit-coach
Rx Refill	https://mobile.va.gov/app/rx-refill
Mindfulness Coach	https://mobile.va.gov/app/mindfulness-coach
CBT-i Coach	https://mobile.va.gov/app/cbt-i-coach
AIMS for Anger Management	https://mobile.va.gov/app/anger-and-irritability-management-skills-aims
VA Online Scheduling	https://mobile.va.gov/app/va-online-scheduling

to patients to obtain information about their conditions and to track information relevant to these conditions. Patient adoption of mobile devices and apps is growing. The informed clinician can utilize these developments to improve her care strategies and provide patients with a richer care experience. (See Table 8.2 for a list of mobile health applications provided by the US Department of Veterans' Affairs.)

2.3 *Telehealth and Virtual Health Care*

Telepsychology is a growing technology area in treating symptoms such as PTSD, depression, anxiety, eating disorders, adjustment disorders, and substance abuse. The virtual component of these visits has been around for years, with the telephonic consultation solution's inception in 1960 as an attempt to connect with hard-to-reach populations. For the behavioral psychologist, telehealth or telepsychology is just one component of the emerging health care technology landscape. The challenge is to have this facet of pertinent patient data readily available to be shared with other care team members.

The COVID-19 pandemic from 2019 to 2021 placed pressure on society to accelerate innovation in the field of digital collaboration. In the health care field, telehealth and digital health (mHealth and health information technologies) saw many improvements. During the spring of 2020, when approximately 90% of the US population was under "stay at home" orders, telepsychology visits were the only option for most individuals seeking treatment. The easing of payment requirements by Medicaid, Medicare, and private insurance carriers along with the easing of licensure requirements by regulatory and state bodies also drove innovation in this field.

A sample visual of a common telehealth-enabled system from the clinician's perspective is presented in Fig. 8.4.

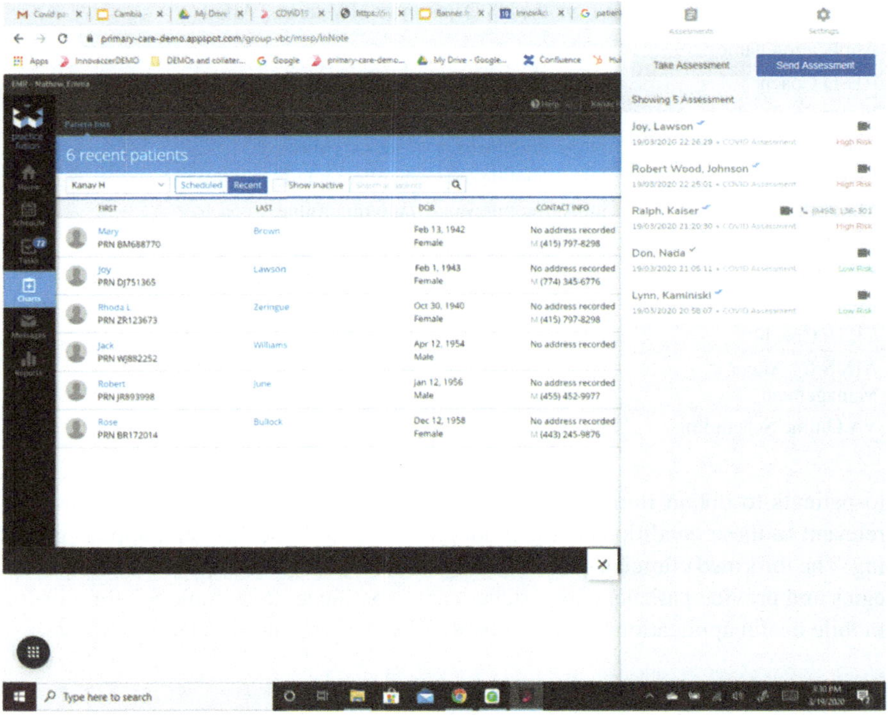

Fig. 8.4 Sample telehealth conferencing system from provider's perspective

The image presents the view from the clinician's side, where access to patient contact information is available through a portal accessible through a web browser. Patients can be ranked based on priority, and teleconference calls to patients can be scheduled and made through the same interface.

Teleconferencing software can be used to schedule patient visits, assign priorities, and keep track of the data generated during the visits all within one system. This software is likely to become increasingly useful, as vendors expand these capabilities to include patient feedback channels, along with data processing, and analytics. In addition, analytical tools can be developed to identify patterns from visits and make suggestions for future scheduling decisions. Strategic issues that will be considered by clinicians using telehealth include:

1. What data generated during the visit are recorded?
2. What information generated from the visit is shared?
3. Who has access to this information?
4. Is the sharing process automated?

Telehealth technology can be coupled with remote monitoring to augment support for aging in place, address home care worker shortages,[2] and reduce the administrative burdens associated with Long-Term Services and Supports by consolidating and automating relevant administrative workflows. In the behavioral psychology field, automated sentiment analysis of patient transcripts can serve as an additional layer of decision support for the health care provider (Provoost et al., 2019; Rajput, 2020).

Modern smartphones are now considered to be as effective for teleconferencing as laptops or desktop computers (Hurst, 2020). How videos are stored, what information is needed prior to a visit, and how visit reports are generated and shared are just a few of the questions that will arise while designing and implementing a data-driven telehealth system. Detailed interactions between clinicians and technology managers will be needed during the planning phase of the technology adoption and implementation process to ensure careful consideration of these issues. Thoughtful decisions are essential to ensure that technology adoption generates a return on investment and strengthens patient health outcomes.

3 Communication Channels

A recurring theme in discussions of health care quality is communication. These discussions traditionally focused on communication between health care providers. However, technological advancements are creating new opportunities for increased connectivity and communication between patients and providers. The successful integration of mobile devices can facilitate increased efficiency within a health care system as patients use these tools to track their own health progress, report information to clinicians, and store data pertaining to their individual health.

This section focuses on analysis of communication channels. Analysis of the flow of information through a set of communication channels provides a useful framework for examination of decisions facing clinicians, as patients increasingly utilize mobile apps, self-diagnosis tools, and telehealth.[3] These technologies introduce new sources of information, new types of data, and potential communication channels that were not included in traditional health care interactions. As clinicians consider strategic options for addressing these new technologies, this framework can help structure their assessments of alternate strategies. This discussion of chan-

[2] A substantive complaint voiced by personal care aides (PCAs) is gaps in communication between health care providers and PCAs. PCAs help patients implement health care recommendations, but they do not always receive information about these recommendations directly. (Osterman, P. [2017] Who will care for us? Long-term care and the long-term workforce. Russell Sage Foundation. 232 pages. ISBN-13: 978-0871546395).

[3] The academic discipline that focuses on the adoption and usage of technology by individuals and organizations is known as Information Systems. University Information Systems departments are typically located within Colleges of Business.

nels is combined with a presentation of five possible health care scenarios. At the conclusion of this section, the reader will have a useful framework to structure assessments of the challenges and opportunities offered by the new technologies. The reader will also be familiar with questions that are likely to arise as provider organizations develop strategic responses to patient engagement with the new technologies. Finally, she will be familiar with evaluation criteria for assessing mobile apps and communicating requirements to developers.

3.1 Scenario 1: Traditional Health Care Model

Prior to the introduction of EHR systems, there was a single communication channel between patients and providers, as illustrated in Fig. 8.5. This channel, denoted here as Channel 1, is the oldest and most established relationship between the patient and the health care provider. Within this channel, the patient provides information to her health care provider and receives feedback, advice, and a treatment plan.

3.2 Scenario 2: Health Care Providers Utilizing EHR Systems

Implementation of EHR systems with patient portals established at least one, and possibly two, additional communication channels, as illustrated in Fig. 8.6. In communication Channel 2, the clinician enters data into the EHR system, and views data stored in the system. The EHR system may also provide information about relevant treatment guidelines and reminders relevant to specific patient care.

3.2.1 Channel 2: Providers and the Database

Implementation of EHR systems generated initial concerns about the impact of this technology on the quality of communications occurring in Channel 1. Clinicians were concerned that time spent sending and receiving information on Channel 2 during visits would restrict the time available for communicating with patients on

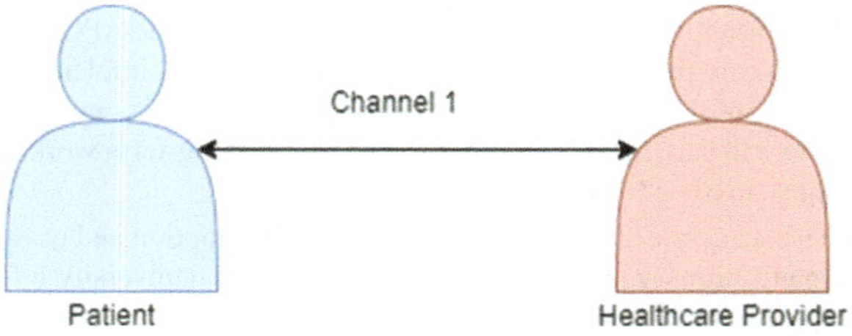

Fig. 8.5 Patient and provider communicate through channel 1

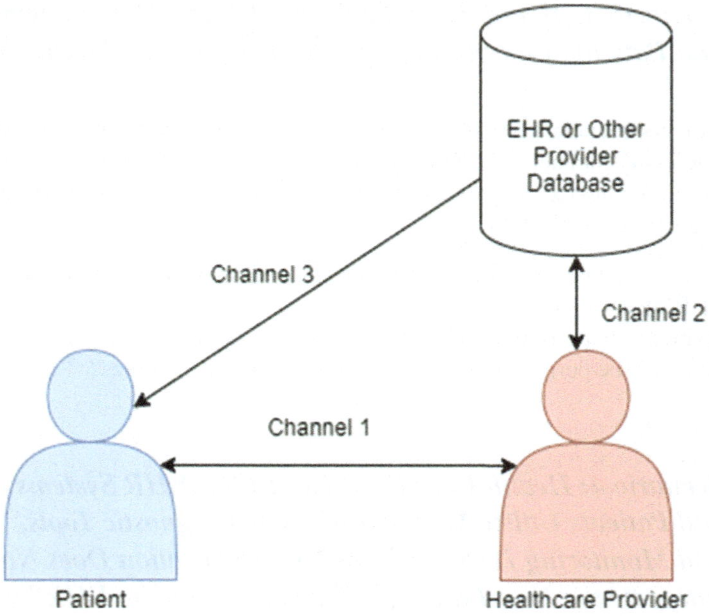

Fig. 8.6 Communication channels through an EHR system

Channel 1. Over time, clinicians and provider organizations have modified workflow patterns to address this issue. For example, some provider organizations use team care models in which medical assistants handle some of the channel 2 communications. (See Chap. 5 for a discussion of issues posed by implementation of EHR systems.)

3.2.2 Channel 3: Patients and the Provider Database

Some provider organizations also implemented patient portals that allow patients to view information stored in the EHR system. In this situation, a third communication channel of information operates between the patient and the EHR system (denoted here as Channel 3). Providing patient access to this data facilitates development of more informed patients and can improve the quality of communication in channel 1. This channel is typically managed by a web portal that grants patients access to information relevant to their treatment, such as lab test results and the status of medication prescriptions. A more thorough discussion of the legal, technological, and ethical environment of patient access to data is available in Chap. 5 of this book.

3.3 Scenario 3: Health Care Providers Utilize EHR Systems and Patients Communicate with Providers via Telehealth

When patients use telehealth to communicate with their established providers, the communication channel structure illustrated in Fig. 8.6 remains unchanged. However, clinicians face questions about the types of data that will be allowed to flow through Channel 3 such as:

- Will patients be permitted to view recordings of the telehealth sessions stored in the EHR database?
- Will patients be permitted to record the sessions as they occur?
- Will patients be permitted to view the clinician's session notes?

3.4 Scenario 4: Health Care Providers Utilize EHR Systems and Patients Utilize Mobile Apps, Self-Diagnostic Tools, and Monitoring Devices: Provider Organization Does Not Integrate the New Types of Information into the EHR System

Clinicians face additional strategic options regarding the channel structure when patients begin using new technologies such as mobile health apps, self-diagnostic tools, and monitoring devices. The provider organization may, or may not, elect to integrate information generated by patient use of these new technologies into the health care setting and into the EHR system. If the provider organization elects to utilize this information during patient visits without integrating the information into the EHR system, the communication channels would be structured as shown in Fig. 8.7.

In this scenario, patient-generated data is not uploaded from the app or mobile device to the provider's EHR system. Therefore, the EHR system is not affected by patient decisions to use the new technologies. Instead, the patient communicates with the health app through the new Channel 4, and the patient communicates with the provider through Channel 1. The patient and provider might jointly examine data generated by the app during visits, but this data is not stored on a provider database. While information generated by the patient's use of the mobile app could strengthen communications in Channel 1, it is also possible that patient difficulties using the app could distract from useful communications in that Channel. This subsection discusses potential impacts of the mobile app on Channel 1 communications, and then it discusses issues relevant to Channel 4.

3.4.1 How Channel 1 Is Affected by Technology

In the context of a technologically integrated environment, this channel provides an opportunity for patients to supplement their communications with clinicians by sharing information. For example, if a medication tracking application shows that a

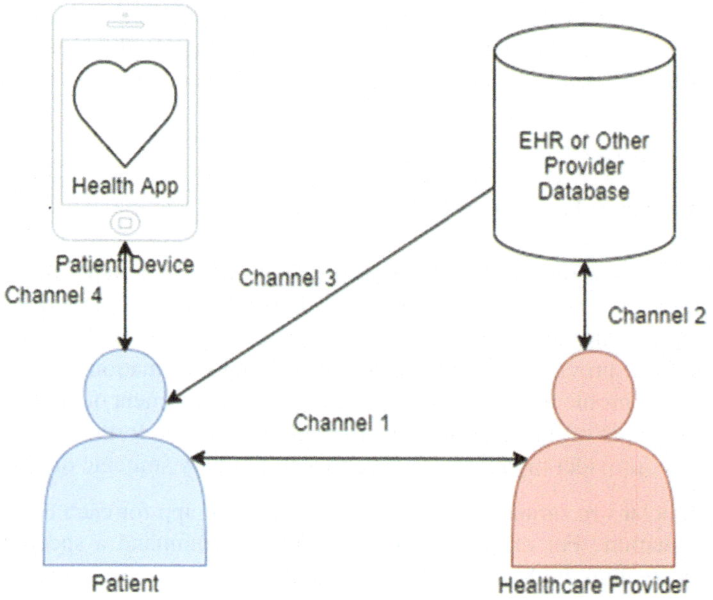

Fig. 8.7 Patient device and health application

patient consistently misses timely doses every Wednesday and Thursday, then channel 1 is where more information can be gathered as to why that is the case.

Integration of technology also changes the typical flow of channel 1. If patients are unable to complete a task on their device, or if they are confused by some aspect of it, then they may need to speak with their health care provider to gain a better understanding of functionalities. Patients need to have a resource in case the help-systems built into the application are unable to address their concerns. Realistically, clinicians are not expected to provide patient support in this regard. Other members of the health care staff could be trained to handle patient requests for IT support, and clinicians can direct patients to this source of assistance, to ensure an orderly integration of systems and transfer of information through channel 1. Ideally, the application provides problem solving steps that users can follow to diagnose common questions or problems. However, if patients still have trouble, successful integration of a technological intervention requires a clear line of communication by which patients can receive help. Recommending a single mobile health application to patients will streamline the effort required to help patients learn how to use the app. With one external channel, responses to data problems and patient concerns can be more standardized and efficient.

Channel 1 provides an opportunity for the health care provider to demonstrate to the patient how to properly access functionality or correctly perform a task such as input data. Within this channel, patients can also communicate the positives from their experiences utilizing an application and potentially generate a source of additional support for their care. To ensure effective communication in this channel, health care providers should be aware of the application's functionalities and the steps to access these. If patients are able to receive the support they need in a timely manner within channel 1, then the data that can be generated from other channels will improve in quality.

3.4.2 Channel 4: Patients and Their Devices

Channel 4 can generate new types of information that can potentially strengthen communications occurring through Channel 1, but it can also potentially distract from important Channel 1 communications if patients have difficulty using the new technology or if providers have difficulty interpreting information provided by the app. This latter problem could occur if patients use an assortment of apps that generate disparate types of information in an array of app-specific formats.

Therefore, provider organizations face two preliminary strategic questions:

- Will clinicians recommend that patients use a single app for each clinically relevant situation? For example, clinicians might recommend a specific app for patients dealing with depression and a different app for patients dealing with PTSD.
- Will the provider organization provide tech support for patients learning to use the recommended apps, and – if so – how will this support be organized and funded?

Patients utilizing a health care application to supplement their care within this system are ideally doing so at the behest of their health care provider. Channel 4 indicates the flow of data between the patient and the application present on her mobile device. Considerations of this channel relate primarily to the planned function of the application and more broadly to the patient's ability to utilize technology. The three goals of this channel are as follows:

1. Accurate, timely data are supplied by a patient.
2. The patient continues to utilize the application.
3. Accurate, timely data are reported back to the patient.

If clinicians will suggest that patients use mobile apps, it may be useful to also provide guidance to help patients select apps with design features that will support achievement of these goals. To achieve goal 1, patients need to first learn how to utilize the application. Any mobile application that will be recommended to patients should account for the average demographic characteristics of potential users. For instance, if a mobile application will be used primarily by elderly individuals (65 and older), or by patients with limited sight or hearing, the application should account for these issues to maximize the app's usability. Research indicates that people exposed to mobile technologies consistently over a period of time are less likely to encounter difficulties pertaining to mobile application usage, particularly if the exposure occurred before the age of 18 (Kerr et al., 2018).

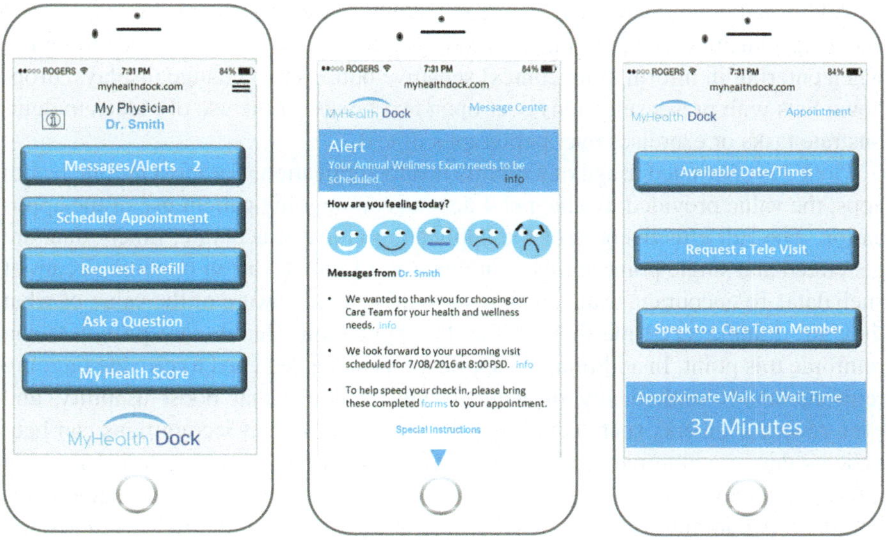

Fig. 8.8 Mockup screens from a patient-facing health care application

Independent of demographic factors, research identifies three key features that improve user experience when utilizing mobile applications: clear screen progression, use of visual information over textual, and clear distinctions between interactive and non-interactive elements (Holzinger & Errath, 2007; Salim et al., 2017). Figure 8.8 contains a mockup of sample screens from a health care application that follows these principles.

The progressions of the screens start on the left and move toward the right. The opening (leftmost) screen displays critical information right away: it identifies the patient's clinician and offers access to five key features via five central buttons. Additional selections are available through the dropdown menu on the upper right corner of the screen. The middle screen is opened when the "messages/alerts" button is selected. The middle screen allows the patient to indicate her health status by selecting one of the facial pictographs. Further information is available to the patient through the "info" links at the end of the bullet points. The text itself is summarized to limit the total amount of information presented at one time. This selective information display gives users the option to select what they wish to read. The rightmost screen is the scheduling screen which can be reached by selecting the "schedule appointment" button on the leftmost screen. The scheduling screen allows patients to schedule an in-person or tele-visit and provides an estimate of the approximate wait time. Throughout the application, the buttons are clearly labeled in contrast to the neutral backdrop. Important information is indicated either through visual representations or by large blocks of text. And the functionalities of each screen and interactive elements are clear. The application screens demonstrate how good design can encourage the flow of information in channel 4.

Additional functionality can be integrated into a system depending on contextual needs of a health care environment. Examples would include large selection areas when entering in information, context sensitive buttons that change displays, drop-down lists with preset selections over open text boxes, or the use of videos to demonstrate tasks or exercises over paragraphs of text.

Goal 2 is continued usage of a mobile health application. For most mobile health apps, the value provided by channel 4 depends on ongoing patient use of the application. The full effectiveness of the application is lost if accurate, timely data are generated at a single point in time, but this is not followed by an ongoing stream of such data. To encourage usage, patients should be made aware of the value of what they are doing every time they utilize the application. Health care providers can reinforce this point. In addition, the application can be designed to provide ongoing reinforcement. Aesthetically pleasing designs, features that boost usability, and even reward elements such as progress bars or achievement recognitions can help patients derive additional extrinsic motivation to continue entering in information into an application. Timely data reported back to the patient also leads to goal number three. A common problem of achieving this goal is keeping patients motivated to continue utilizing the application after the initial novelty period of a new technology has worn off. This novelty period typically lasts between 2 and 4 weeks for mobile applications and wearables (Dinh-Le et al., 2019; Shin et al., 2019). Reinforcement of the benefits of the applications through channel 1 can help patients continue to enter in data to improve the quality of data passing through channel 4.

Providing information back to the patient is goal 3 of channel 4. Over a period of continuous usage, patients should be able to review the information they have supplied and ideally see visualizations of their health progress. Visualization of progress and, ideally, improvements will result in patients becoming less dependent on extrinsic motivators and gradually make the shift to intrinsic motivation (Osborn & Egede, 2010). Once patients have reached this stage, their usage rate and the accuracy of the data that they enter increases and their attrition rate decreases (Mihelj et al., 2012).

In this scenario, there is no integration between the provider database and the mobile health intervention; hence the patient's device's local storage or a third-party database becomes the repository for the patient's data. If data will be stored on the patient's hardware (e.g., cell phone or other device), storage capacity may be a relevant issue. If the patient's data will be stored in cloud-based database, then the patient's ability to connect to the Internet may be a relevant issue.

3.5 Criteria for Evaluating Mobile Health Applications

Clinicians or practice organizations may decide to recommend that patients use a single mobile health app to address each specific patient health issue (such as medication adherence). This strategy can streamline the level of effort required for the health care provider to ensure that use of the app strengthens patient care experiences and patient health outcomes. However, provider organizations implementing this strategy will face the task of evaluating apps in order to select the apps that will be recommended.

Although still evolving, mHealth applications provide patients with support and coping tools, to achieve individual goals and improve efficacy and outcomes. Before implementing a mobile health intervention, however, attention should be paid to the regulatory environment and current guidelines for evaluating mobile health apps. Evidence suggests that a high proportion of mobile health apps do not meet patient and provider expectations.

The Food and Drug Administration (FDA) is one source of guidance on evaluation of mobile health devices and application. As of September 27, 2019, the FDA has categorized mobile health applications into two groups, those definitely subject to oversight by the FDA, and those subject to discretionary oversight, in which the FDA decides on a case-by-case basis whether the app will be subject to oversight. Discretionary oversight is a broad category that is reserved for applications that pose a low risk to patients (see Table 8.3). The main criteria for classifying an app as "subject to oversight" or "discretionary oversight" focuses on the degree to which the FDA assessment indicates that failure of the application would put patients at significant risk of harm (Gruessner, 2015; Sekaran, 2020).

Table 8.3 contains a list of software functions and their current classifications by the FDA (US Food and Drug Administration, 2019). Devices that control medical data, devices that interface with other medical devices directly, and software that provides diagnostic information are subject to oversight. Most mobile health applications fall underneath the category of discretionary oversight.

The FDA acknowledges within the guidance document that the field of mobile health is ever-changing and definitions, along with uses of devices and software, are subject to change. Before implementation of any mobile devices into a health care system, a review of FDA guidelines based on the functionality of the to-be system should be conducted. Mobile health platforms that are registered with the FDA are

Table 8.3 Mobile health devices and software subject to FDA regulatory oversight

Oversight category	Type of software (list is not exhaustive)
Subject to oversight	Extensions of medical devices that can control or analyze medical data
	Software that transforms a mobile platform into a regulated medical device using additional external hardware
	Software that performs patient-specific analysis and provides patient-specific diagnosis or treatment recommendations
Discretionary oversight	Software that provides supplemental information related to treatment
	Software functions that provide access to health information
	Software that assists patients in communicating with health care providers
	Software that performs calculations routinely used in clinical practice
	Software that recommends behavioral coping skills for diagnosed psychiatric conditions
	Software that provides checklists of common signs and symptoms to facilitate care

not necessarily subject to oversight. Prudent health care managers will smooth new implementations by ensuring that the functionalities of proposed mobile health interventions meet the needs of the health care mission and are consistent with FDA guidelines. FDA guidelines and policies are likely to evolve over time. As of this writing, FDA policy is reported in a 2019 document titled *Policy for Device Software Functions and Mobile Medical Applications Guidance for Industry and Food and Drug Administration Staff* (https://www.fda.gov/media/80958/download).

Numerous criteria for evaluation of mobile health applications have been suggested, with no official standard criteria in place that is followed by most developers or evaluators (Dick et al., 2020). HIMMS is an organization that has sought to establish standards in health care data and has presented guidelines pertaining to mobile apps in partnership with Xcertia (2019). These guidelines are consistent with literature on this subject. In addition, this literature indicates that commonalities exist between the HIMMS/XCertia criteria and evaluation criteria proposed by other analysts and entities (Robeznieks, 2019). A compilation of three meta-studies on establishing criteria to evaluate mobile health interventions along with recommendations by the mobile health standards and guidelines body Xcertia, supported by the Health care Information Management Systems Society (HIMMS) is presented in Table 8.4.

A review of these criteria shows that there are three metrics included consistently throughout the sets of evaluation criteria: the *reliability* of the mobile health intervention, the *security* of the data being transferred by the application, and the *usability* of the tool. Studies may differ in terminology or expand on one of the three categories in more elaborate detail, such as aesthetics, networking capacities, and runtime efficiency. However, existing evaluations in the field of mobile health adhere consistently to these three metrics. As the field grows, more metrics of interest will be added and analyzed. However, independent of other developments, the three core criteria will remain a determinant of the potential efficacy of mobile health interventions.

Another ratings system in the mobile health literature is the Mobile Application Rating Scale (MARS) developed in 2016 (Stoyanov et al., 2016). The rating system ranks applications on a scale of 1–5 (5 being highest) and is a popular standard by which academic studies classify the design efficacy of mobile health interventions. Example studies utilize the MARS system to rank applications across four

Table 8.4 Studies and recommendations on mobile health evaluation

Publication	Criteria
Nouri et al. (2018)	Design; Information/Content; Usability; Functionality; Ethical Issues; Security and Privacy; User-Perceived Value
Aungst et al. (2014)	Usefulness; Accuracy; Authority; Objectivity; Timeliness; Functionality; Design; Security
Llorens-Vernet and Miró (2020)	Usability; Privacy; Security; Suitability; Transparency; Safety; Support; Reliability
Xcertia (2019)	Privacy; Security; Operability; Usability; Content
Stoyanov et al. (2016)	Engagement; Functionality; Aesthetics; Information

categories: Engagement, Functionality, Aesthetics, and Information on a scale of 1–5 across a variety of mobile interventions for conditions such as back pain, heart disease, and more (Escriche-Escuder et al., 2020; Knitza et al., 2019).

Commercial applications on app marketplaces will often have user reviews that can serve as an indicator for the reliability and usability facets of the app. For a more thorough examination of an app, the MARS scale or Xcertia recommendations can be applied to determine the functionality of the data side of the application. As an evolving field, new standards for evaluation are being developed and new guidelines are being established as both software and hardware become more advanced

3.6 Scenario 5: Health Care Providers Utilize EHR Systems and Patients Utilize Mobile Apps, Self-Diagnostic Tools and Monitoring Devices: Provider Organization Integrates the New Types of Information into the EHR System

In this scenario, the provider organization implements a fully integrated mobile health system, as illustrated in Fig. 8.9. The diagram shows a setting with four components: the patient, the provider, the patient's mobile computing device, and a provider database. The flow of data and communication (the channels) between the four items within this system are the basis for the following discussion.

In this scenario, the patient's mobile health device sends data to the provider's EHR. The following descriptions assume a fully integrated system wherein the mobile health app utilized by the patient is connected to the provider's EHR and five channels of communication work to support patient care.

Successful implementation of mobile health systems can potentially generate additional benefits. Long-term services and supports and other health care activities conducted by patients and family caregivers can be tracked, and data generated by these care activities can be integrated into the EHR system.[4] These new flows of information can then be utilized to provide relevant feedback to both patients and providers within the technologically enabled health care system. In addition, clinicians can use the information to make timely and informed decisions on care plans.

The decision to integrate data generated through the mobile app into the EHR system can potentially strengthen Channel 1 if the patient consistently enters data into the app, and if frequent communication occurs between patient and provider about the data being stored in the EHR. The decision to integrate can also potentially strengthen the information provided in channel 2 if the EHR system uses the app data to generate useful information to the clinician. Given the potential value of the app data, the provider organization's decision to implement a fully integrated system raises two strategic questions:

[4] See Chap. 5 (Using Computer Technology to Support Clinical Decision Making) for additional discussion of EHR systems and issues posed by patient-generated data and behavioral health data.

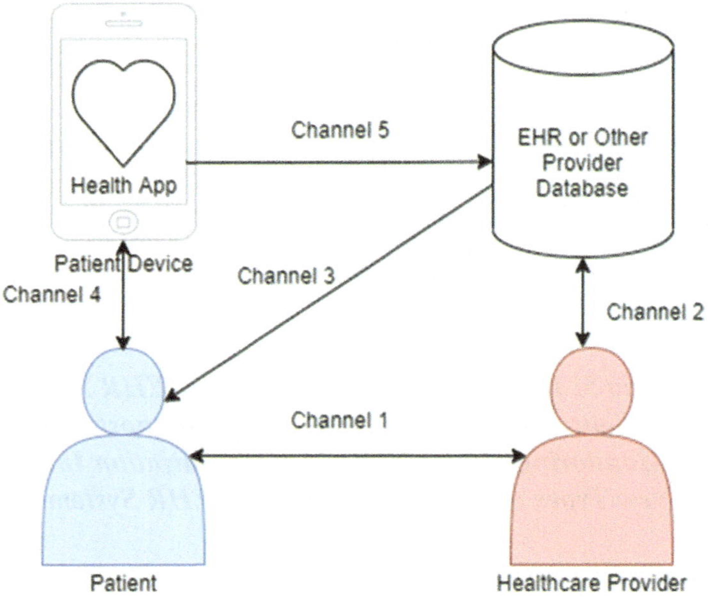

Fig. 8.9 Patient-provider-application data flows in an integrated care setting

- How will the system be designed to ensure that patient-generated data stored by the provider is accurate?
- How will the system report patient-generated data to clinicians? What level of detail and what formats will be useful during a patient visit?

The first question focuses on Channel 5, and the second question focuses on channel 2.

3.6.1 Channel 5: Patient Device and the Provider Database

In channel 5, data generated by the patient are received by the provider's EHR system. Since provider databases are varied, there are many ways for this implementation to occur. When mobile technology data are received and stored by the provider's EHR, this link is typically creating in conjunction with existing health software providers such as Epic, eClinicalWorks, Cerner, or WebPT (Abdolkhani et al., 2019). Examples include integration of existing health care applications into EHR systems, or the creation of new applications along with customized databases to support the new flow of patient data (Dinh-Le et al., 2019; Genes et al., 2018).

New considerations arise if the decision is made to integrate the mobile application with an existing database. Modern networking technology allows for synchronous uploading of data seconds after the user enters it. In theory, if patient data were generated and recorded perfectly, then synchronous connectivity to the EHR would be ideal. However, data collection and transfer is an error-prone process. Having some form of verification system in place can help to alleviate some of these problems. The inclusion of a "delete" or "edit" function for patients can also help alleviate erroneous entries. However, if these functionalities are included, application security becomes a chief concern and some form of verification is needed to ensure that patients or other authorized individuals are the only people editing health records. Most systems will design channel 5 as a one-way transfer of data, meaning that patients can only upload new records to an EHR. However, if patients are permitted to access or modify additional records present in the EHR, stringent security measures will be required to ensure that data breaches do not occur. Channel 4 is where determinants of security and reliability of mobile health information systems primarily take place. Hardware considerations at this stage are also a factor. Depending on how a system is designed, patients may enter information while they are not connected to a network. Once they are connected, that information may then be delayed before sending. Considerations in this channel are data requirements, network connectivity, and the usage of data timestamps to ensure that accurate information is being passed throughout the system.

3.6.2 Channel 2: Using the App Data to Generate Useful Information for Clinicians

In channel 2, the information gathered from treatment of the patient is stored in the provider's EHR and relayed back to the health care provider. If a health app is integrated with a health care provider's system, then it is likely being presented to clinicians as a screen within the EHR. Two important considerations need to be addressed at this stage: (1) The information within the EHR must be accurate; and (2) it needs to be communicated to the health care provider in a useful format. In addition, advances in the field of artificial intelligence can help to detect patterns that may indicate an underlying health problem for a patient that has yet to emerge (Hamet & Tremblay, 2017).

In addition, the advancement of mobile health has occurred in parallel with advances in database management and artificial intelligence. These developments can address the fact that most clinicians would probably not enjoy sorting through raw data from an excel spreadsheet to check on the patient's progress in implementing recommended self-care regimens. While such interfaces exist, most individuals, even if they are subject matter experts, desire more efficient presentations and can make faster decisions if they receive organized recommendations rather than raw data. Visualization of information and clear narrative threads across the data are important for continued and effective usage of a new technology (Munzner, 2014). Integration with existing electronic medical record systems and health care portals and software can limit the difficulties associated with implementation of a new system. Recommending a single mobile health intervention to patients will streamline the process of integrating the mobile health data into the EHR system and providing useful summary information to clinicians.

A proactive manager of these changes will consider the following:

1. The data functionalities of the applications recommended for integration
2. Where the data go
3. The readability of the data
4. How data can be integrated and used in the wider system

The vision of a fully integrated solution includes permitting patients to upload app-generated data and patient-generated data into the EHR system, and then providing useful summaries and visualizations of this data to clinicians. Current EHR systems were not initially designed to perform these functions. Recently, some health care systems and IT system providers are working to address these issues. For example, the company *Innovaccer* offers an EHR system that integrates traditional health care data with behavioral health data, mobile health app data and telehealth capabilities.

Innovaccer is actively addressing issues often raised by individuals working with EHRs. The Innovaccer software platform can integrate several types of data into EHRs, including behavioral health data and data generated from mobile sources. The platform also expands the definition of the health care team to be supported by EHR communications, by allowing for timely information flow to long-term patient support and maintenance caregivers. The data being transferred throughout the systems can then be used to improve patient outcomes. For example, an individual caring for an elderly family member may receive an alert on her phone when that elderly family member has travelled over 50 feet from his home location. This information can then be acted on immediately to ensure that the family member is safe, and relevant information about the event can be recorded for future analysis.

The Innovacer technologies offer the potential to help address limitations of current EHR systems by improving data transformation, decision support, and team-based care by ensuring that team members have ready access to relevant information, including information relevant to the clinical psychologist. Innovaccer is just one of many companies that are capturing the opportunities generated by the growth of information technology in health care.

4 Conclusion

Patient use of mobile devices and mobile applications is increasing. However, the quality of these devices and apps varies. App characteristics that determine their usability, data integrity, and information transparency will determine the success of individual apps.

Some clinicians and some provider organizations are developing strategies for utilizing these apps in clinical settings, to strengthen patient engagement, support behavioral change, and help patients manage chronic conditions. Integrated platforms can import information generated as patients use mobile apps and devices, store the data, and support communication of relevant information between patients and care team members. However, achieving successful integration of information generated by self-diagnostic tools, mobile apps, and telehealth into clinician workflows is not a simple task. Analysis of the structure of communication channels and flows of information through these channels provides a framework for examining strategic options.

As clinicians and provider organizations work to help patients by maximizing the benefits and minimizing the harms of new types of data and communications, they face substantive strategic issues. Health care provider organizations implementing telehealth face a series of strategic questions:

- What information is needed prior to the telehealth visit?
- Will patients be permitted to view recordings of the telehealth sessions stored in the EHR database?
- Will patients be permitted to record the sessions as they occur?
- How will visit reports be generated and shared?
- Will patients be permitted to view the clinician's session notes?

Health care provider organizations considering patient use of mobile apps and devices, and online self-diagnostic tools, face additional questions, including:

- Will clinicians recommend that patients use a single app for each clinically relevant situation (e.g., will clinicians recommend a specific app for patients dealing with depression and a different app for patients dealing with PTSD)? If so, how will these apps be identified and selected? How will these recommendations be updated over time?
- Will the provider organization provide tech support for patients learning to use the recommended apps? If so – how will this support be organized and funded?
- Will patients be permitted to upload app-generated data to the provider organization's EHR system?
  - How will the system be designed to ensure that patient-generated data stored by the provider is accurate?
  - How will the system report patient-generated data to clinicians? What level of detail and what formats will clinicians use to support provider decisions and strengthen communications with patients?

Developing successful strategies for harnessing the benefits offered by these new technologies will require detailed collaboration between the practice organization's Information Technology (IT) professionals and the clinicians who use the organization's EHR system. As the technology continues to advance, the clinical psychologist can play a valuable role by working closely with technology development teams. The psychologist's knowledge and experience will help shape and improve medical technology solutions, which will advance the landscape of population health and patient-centered medical care. Clinicians will fill three roles:

- Clinicians will assess whether specific technologies are likely to be useful for specific patients: Would a virtual cat help a patient manage anxiety? Would a robot be an appropriate monitoring and reminder device?

- To support these decisions, clinicians will also help design studies to evaluate patient satisfaction and outcomes generated by emerging mobile apps and devices.
- Clinicians will work with technology developers and with their organization's IT professionals to specify useful types of app-generated information, useful formats for presenting summarized information to patients and clinicians, and useful types of decision-support tools and automated communications.

References

Abdolkhani, R., Gray, K., Borda, A., & DeSouza, R. (2019). Patient-generated health data management and quality challenges in remote patient monitoring. *JAMIA Open, 2*(4), 471–478. https://doi.org/10.1093/jamiaopen/ooz036

Amisha, P. M., Pathania, M., & Rathaur, V. K. (2019). Overview of artificial intelligence in medicine. *Journal of Family Medicine and Primary Care, 8*(7), 2328. https://doi.org/10.4103/jfmpc.jfmpc_440_19

Aungst, T., Clauson, K., Misra, S., Lewis, T., & Husain, I. (2014). How to identify, assess and utilise mobile medical applications in clinical practice. *International Journal of Clinical Practice, 68*(2), 155–162. https://doi.org/10.1111/ijcp.12375

Beisecker, A. E., & Beisecker, T. D. (1990). Patient information-seeking behaviors when communicating with doctors. *Medical Care, 28*, 19–28. https://doi.org/10.1097/00005650-199001000-00004

Dick, S., O'Connor, Y., Thompson, M. J., O'Donoghue, J., Hardy, V., Wu, T.-S. J., O'Sullivan, T., Chirambo, G. B., & Heavin, C. (2020). Considerations for improved mobile health evaluation: Retrospective qualitative investigation. *JMIR mHealth and uHealth, 8*(1), e12424. https://doi.org/10.2196/12424

Dinh-Le, C., Chuang, R., Chokshi, S., & Mann, D. (2019). Wearable health technology and electronic health record integration: Scoping review and future directions. *JMIR mHealth and uHealth, 7*(9), e12861. https://doi.org/10.2196/12861

Escriche-Escuder, A., De-Torres, I., Roldán-Jiménez, C., Martín-Martín, J., Muro-Culebras, A., González-Sánchez, M., Ruiz-Muñoz, M., Mayoral-Cleries, F., Biró, A., Tang, W., et al. (2020). Assessment of the quality of mobile applications (Apps) for management of low back pain using the mobile app rating scale (MARS). *International Journal of Environmental Research and Public Health, 17*(24), 9209. https://doi.org/10.3390/ijerph17249209

Fan, W., Liu, J., Zhu, S., & Pardalos, P. M. (2020). Investigating the impacting factors for the healthcare professionals to adopt artificial intelligence-based medical diagnosis support system (AIMDSS). *Annals of Operations Research, 294*(1), 567–592. https://doi.org/10.1007/s10479-018-2818-y

Genes, N., Violante, S., Cetrangol, C., Rogers, L., Schadt, E. E., & Chan, Y.-F. Y. (2018). From smartphone to EHR: A case report on integrating patient-generated health data. *NPJ Digital Medicine, 1*(1), 1–6. https://doi.org/10.1038/s41746-018-0030-8

Gruessner, V. (2015). *FDA oversight on high-risk apps in mobile health industry*. mHealth Intelligence. https://mhealthintelligence.com/news/fda-oversight-on-high-risk-apps-in-mobile-health-industry

Hamet, P., & Tremblay, J. (2017). Artificial intelligence in medicine. *Metabolism, 69*, S36–S40. https://doi.org/10.1016/j.metabol.2017.01.011

Hochberg, I., Allon, R., & Yom-Tov, E. (2020). Assessment of the frequency of online searches for symptoms before diagnosis: Analysis of archival data. *Journal of Medical Internet Research, 22*(3), e15065. https://doi.org/10.2196/15065

Holzinger, A., & Errath, M. (2007). Mobile computer Web-application design in medicine: Some research based guidelines. *Universal Access in the Information Society, 6*(1), 31–41.

Hurst, E. J. (2020). Web conferencing and collaboration tools and trends. *Journal of Hospital Librarianship, 20*(3), 266–279. https://doi.org/10.1080/15323269.2020.1780079

Jacobs, W., Amuta, A. O., & Jeon, K. C. (2017). Health information seeking in the digital age: An analysis of health information seeking behavior among US adults. *Cogent Social Sciences, 3*(1), 1302785. https://doi.org/10.1080/23311886.2017.1302785

Jiang, F., Jiang, Y., Zhi, H., Dong, Y., Li, H., Ma, S., Wang, Y., Dong, Q., Shen, H., & Wang, Y. (2017). Artificial intelligence in healthcare: Past, present and future. *Stroke and Vascular Neurology, 2*(4), 230–243. https://doi.org/10.1136/svn-2017-000101

Kerr, D., Serrano, J. A., Ray, P., et al. (2018). The role of a disruptive digital technology for home-based healthcare of the elderly: Telepresence robot. *Digital Medicine, 4*(4), 173.

Knitza, J., Tascilar, K., Messner, E.-M., Meyer, M., Vossen, D., Pulla, A., Bosch, P., Kittler, J., Kleyer, A., Sewerin, P., et al. (2019). German mobile apps in rheumatology: Review and analysis using the Mobile Application Rating Scale (MARS). *JMIR mHealth and uHealth, 7*(8), e14991. https://doi.org/10.2196/14991

Lambert, S. D., & Loiselle, C. G. (2007). Health information—Seeking behavior. *Qualitative Health Research, 17*(8), 1006–1019. https://doi.org/10.1177/1049732307305199

Liu, X., Faes, L., Kale, A. U., Wagner, S. K., Fu, D. J., Bruynseels, A., Mahendiran, T., Moraes, G., Shamdas, M., Kern, C., et al. (2019). A comparison of deep learning performance against health-care professionals in detecting diseases from medical imaging: A systematic review and meta-analysis. *The Lancet Digital Health, 1*(6), e271–e297. https://doi.org/10.1016/S2589-7500(19)30123-2

Llorens-Vernet, P., & Miró, J. (2020). Standards for mobile health–related apps: Systematic review and development of a guide. *JMIR mHealth and uHealth, 8*(3), e13057. https://doi.org/10.2196/13057

Major, I. (2019). Two-sided information asymmetry in the healthcare industry. *International Advances in Economic Research, 25*(2), 177–193. https://doi.org/10.1007/s11294-019-09732-9

Mihelj, M., Novak, D., Milavec, M., Ziherl, J., Olenšek, A., & Munih, M. (2012). Virtual rehabilitation environment using principles of intrinsic motivation and game design. *Presence Teleoperators and Virtual Environments, 21*(1), 1–15. https://doi.org/10.1162/PRES_a_00078

Morgan, A. J., & Trauth, E. M. (2013). Socio-economic influences on health information searching in the USA: The case of diabetes. *Information Technology & People, 26*(4), 324–346. https://doi.org/10.1108/ITP-09-2012-0098

Munzner, T. (2014). *Visualization analysis and design*. CRC Press. https://doi.org/10.1201/b17511

Nouri, R., Niakan Kalhori, S. R., Ghazisaeedi, M., Marchand, G., & Yasini, M. (2018). Criteria for assessing the quality of mHealth apps: A systematic review. *Journal of the American Medical Informatics Association, 25*(8), 1089–1098. https://doi.org/10.1093/jamia/ocy050

Osborn, C. Y., & Egede, L. E. (2010). Validation of an Information–Motivation–Behavioral Skills model of diabetes self-care (IMB-DSC). *Patient Education and Counseling, 79*(1), 49–54. https://doi.org/10.1016/j.pec.2009.07.016

Peek, S. T., Wouters, E. J., Van Hoof, J., Luijkx, K. G., Boeije, H. R., & Vrijhoef, H. J. (2014). Factors influencing acceptance of technology for aging in place: A systematic review. *International Journal of Medical Informatics, 83*(4), 235–248.

Provoost, S., Ruwaard, J., van Breda, W., Riper, H., & Bosse, T. (2019). Validating automated sentiment analysis of online cognitive behavioral therapy patient texts: An exploratory study. *Frontiers in Psychology, 10*, 1065. https://doi.org/10.3389/fpsyg.2019.01065

Rajput, A. (2020). Natural language processing, sentiment analysis, and clinical analytics. In *Innovation in health informatics* (pp. 79–97). Elsevier. https://doi.org/10.1016/B978-0-12-819043-2.00003-4

Robeznieks, A. (2019). *Mobile health gets road map for high-quality apps*. American Medical Association. https://www.ama-assn.org/practice-management/digital/mobile-health-gets-road-map-high-quality-apps

Salim, M. H. M., Ali, N. M., & Noah, S. A. M. (2017). Mobile application on healthy diet for elderly based on persuasive design. *International Journal on Advanced Science, Engineering and Information Technology, 7*(1), 222–227.

Sekaran, R. (2020). *FDA policy for mobile medical applications*. Nossaman LLP. https://www.thehealthlawticker.com/fda-policy-for-mobile-medical-applications

Shin, G., Feng, Y., Jarrahi, M. H., & Gafinowitz, N. (2019). Beyond novelty effect: A mixed-methods exploration into the motivation for long-term activity tracker use. *JAMIA Open, 2*(1), 62–72. https://doi.org/10.1093/jamiaopen/ooy048

Smith, A. (2021). *Mobile fact sheet*. Pew Research Center. https://www.pewresearch.org/internet/fact-sheet/mobile/

Steinhubl, S. R., Muse, E. D., & Topol, E. J. (2015). The emerging field of mobile health. *Science Translational Medicine, 7*(283), 283rv3–283rv3. https://doi.org/10.1126/scitranslmed.aaa3487

Stoyanov, S. R., Hides, L., Kavanagh, D. J., & Wilson, H. (2016). Development and validation of the user version of the Mobile Application Rating Scale (uMARS). *JMIR mHealth and uHealth, 4*(2), e5849. https://doi.org/10.2196/mhealth.5849

US Food and Drug Administration. (2019). *Policy for device software functions and mobile medical applications*. US Department of Health and Human Services. https://www.fda.gov/media/80958/download

Varshney, U. (2014). Mobile health: Four emerging themes of research. *Decision Support Systems, 66*, 20–35. https://doi.org/10.1016/j.dss.2014.06.001

Xcertia. (2019). *MHealth app guidelines*. Xcertia Board of Directors. https://www.himss.org/sites/hde/files/media/file/2020/04/17/xcertia-guidelines-2019-final.pdf

Part II
Innovative Clinical Applications in the Military & Veteran Health Clinics

Chapter 9
Assessment and Treatment of Chronic Pain in the Military: Current Practices and Future Directions for Clinical Health Psychologists

Justin T. Matsuura, Jill S. Panos, and Jay Earles

1 Introduction

1.1 Chronic Pain Problem in the US Military

Chronic pain has been defined as "pain that persists beyond the normal time of healing and as a result, lacks the typical warning function of physiological nociception" (Treede et al., 2015, p. 1003). Additionally, chronic pain is characterized as pain that persists beyond 3–6 months. Unrelieved and persistent pain results in numerous negative consequences, particularly for military populations, which include: depression, anxiety, poor sleep patterns, decreased quality of life, substance use disorder and suicide (Department of Veteran Affairs, 2017). The most frequently seen chronic pain conditions in the US military include: peripheral/central nervous system, osteoarthritis, back and neck pain, headaches, non-traumatic joint disorders, other musculoskeletal, and visceral/pelvic (Rief et al., 2018).

The prevalence of chronic pain in the US Military is particularly high. In 2012, approximately 63% of Army soldiers had at least one diagnosis of pain and 59% had a primary pain diagnosis (Rief et al., 2018). More recent data on service members (SM)s, across all branches of service, found that approximately 34% of SMs seen

The views expressed in this publication are those of the authors and do not necessarily reflect the official policy of the Department of Defense, Department of Army, US Army Medical Department, or the US Government.

J. T. Matsuura (✉) · J. S. Panos
Interdisciplinary Pain Management Center, Tripler Army Medical Center, Honolulu, HI, USA
e-mail: justin.t.matsuura.civ@health.mil; jill.s.panos.civ@mail.mil

J. Earles
Midland Valley Behavioral Health LLC, Graniteville, SC, USA

L. C. James et al. (eds.), *Clinical Health Psychology in Military and Veteran Settings*, https://doi.org/10.1007/978-3-031-12063-3_9

for medical treatment in 2018 had chronic pain concerns (Smith et al., 2020). Unfortunately, true prevalence numbers of SMs struggling with chronic pain may be difficult to obtain as underreporting of injuries and medical problems frequently occur. Smith et al. (2016) evaluated a large sample of SMs and found that almost half did not report their acute and chronic injuries to medical personnel in order to avoid mandated physical restrictions or "profiles."

Chronic pain has exacted enormous healthcare costs for the military which include: direct medical costs, costs due to disability or limited duty, and medical separation. In 2018, the US Army spent approximately $434 million in direct patient care costs to address musculoskeletal related conditions among soldiers (Molloy et al., 2020). Additionally, chronic pain often results in SMs receiving limited duty restrictions. For instance, among soldiers who had a primary pain diagnosis, 55% reported having moderate to severe pain resulting in approximately 44% of these individuals having military work restrictions (Rief et al., 2018). Further, chronic pain conditions are often the reasons for medical discharges among SMs. Data between 1981 and 2005 suggest an increasing trend which places musculoskeletal disability as the most frequent cause of disability for SMs within the Army (Bell et al., 2008). Similarly, a Department of Defense (DOD) report, which evaluated active duty personnel across all branches of service; found that SMs with musculoskeletal conditions were more likely to result in a disability discharge compared to other medical conditions (Maby et al., 2017).

Prescription medication has been the most frequently used treatment modality for chronic pain. The total cost of prescribed pain medication in the United States is approximately $17.8 billion annually, in which opioids contribute to a significant portion of these costs ($3.6 billion or 20% of annual drug costs) (Rasu et al., 2014). Opioid use, which exhibits a high propensity for misuse, has been found to be much more frequently prescribed among SMs (14%) compared to the civilian population (4%) (Toblin et al., 2014). In 2010, approximately 32% of military personnel were given a prescription of opioids (Jeffery et al., 2014). In response to the opioid crisis, there have been recent efforts to reduce opioid prescriptions in the military. Opioid prescriptions among SMs were found to have decreased in 2012 and 2013 by 1% and 15%, respectively (Kazanis et al., 2018). Although encouraging, efforts to reduce opioid prescriptions should continue as opioid misuse (e.g., continuing to use expired prescriptions) remains a problem for the military (Ramirez et al., 2017).

1.2 Paradigm Shift in Pain Treatment in the Military

Given the deleterious effects of chronic pain on SM return to duty readiness and risks associated with frequently prescribed medical treatments for pain, the development of effective and low-risk treatment modalities to address chronic pain has been a high priority for the US military (Vallerand et al., 2015). In 2010, the Office of the Army Surgeon General disseminated the US Army's Pain Management Task Force report, which helped to standardize the US Army's approach to addressing chronic pain and provided a framework to guide stakeholders on the implementation of evidence-based clinical practices, research, and training (Office of the Army Surgeon General, 2010). The US Army Surgeon General's office followed the Pain Management Task Force report with an Operational Order, OPORD 10–76 USAMEDCOM Surgeon General's Comprehensive Pain Management Campaign Plan, to establish Interdisciplinary Pain Management Centers (IPMC) in all Army Medical Centers and several smaller Army hospitals. The OPORD emphasized a holistic approach to pain medicine and placed interdisciplinary care as the gold standard of treatment for chronic pain. The IPMC mission is to provide acute and chronic pain care services, help identify and manage patients with complex pain related issues (e.g. functioning issues, polypharmacy, other co-morbid conditions, etc.), and provide education to primary care clinics. In addition, the OPORD mandates specific provider types for IPMCs, one of which is a clinical health psychologist. In at least one IPMC, a clinical health psychologist is the Director of the IPMC.

The shift in treatment approach for chronic pain in the US military have placed clinical health psychologists in critical roles to address chronic pain. Since the DOD Pain Management Task Force report was introduced, clinical health psychologists, working in the subspecialty of chronic pain, have utilized tools to assess and treat biopsychosocial concerns related to chronic pain conditions. Such clinical tools have helped to define the role clinical health psychologists have as essential members of interdisciplinary pain management teams (Wandner et al., 2018).

The goal of this chapter is to provide an overview of current assessment and treatment practices for clinical health psychologists working in pain treatment teams in the US military. Additionally, we discuss recent clinical trends that may further improve the practice of chronic pain treatment among SMs. Finally, a clinical case is presented to demonstrate how current assessment and treatment practices are implemented in an interdisciplinary pain treatment center.

2 Pain Assessment and Treatment Approaches

2.1 Biopsychosocial Assessment

A biopsychosocial assessment is an essential component of clinical care for patients with chronic pain. Biopsychosocial assessments seek to provide a thorough understanding of factors contributing to chronic pain among SMs, which serves to conceptually bridge biological and contextual elements related to one's pain. For clinical health psychologists, biopsychosocial assessments are considered to be a standard of care across all levels of care (e.g., primary vs. tertiary). For example, a clinical health psychologist may conduct a biopsychosocial assessment in the same session as the team's pain physician to determine which evidence-based behavioral treatments to utilize as part of the interdisciplinary pain treatment. Whereas a primary care manager may refer a patient for an evaluation with a clinical health psychologist, embedded in the primary care unit, to help improve their patient's compliance with medical regimens .

Having a thorough understanding of the biopsychosocial model is critical to effectively complete biopsychosocial assessments. A biopsychosocial framework posits that pain and disability develop from a "complex and dynamic interaction among physiological, psychological, and social factors that perpetuate chronic and complex pain syndromes" (Gatchel et al., 2014, p. 120). Now widely accepted, the biopsychosocial model for chronic pain addresses shortcomings inherent in the biomedical model as it is now understood that pain does not develop from biological pathways alone (Gatchel et al., 2007).

Wandner et al. (2018) assert that biopsychosocial assessments in chronic pain should include three essential components. These components include: selecting appropriate assessment instruments for the evaluation (e.g., clinical interview, self-report instruments, personality tests, etc.), awareness of contextual factors (e.g., poor social support from family, secondary gain issues, etc.) that may impact the validity of the assessment, and effective communication with relevant stakeholders (e.g., patient, support network, treatment team, etc.) to inform clinical care.

The biopsychosocial approach provides a framework to guide clinical health psychologists in selecting appropriate assessment and treatment tools for each patient struggling with chronic pain. The following section describes pain assessment tools currently used by clinical health psychologists in the military to evaluate chronic pain, particularly the impact pain has on psychological wellbeing and daily functioning.

2.1.1 Clinical Interview

A clinical interview is a core component of a biopsychosocial assessment for chronic pain and a critical part of the treatment process. In addition to gathering data on the patient's condition, a clinical interview is an opportunity to build rapport with the patient, provide psychoeducation on their pain condition and discuss relevant treatment options. Clinical interviews to assess chronic pain may include: pain history, current pain location, description of pain sensations, pain ratings, last pain-free day, pain modifiers, pain's impact on functioning and quality of life, and pain medication use. The clinical interview session is also an opportunity for the clinician to complete goal setting with the patient. Setting functional goals serves as a collaborative tool to assess a patient's readiness for pain rehabilitation and determine the course of treatment based on the patient's values and goals. Additionally, a thorough review of the patient's medical chart should be conducted to understand the patient's medical and psychiatric history. Co-morbid psychiatric conditions (e.g., substance use disorders, depression, etc.) as well as other medical problems (e.g., sleep disorders, etc.) often occur with chronic pain and should be evaluated (Wandner et al., 2018).

2.1.2 Self-Report Instruments

Self-report instruments are critical to effective chronic pain assessment and treatment planning among SMs. Consistent with recommendations from the VA/DOD Clinical Practice Guideline for Low Back Pain to screen for co-morbid mental health concerns and assist with treatment selection, a variety of tools are used by clinical health psychologists to assess pain severity, relative impairment, depression and anxiety, pain coping style and pain acceptance (Department of Veterans Affairs & Department of Defense, 2017).

The Defense and Veterans Pain Rating Scale (DVPRS 2.0), jointly developed by the DOD and the Department of Veterans Affairs (VA), is a brief 5-item pain assessment instrument that is widely used among DOD and veteran populations. The DVPRS is easy to use and can be administered at each medical appointment in most settings, including those in austere environments. The DVPRS 2.0 includes items that assess pain severity and the impact of pain on life domains such as activity level, sleep, mood, and level of stress. Most importantly, the pain rating scale is enhanced with matching pain descriptions, color coding, and facial expressions. The DVPRS 2.0 has been found to be a valid and highly reliable measure for pain among both SMs and veterans (Polomano et al., 2016).

Other multidimensional pain instruments that are frequently used include the Pain Outcomes Questionnaire-Short Form (POQ-SF; Clark et al., 2003) and the West Haven-Yale Multidimensional Pain Inventory (WHYMPI/MPI; Kerns et al., 1985), especially when a more comprehensive understanding of the impact chronic pain has on one's life is desired. These measures are frequently used as a standard of care for chronic pain assessment at military treatment facilities (MTFs) and assist in guiding interdisciplinary pain treatment. Although these pain measures are relatively brief in length, it is imperative that adequate time be given to patients to complete these measures as they are more time-consuming to administer and score than the DVPRS.

The Pain Outcomes Questionnaire-Short Form (POQ-SF) is a 19-item self-report questionnaire used to address the multifaceted nature of pain among veterans and SMs (Clark et al., 2003). This measure assesses clinical domains related to pain which include: pain severity, mobility issues, activities of daily living, vitality, mood, and pain-related anxiety. The POQ-SF has been used frequently in military hospital settings as a brief, easy to administer, tool for pain assessment. Interpretation of scores are often discussed in session with patients in order to increase collaboration in treatment planning.

An alternative comprehensive pain measure is the West Haven-Yale Multidimensional Pain Inventory (WHYMPI; Kerns et al., 1985). This measure is divided into three sections which include: assessing important dimensions of one's own pain experience, patient's perceptions on how spouses respond to their pain, and activity engagement. In addition, the WHYMPI has been found to be sensitive to change in pain and functioning among patients undergoing treatment (Kerns & Haythornthwaite, 1988).

Disability is often a consequence of chronic pain, particularly for SMs. As a result, finding resolutions related to an SM's likelihood of return to duty is often an undeniable part of pain treatment. Therefore, tools to assist in understanding a patient's impairment due to pain are essential. The Pain Disability Index (PDI; Pollard, 1984), is used to assess the degree to which pain interferes with functioning in a number of domains which include: family/home responsibilities, recreation, social activity, occupation, sexual behavior, self-care, and life support activity. Normative data suggests that PDI scores are moderated by work compensation status, litigation, and circumstances of pain onset (i.e., injured at work vs. non work-related injury) (Chibnall & Tait, 1994).

Symptoms of depression and anxiety are highly comorbid with chronic pain and may impede on pain rehabilitation (Miller & Kaiser, 2018). For instance, pain-related symptoms of anxiety have been found to impact physical functioning, such as weight-lifting capacity, which is highly relevant to performance in the military (Burns et al., 2000). As a result, symptom specific measures targeting pain-related anxiety and depression have become essential components of a biopsychosocial evaluation and are routinely assessed in military pain management centers.

The Pain Anxiety Symptoms Scale (PASS) is used to assess pain-related anxiety and fear (McCracken et al., 1992; McCracken & Dhingra, 2002). The PASS is a psychometrically sound instrument demonstrating strong correlations with pain outcome variables on the WHYMPI and PDI (McCracken et al., 1992). A short form version, the PASS-20, which contains 20 items, is also available for brief clinical encounters (McCracken & Dhingra, 2002).

Well-established measures of depression, such as the Patient Health Questionnaire-9 (PHQ-9; Kroenke et al., 2001) and the Beck Depression Inventory – Second Edition (BDI-II; Beck et al., 1996), are frequently used to assess depression related to chronic pain within MTFs. The PHQ-9 and the BDI-II are brief measures and can easily be administered in most settings. Studies have demonstrated that both measures are highly reliable and valid tools to assess depression among patients with chronic pain (Seo & Park, 2015; Harris & D'Eon, 2008).

Chronic pain is also highly comorbid with post-traumatic stress disorder (PTSD). One study found that among veterans with chronic pain, about 49% of those individuals also met criteria for PTSD (Otis et al., 2010). That same study also found that individuals with both chronic pain and PTSD exhibited higher levels of pain-related distress compared to patients with chronic pain alone. The Post-traumatic Stress Disorder Checklist (PCL-5) is the primary tool used to assess the severity of PTSD symptoms as reflected in the fifth edition of the Diagnostic and Statistical Manual of Mental Disorders (DSM-5) (Weathers et al., 2013).

Certain pain-coping styles have been associated with poor pain control. Pain catastrophizing, the tendency to ruminate and exaggerate about negative aspects of one's pain, is primarily assessed by using the Pain Catastrophizing Scale (PCS; Sullivan et al., 1995). The PCS evaluates three components of catastrophizing which include: rumination, magnification, and helplessness. Pain catastrophizing, assessed by the PCS, has been found to be a significant predictor of pain-related disability (Osman et al., 1997; Arnow et al., 2011).

Acceptance of chronic pain has recently become a construct of interest for pain treatment in military medicine as pain treatments continue to focus on functional restoration. Reneman et al. (2010) defined pain acceptance as an "underlying psychological state of willingness to experience chronic pain and its cognitive and emotional facets while continuing life as normal as possible (p. 458)." Pain acceptance has been identified as a key treatment process variable linked to improvements in adjustment and functioning despite persistent pain (Miller & Kaiser, 2018; Baranoff et al., 2013). Pain acceptance has also been found to be negatively correlated with factors associated with poor pain coping, such as depressive symptoms, anxiety, and pain-related disability (Baranoff et al., 2013; Bernini et al., 2014).

The Chronic Pain Acceptance Questionnaire – Revised (CPAQ-R; McCracken et al., 2004) is a brief 20-item measure of pain acceptance, following a full revision of the original CPAQ measure. Activity engagement and pain willingness are two factors that have been identified on the CPAQ-R. Changes in activity engagement and pain willingness factors, due to pain treatment, have been linked to changes in pain treatment outcome variables such as pain related anxiety, disability, and function (i.e., sitting-to-standing movements) (McCracken et al., 2005).

Comprehensive personality assessment measures may also provide useful information regarding a patient's likelihood of success in pain rehabilitation. Perhaps the most feasible assessment tool is the Millon Behavioral Medicine Diagnostic (MBMD; Millon et al., 2001). The MBMD was developed to assess personality and psychopathology factors that are relevant to medical populations as opposed to concerns that are mostly associated with psychiatric populations (Lattie et al., 2013). The MBMD has established chronic pain norms and can help predict success among patients undergoing multidisciplinary pain treatments (Lattie et al., 2013).

2.2 *Behavioral Treatment Approaches*

Evidence-based behavioral interventions typically operate within a biopsychosocial framework highlighting the multidimensional nature of chronic pain (Gatchel et al., 2014; Wandner et al., 2018). Consistent with a biopsychosocial model, other integrative models of pain, such as the gate-control-neuromatrix model of pain and the fear-avoidance model, have been frequently used to further describe the specific contribution of brain and behavioral processes on the sequela of chronic pain (Melzack, 1999; Crombez et al., 2012). The gate-control-neuromatrix model posits that sensory inputs (e.g., injury) interact with cognitive-emotional regions of the brain creating a "neurosignature," resulting in a unique neural network output pattern impacting pain perception, behavior, and stress regulation (Melzack, 1999). Whereas the fear-avoidance model of chronic pain provides a useful description on how pain can be perpetuated by a vicious cycle of pain-related fear, avoidance of physical activity, and physical deconditioning (Crombez et al., 2012). Both models can be used to describe precipitating and perpetuating factors related to each patient's experience of pain and can be integrated with many evidence-based behavioral treatments for chronic pain.

2.2.1 Motivational Interviewing

Over the past decade, the military and VA health systems have initiated training in motivational interviewing (MI) strategies among medical providers to more effectively address medical problems including chronic pain (Midboe et al., 2011). MI is a "client-centered, directive method for enhancing an individual's intrinsic motivation to change by exploring and resolving ambivalence" (Miller et al., 2002, p. 25). MI is applied by actively eliciting and reinforcing change talk (e.g., "I want to play sports with my kids") and helping patients to quickly develop an awareness of discrepancies that exist between continuing maladaptive behaviors (e.g., avoidance) and achieving one's personal goals (Miller et al., 2002). Clinicians using an MI approach may draw on specific skills such as asking open-ended questions, listening reflectively, and exploring goals; to build a patient's motivation to change (Miller et al., 2002). The transtheoretical model of behavioral change may help healthcare stakeholders understand a patient's readiness to change as they move through discrete stages which include: precontemplation, contemplation, preparation, action, and maintenance (Alperstein & Sharpe, 2016).

Although MI may be applied as a standalone intervention, MI is considered to be most effective when implemented in conjunction with other behavioral interventions, as it is purported to increase adherence to those treatments. A recent meta-analysis evaluating the effects of MI on chronic pain treatment adherence found small to moderate treatment effects of MI on adherence to other pain treatments and pain intensity reduction (Alperstein & Sharpe, 2016). That same study also found that MI was only effective in improving adherence to pain treatments in the short term (i.e., post-treatment) rather than for extended periods or time (i.e., 6 months' follow-up), suggesting that other treatment approaches may be necessary to maintain commitment to behavioral change in the long term. MI can be easily applied in most treatment settings (e.g., primary care visits) since it can be completed in as little as 10 minutes (Jones et al., 2004).

2.2.2 Cognitive-Behavioral Therapy for Chronic Pain

Cognitive-behavioral therapy for chronic pain (CBT-CP) is considered to be the sine qua non among behavioral interventions for pain. There is a plethora of evidence to suggest that CBT-CP is effective in helping patients manage chronic pain. Meta-analytic studies, have been conducted on the efficacy of CBT-CP and have found that CBT-CP demonstrates medium effect sizes of 0.5 (Morley et al., 1999). CBT-CP programs primarily focus on skills acquisition and teaching patients to apply these skills into their daily routine. Functional restoration and improvements in quality of life are primary objectives of CBT (Kerns et al., 2011).

There are many CBT-CP strategies that have been included in treatment protocols. CBT-CP strategies may include: education on chronic pain (e.g., gate control theory), self-regulation, behavioral activation/pleasurable activity scheduling, activity pacing, cognitive restructuring, effective communication training, and problem solving. However, there is considerable variability in which skills are included in each CBT program (Knoerl et al., 2016). A recent comprehensive review on CBT-CP found that the most frequently used treatment strategies include: cognitive restructuring, psychoeducation, activity pacing, and self-regulation (Knoerl et al., 2016).

In addition to psychoeducation, which can provide SMs with a more accurate understanding of chronic pain in general, cognitive restructuring is a behavioral intervention that can teach individuals to effectively target maladaptive thoughts related to pain (e.g., "Nothing helps my pain") and modify such thinking into more realistic beliefs. Maladaptive thinking can be processed with therapists either through discussion or using tools such as thought logs. Cognitive restructuring effectively addresses negative thinking patterns such as pain catastrophizing and pain helplessness, which have been found to be significant predictors of pain-related disability (Burns et al., 2003).

Activity pacing focuses on helping patients develop activity schedules that will allow them to perform tasks based on time or quotas rather than pain intensity (Nielson et al., 2013). For example, SMs are encouraged to set time limits on their exercises (e.g., running) in order to keep their pain below pain tolerance levels, as opposed to just "pushing through the pain." Therapists may systematically increase activity time frames as a patient's pain tolerance improves over the course of treatment. Activity pacing is an essential component of CBT-CP for SMs as it directly targets behavioral avoidance and may increase their activity level (e.g., exercise). Such improvements in physical functioning may increase the likelihood of SMs returning to full duty.

CBT-CP programs often include self-regulation training to help individuals address difficulties controlling psychophysiological arousal, which could impact coping with chronic pain (Kerns et al., 2011). Self-regulation strategies may include: diaphragmatic breathing, progressive muscle relaxation, and visualization techniques (Knoerl et al., 2016). Biofeedback therapy is frequently integrated into self-regulation programs as a tool to increase awareness in autonomic processes and to reinforce physiological control. Biofeedback utilizes technology in the form of devices and computer software to assess autonomic arousal processes (e.g., respiration rate, heart rate variability, muscle tension, etc.) and provide "feedback" (e.g. visual cues) to the patient (Schwartz & Andrasik, 2003). Clinical health psychologists may choose to implement self-regulation and biofeedback strategies during CBT-CP sessions or utilize technicians trained in biofeedback to teach these skills in sessions separate from CBT-CP.

Most research examining the effectiveness of CBT-CP in military populations (i.e., SMs and veterans) have been conducted only on veterans. A recent comprehensive review of the treatment literature, published between 2009 and 2015, included only two randomized controlled trials of CBT-CP conducted on military populations, which focused only on veterans (Knoerl et al., 2016). Otis et al. (2013)

examined the efficacy of CBT-CP among veterans with painful diabetic peripheral neuropathy, comparing CBT to treatment as usual (TAU). They found that veterans completing CBT-CP demonstrated significant decreases in both pain severity and pain interference from pretreatment to 4-month follow-up, compared to TAU which did not demonstrate any significant improvements on the same outcomes. Carmody et al. (2013) compared CBT-CP delivered through telephone to pain education delivered through telephone, among older veterans seeking treatment for chronic pain. They found that both treatments, when delivered through a telehealth format, were slightly effective in improving pain treatment outcomes with no differences between the interventions in terms of treatment effects.

While less is known on how SMs respond to CBT-CP, uncontrolled studies provide some evidence to suggest CBT-CP may be helpful for SMs. An early pilot study evaluated the effectiveness of a multicomponent CBT program for chronic pain among SMs seeking treatment in a military tertiary care center (Peters et al., 2000). That study found that CBT demonstrated significant improvements in quality of life and reduction in utilization and costs. A more recent qualitative analysis of a CBT-CP program, implemented at an interdisciplinary pain management center for SMs, found that patients who completed the program reported a high degree of satisfaction with their treatment. However, they reported that SMs also exhibited challenges adhering to CBT due to perceived stigma of being seen as "weak" by engaging in behavioral health treatment (Coulter et al., 2016).

2.2.3 Contextual Cognitive Behavioral Therapy Approaches

Contextual CBT approaches fall under the family of CBT interventions. Among these, mindfulness-based stress reduction (MBSR) and acceptance and commitment therapy (ACT) are the most frequently used of these treatments for chronic pain (Veehof et al., 2016). Contextual CBT approaches distinguish themselves from earlier CBT treatments by applying experiential interventions (e.g., mindfulness meditation) as opposed to didactic experiences, and target one's response to symptoms rather than focusing on symptom reduction (McCracken & Vowles, 2014). Additionally, contextual CBT interventions seek to cultivate a greater awareness of moment-to-moment experiences and develop a greater flexibility or openness to experience despite pain (Veehof et al., 2016).

Mindfulness-based interventions utilize targeted mindfulness meditation skills such as focused breathing, mindful hearing and thinking, body scan, mindful eating, and mindful walking exercises to increase moment-to-moment awareness and reduce ruminative thinking throughout the day (Williams et al., 2007). An alternative to traditional cognitive restructuring strategies used in CBT, the process of increasing moment-to-moment awareness, results in both decreases in attempts to control thinking and reductions in pain-related distress (Wong et al., 2011).

More recently, MBSR interventions for chronic pain have been adapted for use in the military. Brintz et al. (2020) proposed an MBSR program for chronic pain that is better suited for SMs. Although most mindfulness meditation skills in their program were consistent with previous MBSR interventions, training objectives were presented to SMs in terms of "performance enhancement techniques," particularly for tasks such as physical fitness training. Unlike traditional MBSR programs, a didactic format using slide presentations and a smartphone app was adopted in order to be consistent with other instructional programs within the military system. Although efforts to develop MBSR programs in the military have been initiated, evaluations of these programs have yet to be undertaken.

ACT has also emerged as an effective behavioral intervention for chronic pain. Unlike other cognitive behavioral interventions, the primary focus of ACT is not symptom control or reduction. Although symptom reduction may occur, patients learn skills to help them shift their focus away from symptom control and toward committed action (e.g., progressing toward functional goals) based on their freely chosen values (Feliu-Soler et al., 2018). In order to achieve this, ACT therapists utilize a psychological flexibility framework and guide patients through mindfulness, acceptance, and behavioral activation processes (Hayes et al., 2012). Similar to MBSR, there is a strong emphasis on applying experiential exercises to help patients change their relationship with thoughts and language, in general, as opposed to directly targeting the content of maladaptive thinking patterns.

Research suggests that ACT is an effective treatment for chronic pain and comparable to CBT overall (Veehof et al., 2016; Wetherell et al., 2011). Although ACT has been found to be generally effective for chronic pain, not all individuals may respond to ACT in the same way. Research has found that older individuals are more likely to respond positively to ACT for chronic pain than younger individuals (Wetherell et al., 2016). Understanding the impact one's age may have on ACT is of particular importance among active-duty populations, as SMs tend to be significantly younger than the community as a whole (Wetherell et al., 2011). According to recent DOD data, approximately 66% of all SMs are age 30 years or younger, and 45% of all SMs are younger than 25 years of age (DOD, 2017).

3 Future Directions

There are a number of innovative developments that have the potential to improve military pain medicine in the future. First, a high priority for the military has been to develop innovative technologies to increase the efficiency of assessment tools for pain (Cook et al., 2014). There have also been improvements in CBT interventions for chronic pain as protocols have been enhanced to effectively address other chronic conditions that are linked to pain, such as insomnia. Additionally, interdisciplinary pain centers within the military continue to develop integrative programs that help patients progress toward functional restoration (Flynn et al., 2017).

3.1 Assessment

Although there may be benefits to having many pain assessment instruments to choose from, certain limitations exist. Specifically, heterogeneity among applied assessments may lead to confusion as they limit the ability for comparisons to be made between assessment measures. In order to address this concern, the US Army Pain Management Task Force (PMTF) has developed a standard assessment program to be used across the DOD (Cook et al., 2014).

The PMTF developed the Pain Assessment Screening Tool and Outcomes Registry (PASTOR), which is a web-based self-report assessment that is derived from the National Institutes of Health (NIH) Patient-Reported Outcomes Measurement Information System (PROMIS®) initiative. The PROMIS® initiative is a data bank of health outcome measures that administers questionnaire items through an electronic platform using computer adaptive testing (CAT) (Cook et al., 2014). CAT systems offer a significant advantage over traditional self-report measures since it uses a computer algorithm to select test items based on an individual's response to previous test questions. Further, such assessment tools are considered to be more precise and less burdensome for individuals, as they tend to generate shorter series of focused questions compared to standard self-report measures (Cook et al., 2014).

PASTOR is an efficient and comprehensive pain assessment tool that evaluates pain-related areas of concern, including pain interference, neuropathic pain, headache, activity goals and limitations, post-traumatic stress disorder (PTSD), anxiety, depression, alcohol misuse, global health, fatigue, satisfaction with social roles, anger, sleep dysfunction, and physical impairment. Most outcomes being assessed on PASTOR are standardized to *T*-scores with a mean score of 50 and a standard deviation of 10 (Flynn et al., 2017). Thus, PASTOR allows for clinicians and researchers to compare data collected to a reference population (Cook et al., 2014). Additionally, once SMs complete their assessment on PASTOR, a clinical report is generated as an efficient summary of a patient's current clinical status to be reviewed with the patient or other treatment team members (Cook et al., 2014).

Initial evaluation studies of PASTOR within the military are currently underway. So far, pilot study results suggest that PASTOR can be administered to most SMs being seen in large interdisciplinary pain management centers within the DOD. PASTOR may be a useful tool to assess treatment outcome in focused integrative pain treatment programs to improve functional outcomes among SMs (Flynn et al., 2017). However, further evaluation should be conducted to determine the utility of PASTOR within pain treatment programs using controlled studies.

3.2 Treatment Programs

Chronic pain is often associated with a number of physical and psychological comorbidities, particularly sleep disturbances. The relationship between chronic pain and sleep problems is reciprocal, often resulting in a self-perpetuating cycle (Smith & Haythornthwaite, 2004). Furthermore, the interaction between sleep and chronic pain for SMs may be further exacerbated by unique circumstances that are endemic to life in the military (e.g., shiftwork, moving to different duty stations, etc.) (Pruiksma et al., 2020). Therefore, as CBT treatments for chronic pain continue to be refined, it is essential for clinical health psychologists to be trained to address both chronic pain and sleep disturbances, particularly insomnia.

The effectiveness of CBT-CP and cognitive behavioral therapy for insomnia (CBTi) is well known; however, efforts to integrate both treatments into a "hybrid" intervention has been a more recent undertaking (Tang, 2018). Hybrid CBTi/CBT-CP programs place an equal emphasis on interventions for chronic pain and insomnia. Strategies within hybrid programs include: psychoeducation on sleep and pain, cognitive restructuring techniques to address maladaptive thinking related to sleep and pain, and behavioral strategies (i.e., sleep restriction/stimulus control and activity pacing/behavioral activation) (Tang, 2018). Preliminary studies have found hybrid CBT programs for pain and sleep to be effective in improving sleep, pain interference, mood, and fatigue (Tang et al., 2012). Such programs appear to be more efficient (approximately 4–10 weekly sessions) than implementing two separate protocols, which may have cost savings implications for the military (Tang, 2018; Tang et al., 2012). Improvements in one medical condition may help to increase SM "buy in" and mastery in CBT skills throughout the program. Clinical health psychologists are well positioned to develop hybrid CBT-CP/CBTi programs throughout the military system, given their training in assessment and CBT for pain and sleep.

As CBT programs continue to be refined, interdisciplinary pain management centers have focused on developing functional restoration programs (FRP) with the goal of returning SMs to full duty. Functional restoration programs typically consist of an interdisciplinary team which include: clinical health psychology, medicine, nursing, physical therapy, occupational therapy, and vocational rehabilitation. The schedule and time commitment requirements for FRPs are similar to intensive outpatient programs within behavioral health, which can require patients to spend a full work day in the program, over the course of several weeks.

FRP programs have been operating within the military for over a decade. Initial data on FRPs in the military is promising, since such programs results in greater functional improvements for patients compared to standard medical treatment alone (Gatchel et al., 2009). However, data on the effectiveness of specific FRP programs within the military has yet to be conducted, as subsequent research has been mostly descriptive rather than evaluative (Pujol et al., 2015).

As FRPs in the military continue to be developed, clinical health psychologists have a key role to play throughout this process. In addition to providing didactic components in these programs, clinical health psychologists should focus on developing evidence-based behavioral interventions that are highly effective in targeting the critical treatment processes necessary to sustain pain rehabilitation. Such processes include motivational enhancement, present moment focus, and acceptance, to name a few. Therefore, as clinical health psychologists continue to improve CBT programs as a standalone treatment for pain, psychologists should continue to focus on developing FRPs by further integrating evidence-based behavioral interventions into these programs.

4 Case Study

4.1 Biopsychosocial Assessment

SM is a 35-year-old married woman who served as a helicopter pilot in the US Army. She was referred to interdisciplinary pain treatment to address chronic neck pain, upper back pain, and headaches. At her initial evaluation, she reported that her pain began 5 years prior to being seen in the pain center and she attributed the development of her pain condition to the repetitive high impact nature of her work as a pilot. SM reported pain and limited range of motion in her neck while sitting, standing, and in various sleeping positions. She also indicated that while the pain began at the back of her neck, it would radiate up towards the back of her head causing headaches. She described her headaches as a stabbing sensation and feeling as if a "rubber band" was around her head. SM reported her headaches occurred 1-2 times a week and her pain severity level was a 10/10 (0 being *no pain* and 10 being the *worst pain*), pain as usual was a 7.5/10, and the lowest possible pain was a 7/10. Previous pain treatments included pain medications (nonsteroidal anti-inflammatory drugs) and physical therapy, both of which resulted in little benefit to SM. C-spine MRI and X-rays in SM's medical record indicated that she had cervical degenerative disc disease. SM indicated that her neck pain and headaches were significantly impacting her ability to perform her job and carry out activities of daily living (e.g. driving). Additionally, her sleep had been significantly impacted by pain, resulting in symptoms of insomnia. She reported an average total sleep time of 5 hours each night. Her average initial sleep onset, each night, was 180 min, due to worry and psychophysiological arousal. Her wakefulness after sleep onset was approximately 180 min due to pain and arousal. Her pain had resulted in significant depressive symptoms including suicidal ideation, which resulted in a brief hospital stay on an inpatient unit prior to being seen at the pain center. No imminent safety concerns were noted at the time of evaluation. She had no significant behavioral health history prior to her chronic pain. She reported that only medications and stretching were palliative factors for her pain. SM's goals for treatment included the following: pain relief, improving her sleep, increasing her level of exercise/activity and learning emotional coping strategies.

4.1.1 Treatment

A treatment plan was collaboratively developed with the patient to proceed with an integration of cognitive behavioral therapy for insomnia (CBTi), biofeedback/self-regulation, and cognitive behavioral therapy for chronic pain (CBT-CP). Complementary and alternative medicine treatments were recommended by her pain physician, which included battlefield acupuncture with an acupuncturist and myofascial release with a medical massage specialist.

SM was seen for seven individual sessions of CBTi with her psychologist in the pain center to address symptoms of insomnia. She was first provided with psychoeducation on normal sleep and insomnia (e.g., the definition of insomnia and understanding the precipitating and perpetuating factors of insomnia). A review of SM's understanding of sleep hygiene was also conducted and deficiencies in these skills were addressed. In subsequent sessions, a strong emphasis was placed on self-monitoring (i.e., sleep diary) and making behavioral changes through sleep restriction therapy and stimulus control. SM responded well to sleep restriction therapy and was able to increase her sleep efficiency by 46% and significantly decrease her initial sleep onset time. She was also taught cognitive restructuring techniques and mindfulness-based stress reduction techniques in order to address both the content and process of negative cognitions related to poor sleep.

While completing CBTi sessions, SM engaged in biofeedback guided self-regulation with a biofeedback therapist to directly address her headaches and psychophysiological arousal. During baseline evaluations, she exhibited both elevations in respiration rate and muscle tension in her trapezius (>10–15 mv) as well as a delay in physiological recovery. She completed five sessions of biofeedback that addressed respiration, heart rate variability, and muscle tension in her shoulders. At the conclusion of her biofeedback sessions, SM was able to maintain a respiration rate of six breaths per minute without any difficulty or symptoms. She also demonstrated significant control of her muscle tension (maintaining <5 mv) while practicing progressive muscle relaxation. At the end of treatment, she demonstrated a significant decrease in the severity of her headaches, as she reported her headache severity to be a 2.5/10 (0–10 scale) on average each day.

After completing CBTi focused sessions, SM completed five sessions of CBT for chronic pain with her psychologist. Her sleep diary continued to be evaluated during these sessions. Her treatment consisted of goal setting, psychoeducation on the pain cycles and the gate control theory/neuromatrix model, pleasurable activity scheduling, activity pacing, cognitive restructuring, effective communication training, and relapse prevention. She demonstrated a decrease in her depressive symptoms as a result of increasing pleasurable activities, such as her hobbies. She was also effective in applying activity pacing strategies, while engaging in activities such as yoga, walking, and using her myofascial roller. She was also effective in identifying negative automatic thoughts related to situations associated with her pain and able to reframe negative thinking patterns related to these situations. Additionally, she reported that complementary and alternative medicine treatments such as battlefield acupuncture and myofascial release treatments also contributed to improvements in her headaches.

SM's pain treatment was also closely coordinated with the care she received from her behavioral health team in order to prevent relapse of severe depressive symptoms. Her depressive symptoms were closely monitored and her treatment was selected in coordination with both teams. Multidisciplinary meetings were conducted between her treatment teams to ensure communication on her care was optimal. Over the course of 2–3 months, her depressive symptoms significantly improved.

4.1.2 Discussion

This is a typical case seen in interdisciplinary pain centers across the DOD. SM's case highlights the complexity on how chronic pain and behavioral health concerns are intertwined and must be treated in close coordination with medical teams. Improvement in SM's mood and functioning were highly dependent on closely coordinated interdisciplinary care. In terms of SM's pain psychology treatment, a biopsychosocial assessment was critical in determining both the type of evidence-based interventions to be implemented and the timing in which to implement each intervention in the larger context of her care. Combined CBT-CP and CBTi were selected to improve sleep and coping with pain. SM's treatment also included complementary and alternative medicine interventions (e.g., acupuncture). At the end of her treatment, SM medically retired from the Army; however, she demonstrated significant improvements in daily functioning, mood, and overall quality of life at her discharge.

5 Discussion

As the need for effective treatments for chronic pain continues to grow, clinical health psychologists are well positioned to address many of the biopsychosocial concerns related to this complex condition. Since the initiation of the Pain Management Task Force, the US military has prioritized the development of effective behavioral tools to address chronic pain at all levels of medical care (Vallerand et al., 2015). This chapter highlights the most effective assessment and behavioral treatment tools used by clinical health psychologists in order to address chronic pain, from a biopsychosocial perspective. Further, we also discussed the development of recent behavioral programs that may help to improve the efficiency in addressing chronic pain concerns. Lastly, as behavioral programs used to address chronic pain continue to be developed, it is imperative that military-related contextual factors that may directly impact therapeutic change are explored.

References

Alperstein, D., & Sharpe, L. (2016). The efficacy of motivational interviewing in adults with chronic pain: A meta-analysis and systematic review. *The Journal of Pain, 17*(4), 393–403. https://doi.org/10.1016/j.jpain.2015.10.021

Arnow, B. A., Blasey, C. M., Constantino, M. J., Robinson, R., Hunkeler, E., Lee, J., ... Hayward, C. (2011). Catastrophizing, depression and pain-related disability. *General Hospital Psychiatry, 33*(2), 150–156. https://doi.org/10.1016/j.genhosppsych.2010.12.008

Baranoff, J., Hanrahan, S. J., Kapur, D., & Connor, J. P. (2013). Acceptance as a process variable in relation to catastrophizing in multidisciplinary pain treatment. *European Journal of Pain, 17*(1), 101–110. https://doi.org/10.1002/j.1532-2149.2012.00165.x

Beck, A. T., Steer, R. A., & Brown, G. K. (1996). Manual for the beck depression inventory-II. *San Antonio, TX: Psychological Corporation, 1*, 82.

Bell, N. S., Schwartz, C. E., Harford, T., Hollander, I. E., & Amoroso, P. J. (2008). The changing profile of disability in the US Army: 1981–2005. *Disability and Health Journal, 1*(1), 14–24. https://doi.org/10.1016/j.dhjo.2007.11.007

Bernini, O., Rivas, T., & Berrocal, C. (2014). The chronic pain acceptance questionnaire: Preliminary evidence for the predictive validity of patients' subgroups. *Journal of Evidence-Based Psychotherapies, 14*(1), 3–20.

Brintz, C. E., Miller, S., Olmsted, K. R., Bartoszek, M., Cartwright, J., Kizakevich, P. N., ... Gaylord, S. A. (2020). Adapting mindfulness training for military service members with chronic pain. *Military Medicine, 185*(3–4), 385–393. https://doi.org/10.1093/milmed/usz312

Burns, J. W., Mullen, J. T., Higdon, L. J., Wei, J. M., & Lansky, D. (2000). Validity of the pain anxiety symptoms scale (PASS): Prediction of physical capacity variables. *Pain, 84*(2–3), 247–252. https://doi.org/10.1016/s0304-3959(99)00218-3

Burns, J. W., Glenn, B., Bruehl, S., Harden, R. N., & Lofland, K. (2003). Cognitive factors influence outcome following multidisciplinary chronic pain treatment: A replication and extension of a cross-lagged panel analysis. *Behaviour Research and Therapy, 41*(10), 1163–1182. https://doi.org/10.1016/s0005-7967(03)00029-9

Carmody, T. P., Duncan, C. L., Huggins, J., Solkowitz, S. N., Lee, S. K., Reyes, N., ... Simon, J. A. (2013). Telephone-delivered cognitive–behavioral therapy for pain management among older military veterans: A randomized trial. *Psychological Services, 10*(3), 265. https://doi.org/10.1037/a0030944

Chibnall, J. T., & Tait, R. C. (1994). The pain disability index: Factor structure and normative data. *Archives of Physical Medicine and Rehabilitation, 75*(10), 1082–1086. https://doi.org/10.1016/0003-9993(94)90082-5

Clark, M. E., Gironda, R. J., & Young, R. W. (2003). Development and validation of the pain outcomes questionnaire-VA. *Journal of Rehabilitation Research and Development, 40*(5), 381–396. https://doi.org/10.1682/jrrd.2003.09.0381

Cook, K. F., Buckenmaier, C., 3rd, & Gershon, R. C. (2014). PASTOR/PROMIS® pain outcomes system: What does it mean to pain specialists? *Pain Management, 4*(4), 277–283. https://doi.org/10.2217/pmt.14.25

Coulter, I. D., Hilton, L., Walter, J., & Brown, K. S. (2016). Integrative pain management centers in the military: The challenges. *Military Medicine, 181*(9), 1033–1039. https://doi.org/10.7205/MILMED-D-15-00317

Crombez, G., Eccleston, C., Van Damme, S., Vlaeyen, J. W., & Karoly, P. (2012). Fear-avoidance model of chronic pain: The next generation. *The Clinical Journal of Pain, 28*(6), 475–483. https://doi.org/10.1097/AJP.0b013e3182385392

Department of Veterans Affairs & Department of Defense. (2017). VA/DOD Clinical Practice Guideline for diagnosis and treatment of low back pain. https://www.healthquality.va.gov/guidelines/Pain/lpb/VADoDLBPCPG092917.pdf

Feliu-Soler, A., Montesinos, F., Gutiérrez-Martínez, O., Scott, W., McCracken, L. M., & Luciano, J. V. (2018). Current status of acceptance and commitment therapy for chronic pain: A narrative review. *Journal of Pain Research, 11*, 2145. https://doi.org/10.2147/JPR.S144631

Flynn, D. M., Cook, K., Kallen, M., Buckenmaier, C., Weickum, R., Collins, T., … Joltes, K. (2017). Use of the pain assessment screening tool and outcomes registry in an army interdisciplinary pain management center, lessons learned and future implications of a 10-month beta test. *Military Medicine, 182*(suppl_1), 167–174. https://doi.org/10.7205/MILMED-D-16-00212

Gatchel, R. J., Peng, Y. B., Peters, M. L., Fuchs, P. N., & Turk, D. C. (2007). The biopsychosocial approach to chronic pain: Scientific advances and future directions. *Psychological Bulletin, 133*(4), 581. https://doi.org/10.1037/0033-2909.133.4.581

Gatchel, R. J., McGeary, D. D., Peterson, A., Moore, M., LeRoy, K., Isler, W. C., … Edell, T. (2009). Preliminary findings of a randomized controlled trial of an interdisciplinary military pain program. *Military Medicine, 174*(3), 270–277. https://doi.org/10.7205/milmed-d-03-1607

Gatchel, R. J., McGeary, D. D., McGeary, C. A., & Lippe, B. (2014). Interdisciplinary chronic pain management: Past, present, and future. *American Psychologist, 69*(2), 119. https://doi.org/10.1037/a0035514

Harris, C. A., & D'Eon, J. L. (2008). Psychometric properties of the Beck Depression Inventory-(BDI-II) in individuals with chronic pain. *Pain, 137*(3), 609–622. https://doi.org/10.1016/j.pain.2007.10.022

Hayes, S. C., Strosahl, K. D., & Wilson, K. G. (2012). *Acceptance and commitment therapy: The process and practice of mindful change*. Guilford Press.

Jeffery, D. D., May, L., Luckey, B., Balison, B. M., & Klette, K. L. (2014). Use and abuse of prescribed opioids, central nervous system depressants, and stimulants among US active duty military personnel in FY 2010. *Military Medicine, 179*(10), 1141–1148. https://doi.org/10.7205/MILMED-D-14-00002

Jones, K. D., Burckhardt, C. S., & Bennett, J. A. (2004). Motivational interviewing may encourage exercise in persons with fibromyalgia by enhancing self efficacy. *Arthritis Care and Research, 51*(5), 864–867. https://doi.org/10.1002/art.20684

Kazanis, W., Pugh, M. J., Tami, C., Maddry, J. K., Bebarta, V. S., Finley, E. P., … Potter, J. S. (2018). Opioid use patterns among active duty service members and civilians: 2006–2014. *Military Medicine, 183*(3–4), e157–e164. https://doi.org/10.1093/milmed/usx014

Kerns, R. D., & Haythornthwaite, J. A. (1988). Depression among chronic pain patients: Cognitive-behavioral analysis and effect on rehabilitation outcome. *Journal of Consulting and Clinical Psychology, 56*(6), 870. https://doi.org/10.1037//0022-006x.56.6.870

Kerns, R. D., Turk, D. C., & Rudy, T. E. (1985). The west haven-yale multidimensional pain inventory (WHYMPI). *Pain, 23*(4), 345–356. https://doi.org/10.1016/0304-3959(85)90004-1

Kerns, R. D., Sellinger, J., & Goodin, B. R. (2011). Psychological treatment of chronic pain. *Annual Review of Clinical Psychology, 7*, 411–434. https://doi.org/10.1146/annurev-clinpsy-090310-120430

Knoerl, R., Lavoie Smith, E. M., & Weisberg, J. (2016). Chronic pain and cognitive behavioral therapy: An integrative review. *Western Journal of Nursing Research, 38*(5), 596–628. https://doi.org/10.1177/0193945915615869

Kroenke, K., Spitzer, R. L., & Williams, J. B. (2001). The PHQ-9: Validity of a brief depression severity measure. *Journal of General Internal Medicine, 16*(9), 606–613. https://doi.org/10.1046/j.1525-1497.2001.016009606.x

Lattie, E. G., Antoni, M. H., Millon, T., Kamp, J., & Walker, M. R. (2013). MBMD coping styles and psychiatric indicators and response to a multidisciplinary pain treatment program. *Journal of Clinical Psychology in Medical Settings, 20*(4), 515–525. https://doi.org/10.1007/s10880-013-9377-9

Maby, J. I., Kwon, P. O., Washington, W., Cowan, D. N., Toolin, C., Pearce, T. D., Kelley, A. I., & Campbell, C. K. (2017). *Disability evaluation system analysis and research annual report 2017*. Accession Medical Standards Analysis and Research Activity (AMSARA) Silver Spring United States.

McCracken, L. M., & Dhingra, L. (2002). A short version of the Pain Anxiety Symptoms Scale (PASS-20): Preliminary development and validity. *Pain Research and Management, 7*, 45–50. https://doi.org/10.1155/2002/517163

McCracken, L. M., & Vowles, K. E. (2014). Acceptance and commitment therapy and mindfulness for chronic pain: Model, process, and progress. *American Psychologist, 69*(2), 178. https://doi.org/10.1037/a0035623

McCracken, L. M., Zayfert, C., & Gross, R. T. (1992). The Pain Anxiety Symptoms Scale: Development and validation of a scale to measure fear of pain. *Pain, 50*(1), 67–73. https://doi.org/10.1016/0304-3959(92)90113-p

McCracken, L. M., Vowles, K. E., & Eccleston, C. (2004). Acceptance of chronic pain: Component analysis and a revised assessment method. *Pain, 107*(1–2), 159–166. https://doi.org/10.1016/j.pain.2003.10.012

McCracken, L. M., Vowles, K. E., & Eccleston, C. (2005). Acceptance-based treatment for persons with complex, long standing chronic pain: A preliminary analysis of treatment outcome in comparison to a waiting phase. *Behaviour Research and Therapy, 43*(10), 1335–1346. https://doi.org/10.1016/j.brat.2004.10.003

Melzack, R. (1999). From the gate to the neuromatrix. *Pain, 82*, S121–S126. https://doi.org/10.1016/s0304-3959(99)00145-1

Midboe, A. M., Cucciare, M. A., Trafton, J. A., Ketroser, N., & Chardos, J. F. (2011). Implementing motivational interviewing in primary care: The role of provider characteristics. *Translational Behavioral Medicine, 1*(4), 588–594. https://doi.org/10.1007/s13142-011-0080-9

Miller, R. M., & Kaiser, R. S. (2018). Psychological characteristics of chronic pain: A review of current evidence and assessment tools to enhance treatment. *Current Pain and Headache Reports, 22*(3), 22. https://doi.org/10.1007/s11916-018-0663-y

Miller, W. R., Rollnick, S., & Conforti, K. (2002). Preparing people for change. *Motivational Interviewing*.

Millon, T., Antoni, M. H., Millon, C., Minor, S., & Grossman, S. (2001). *Test manual for the Millon Behavioral Medicine Diagnostic (MBMD)*. National Computer Services.

Molloy, J. M., Pendergrass, T. L., Lee, I. E., Chervak, M. C., Hauret, K. G., & Rhon, D. I. (2020). Musculoskeletal injuries and United States Army readiness part I: Overview of injuries and their strategic impact. *Military Medicine, 185*, e1461–e1471. https://doi.org/10.1093/milmed/usaa027

Morley, S., Eccleston, C., & Williams, A. (1999). Systematic review and meta-analysis of randomized controlled trials of cognitive behaviour therapy and behaviour therapy for chronic pain in adults, excluding headache. *Pain, 80*(1–2), 1–13. https://doi.org/10.1016/s0304-3959(98)00255-3

Nielson, W. R., Jensen, M. P., Karsdorp, P. A., & Vlaeyen, J. W. (2013). Activity pacing in chronic pain: Concepts, evidence, and future directions. *The Clinical Journal of Pain, 29*(5), 461–468. https://doi.org/10.1097/AJP.0b013e3182608561

Office of the Army Surgeon General. (2010). *Pain management task force report: Providing a standardize DoD and VHA vision and approach to pain management to optimize the care of warriors and their families*. U.S. Department of Defense. www.dvcipm.org/clinical-resources/pain-management-task-force

Osman, A., Barrios, F. X., Kopper, B. A., Hauptmann, W., Jones, J., & O'neill, E. (1997). Factor structure, reliability, and validity of the Pain Catastrophizing Scale. *Journal of Behavioral Medicine, 20*(6), 589–605. https://doi.org/10.1023/a:1025570508954

Otis, J. D., Gregor, K., Hardway, C., Morrison, J., Scioli, E., & Sanderson, K. (2010). An examination of the co-morbidity between chronic pain and posttraumatic stress disorder on US veterans. *Psychological Services, 7*(3), 126. https://doi.org/10.1037/a0020512

Otis, J. D., Sanderson, K., Hardway, C., Pincus, M., Tun, C., & Soumekh, S. (2013). A randomized controlled pilot study of a cognitive-behavioral therapy approach for painful diabetic peripheral neuropathy. *The Journal of Pain, 14*(5), 475–482. https://doi.org/10.1016/j.jpain.2012.12.013

Peters, L., Simon, E. P., Folen, R. A., & Umphress, V. (2000). The COPE program: Treatment efficacy and medical utilization outcome of a chronic pain management program at a major military hospital. *Military Medicine, 165*(12), 954–960. https://doi.org/10.1093/milmed/165.12.954

Pollard, C. A. (1984). Preliminary validity study of the pain disability index. *Perceptual and Motor Skills, 59*, 974. https://doi.org/10.2466/pms.1984.59.3.974

Polomano, R. C., Galloway, K. T., Kent, M. L., Brandon-Edwards, H., Kwon, K. N., Morales, C., & Buckenmaier, C. T., III. (2016). Psychometric testing of the Defense and Veterans Pain Rating Scale (DVPRS): A new pain scale for military population. *Pain Medicine, 17*(8), 1505–1519. https://doi.org/10.1093/pm/pnw105

Pruiksma, K. E., Hale, W. J., Mintz, J., Peterson, A. L., Young-McCaughan, S., Wilkerson, A., … Roache, J. D. (2020). Predictors of Cognitive Behavioral Therapy for Insomnia (CBTi) outcomes in active-duty US Army personnel. *Behavior Therapy, 51*(4), 522–534. https://doi.org/10.1016/j.beth.2020.02.001

Pujol, L. A., Sussman, L., Clapp, J., Nilson, R., Gill, H., Boge, J., & Goff, B. (2015). Functional restoration for chronic pain patients in the military: Early results of the San Antonio Military Medical Center functional restoration program. *U.S. Army Medical Department Journal*, 1–7.

Ramirez, S., Bebarta, V. S., Varney, S. M., Ganem, V., Zarzabal, L. A., & Potter, J. S. (2017). Misuse of prescribed pain medication in a military population—A self-reported survey to assess a correlation with age, deployment, combat illnesses, or injury? *American Journal of Therapeutics, 24*(2), e150–e156. https://doi.org/10.1097/MJT.0000000000000141

Rasu, R. S., Vouthy, K., Crowl, A. N., Stegeman, A. E., Fikru, B., Bawa, W. A., & Knell, M. E. (2014). Cost of pain medication to treat adult patients with nonmalignant chronic pain in the United States. *Journal of Managed Care Pharmacy, 20*(9), 921–928. https://doi.org/10.18553/jmcp.2014.20.9.921

Reneman, M. F., Dijkstra, A., Geertzen, J. H., & Dijkstra, P. U. (2010). Psychometric properties of chronic pain acceptance questionnaires: A systematic review. *European Journal of Pain, 14*(5), 457–465. https://doi.org/10.1016/j.ejpain.2009.08.003

Rief, S., Adams, R. S., Ritter, G. A., Williams, T. V., & Larson, M. J. (2018). Prevalence of pain diagnoses and burden of pain among active duty soldiers, FY2012. *Military Medicine, 183*(9–10), e330–e337. https://doi.org/10.1093/milmed/usx200

Schwartz, M. S., & Andrasik, F. (Eds.). (2003). *Biofeedback: A practitioner's guide*. Guilford Publications.

Seo, J. G., & Park, S. P. (2015). Validation of the Patient Health Questionnaire-9 (PHQ-9) and PHQ-2 in patients with migraine. *The Journal of Headache and Pain, 16*(1), 65. https://doi.org/10.1186/s10194-015-0552-2

Smith, M. T., & Haythornthwaite, J. A. (2004). How do sleep disturbance and chronic pain interrelate? Insights from the longitudinal and cognitive-behavioral clinical trials literature. *Sleep Medicine Reviews, 8*(2), 119–132. https://doi.org/10.1016/S1087-0792(03)00044-3

Smith, L., Westrick, R., Sauers, S., Cooper, A., Scofield, D., Claro, P., & Warr, B. (2016). Underreporting of musculoskeletal injuries in the US Army: Findings from an infantry brigade combat team survey study. *Sports Health, 8*(6), 507–513. https://doi.org/10.1177/1941738116670873

Smith, H. J., Taubman, S. B., & Clark, L. L. (2020). A burden and prevalence analysis of chronic pain by distinct case definitions among active duty US military service members, 2018. *Pain Physician, 23*, E429–E439.

Sullivan, M. J., Bishop, S. R., & Pivik, J. (1995). The pain catastrophizing scale: Development and validation. *Psychological Assessment, 7*(4), 524. https://doi.org/10.1037/1040-3590.7.4.524

Tang, N. K. (2018). Cognitive behavioural therapy in pain and psychological disorders: Towards a hybrid future. *Progress in Neuro-Psychopharmacology and Biological Psychiatry, 87*, 281–289. https://doi.org/10.1016/j.pnpbp.2017.02.023

Tang, N. K., Goodchild, C. E., & Salkovskis, P. M. (2012). Hybrid cognitive-behaviour therapy for individuals with insomnia and chronic pain: A pilot randomized controlled trial. *Behaviour Research and Therapy, 50*(12), 814–821. https://doi.org/10.1016/j.brat.2012.08.006

Toblin, R. L., Quartana, P. J., Riviere, L. A., Walper, K. C., & Hoge, C. W. (2014). Chronic pain and opioid use in US soldiers after combat deployment. *JAMA Internal Medicine, 174*(8), 1400–1401. https://doi.org/10.1001/jamainternmed.2014.2726

Treede, R. D., Rief, W., Barke, A., Aziz, Q., Bennett, M. I., Benoliel, R., ... Giamberardino, M. A. (2015). A classification of chronic pain for ICD-11. *Pain, 156*(6), 1003. https://doi.org/10.1097/j.pain.0000000000000160

Vallerand, A. H., Cosler, P., Henningfield, J. E., & Galassini, P. (2015). Pain management strategies and lessons from the military: A narrative review. *Pain Research and Management, 20*, 261–268. https://doi.org/10.1155/2015/196025

Veehof, M. M., Trompetter, H. R., Bohlmeijer, E. T., & Schreurs, K. M. G. (2016). Acceptance- and mindfulness-based interventions for the treatment of chronic pain: A meta-analytic review. *Cognitive Behaviour Therapy, 45*(1), 5–31. https://doi.org/10.1080/16506073.2015.1098724

Wandner, L. D., Prasad, R., Ramezani, A., Malcore, S. A., & Kerns, R. D. (2018). Core competencies for the emerging specialty of pain psychology. *American Psychologist, 74*(4), 432. https://doi.org/10.1037/amp0000330

Weathers, F. W., Litz, B. T., Keane, T. M., Palmieri, P. A., Marx, B. P., & Schnurr, P. P. (2013). *The PTSD checklist for DSM-5 (PCL-5)–standard [measurement instrument]*. Retrieved from http://www.ptsd.va.gov

Wetherell, J. L., Afari, N., Rutledge, T., Sorrell, J. T., Stoddard, J. A., Petkus, A. J., ... Atkinson, J. H. (2011). A randomized, controlled trial of acceptance and commitment therapy and cognitive-behavioral therapy for chronic pain. *Pain, 152*(9), 2098–2107. https://doi.org/10.1016/j.pain.2011.05.016

Wetherell, J. L., Petkus, A. J., Alonso-Fernandez, M., Bower, E. S., Steiner, A. R., & Afari, N. (2016). Age moderates response to acceptance and commitment therapy vs. cognitive behavioral therapy for chronic pain. *International Journal of Geriatric Psychiatry, 31*(3), 302–308. https://doi.org/10.1002/gps.4330

Williams, M., Teasdale, J. D., Segal, Z. V., & Kabat-Zinn, J. (2007). *The mindful way through depression: Freeing yourself from chronic unhappiness*. Guilford Press.

Wong, S. Y. S., Chan, F. W. K., Wong, R. L. P., Chu, M. C., Lam, Y. Y. K., Mercer, S. W., & Ma, S. H. (2011). Comparing the effectiveness of mindfulness-based stress reduction and multidisciplinary intervention programs for chronic pain: A randomized comparative trial. *The Clinical Journal of Pain, 27*(8), 724–734. https://doi.org/10.1097/AJP.0b013e3182183c6e

Chapter 10
Post-traumatic Stress Disorder and Chronic Pain Among Military Members and Veterans

Jeremiah A. Schumm, Leanna J. Pittsenbarger, and Caroline A. McClellan

Post-traumatic stress disorder (PTSD) and chronic pain are debilitating conditions that commonly co-occur in military members and veterans (Lew et al., 2009; Shipherd et al., 2007; Stratton et al., 2014). The co-occurrence of these conditions has important implications to the military, since these conditions increase risk for medical discharge from military service. Although PTSD and chronic pain independently increase risk for military medical discharge, the co-occurrence of these conditions compound this risk (Benedict et al., 2019). Compared to veterans with only one of these conditions, veterans with co-occurring PTSD and chronic pain are also shown to utilize more primary care and pain-related specialty care visits. In addition, veterans with co-occurring PTSD and chronic pain use more medications, including opioids, benzodiazepines, non-opioid analgesics, and antidepressants, when compared to those with only one of these conditions (Outcalt et al., 2014). Overall, these findings demonstrate that PTSD and chronic pain are substantial burdens to the military, the military and veteran health care systems, and the military members and veterans afflicted with these conditions.

The purpose of this chapter is to describe PTSD and chronic pain and interventions that can be used to address these conditions among military members and veterans. We begin by defining PTSD and chronic pain and describing the prevalence of these conditions among the military and veteran population. We next

J. A. Schumm (✉)
School of Professional Psychology, College of Health, Education, and Human Services, Wright State University, Dayton, OH, USA
e-mail: Jeremiah.schumm@wright.edu

L. J. Pittsenbarger
Counseling and Psychiatric Services, University of Colorado Boulder, Boulder, CO, USA

C. A. McClellan
Counseling and Psychological Services, The Ohio State University, Columbus, OH, USA
e-mail: lpittsenbarger@ohio.edu

L. C. James et al. (eds.), *Clinical Health Psychology in Military and Veteran Settings*, https://doi.org/10.1007/978-3-031-12063-3_10

discuss how traumatic events and other risk factors might explain the high co-occurrence of these conditions. The chapter then describes treatments for PTSD and chronic pain, with particular attention to Department of Veterans Affairs and Department of Defense (VA/DoD) guidelines that have been developed to guide clinicians who are working with military members and veterans. We provide two case examples of how treatments might be implemented and typical challenges that might be faced in the context of treating these comorbid conditions. Finally, we discuss recommendations for future directions in diagnosing and treating PTSD and chronic pain in military members and veterans.

1 Definitions of PTSD and Chronic Pain

To qualify for a diagnosis of PTSD according to the *Diagnostic and Statistical Manual of Mental Disorders*, 5th edition (DSM-5; American Psychiatric Association, 2013), individuals must have been exposed to situations that involved actual or threatened serious injury, or sexual violence. The diagnosis requires that in response to these types of traumatic events, the individual exhibits symptoms of intrusions related to the events, avoidance of reminders of the event, negative alterations in cognition and mood following the event, and increased arousal following the event. Regarding intrusive symptoms, individuals must experience one or more of the following: unwanted thoughts in relation to the traumatic event, nightmares surrounding the trauma, flashbacks, emotional reactions in response to trigger to the event, or physical reactivity after being exposed to something that reminds the individual of the event. Additionally, the individual must experience avoidance surrounding trauma stimuli, which can be trauma-related thoughts or feelings. Avoidance may also involve avoiding situations, people, or places that serve as reminders of the traumas. Additionally, negative alterations in cognition and mood must occur in response to the trauma. Examples of these symptoms involve feeling isolated, negative affect, difficulty experiencing positive affect, inability to recall key features of the trauma, exaggerated blame of self or others, or overly negative thoughts and assumptions about the world or themselves. Finally, the diagnosis requires that individuals exhibit increased arousal and reactivity following the trauma. These symptoms may include irritable or angry behaviors, risky behaviors, hypervigilance, heightened arousal, difficulty concentrating, or difficulty sleeping. These symptoms must be present for at least 1 month, cause distress or functional impairment, and not be due to another condition.

Like PTSD, chronic pain is a condition that has both physical and psychological symptoms. According to the International Association for the Study of Pain (2017), pain includes both unpleasant physical and emotional responses to bodily injury. However, unlike evaluation of PTSD, pain does not require that the person who is experiencing it is able to verbalize the experiences, and pain reactions can be determined in those who are verbal and non-verbal. Although there are no universally agreed-upon definitions of when pain can be considered to be "chronic," an older version of the chronic pain classification guidelines suggest that a duration of approximately 3 months can be used to differentiate chronic from more acute pain (International Association for the Study of Pain, 1986).

2 Prevalence of PTSD and Chronic Pain

Prevalence of PTSD in active duty military members and veterans varies across wars and generations. According to medical archive data from the Department of Defense Health Care System, 2.2% of active duty population accessed PTSD-related care. That data was further broken down by gender and if the individual was deployed. Prevalence was higher for female Service Members (3.2%) than male Service Members (2.0%). Additionally, rates of PTSD were higher for those who had deployed (3.6%) as compared to those who had not deployed (0.8%) (Armed Forces Health Surveillance Branch, 2017). Further, the Army Study to Assess Risk and Resilience in Service Members (ARMYSTARRS) found a PTSD prevalence of 8.6% of active study personnel, which is consistent with estimates of younger veteran cohorts (Kessler et al., 2014). That said, given a variety of reasons, including stigma, job loss, barriers to treatment, it is likely that these numbers underrepresent the prevalence of PTSD among Active Duty Military.

In regard to prevalence of PTSD among Veteran populations, as mentioned above, numbers can vary greatly based on war and era. Results from the national health and resilience in veterans study showed that 8% of veterans screen positive for lifetime PTSD. It was noted that lifetime prevalence was higher in women veterans when compared to male Veterans as well as being higher in younger veterans as compared with older veterans (Wisco et al., 2014). A Veterans Health Administration data sheet produced by the VA's Northeast Program Evaluation Center, provided a snapshot of the patient populations receiving PTSD treatment in the VA. In 2016, there were 5,841,668 total veterans served. Of those veterans, 10.6% were diagnosed with PTSD; 10.2% were men and 15.5% were women. In 2015, prevalence data showed that the highest rates of PTSD were in veterans who served in Iraq or Afghanistan at 26.7%, with 27.3% being men and 22.5% women (Greenberg & Hoff, 2016; Harpaz-Rotem & Hoff, 2015).

Prevalence of PTSD also varies based upon service era. As reported by the National Vietnam Veterans Readjustment Study, 30% of Vietnam Veterans have had PTSD in their lifetime. When reassessed in the 1980s, 15% of Vietnam Era Veterans still had a PTSD diagnosis. It is estimated that 12% of Gulf War Veterans have PTSD in a given year. Veterans of Iraq and Afghanistan are estimated to have a prevalence of 11–20% in a given year (Eber et al., 2013; Tanielian & Jaycox, 2008; U.S. Department of Veterans Affairs PTSD in Iraq and Afghanistan veterans, 2015). In all eras, a higher prevalence of PTSD was found for women, Veterans who faced combat, and younger veterans. Finally, women were at higher risk of experiencing sexual harassment and military sexual trauma, which increased their likelihood of developing PTSD (Magruder & Yeager, 2019; Wisco et al., 2014).

Studies using VA medical record review provide a basis for estimating prevalence of chronic pain among veterans. These studies have found that 43–47% of veterans exhibit some degree of current pain (Gironda et al., 2006; Haskell et al., 2009). Of those reporting at least some pain, 57–63% report pain ratings that are moderate-to-severe. The ability to categorize pain as chronic has been limited in these studies by missing medical chart descriptions of whether the pain is considered by providers or patients to be chronic and by missing longitudinal assessment of pain ratings to determine persistence of the pain. In a large-scale cohort study of Operation Iraqi Freedom/Operation Enduring Freedom (OIF/OEF) veterans, Haskell et al. (2009) found that pain ratings were not assessed in 41% of the charts reviewed in their sample. In a smaller study sample from a single VA medical center location, Gironda et al. (2006) found that 21% of Veteran charts had missing information about duration of pain and 18% had documentation describing the pain as "chronic," but without the duration being specified. In this same study, more than 80% had pain lasting more than 1 month, and the average duration of pain was 19.2 months, which is well beyond a suggested 3-month duration for classifying pain as "chronic" (International Association for the Study of Pain, 1986). Haskell et al. (2009) defined "persistent" pain as having chart documentation of moderate-to-severe pain ratings on at least three separate months, which is consistent with the previously noted manner of classifying pain as being chronic if it lasts at least 3 months. They found that 20.6% of veterans met this definition of exhibiting persistent pain. However, the authors note that this may be an underestimation, given that earlier work on pain rating scales have shown that these scales tend to underestimate true prevalence of pain. Although the prevalence rate estimates vary, we can still conclude from these studies that chronic or persistent pain is a relatively common condition among veterans presenting for treatment.

It is also important to consider where the pain is located in the body. Among OEF/OIF veterans, Gironda et al. (2006) found that back or neck pain was most frequent (52.4%), followed by lower extremities (31.3%), and upper extremities (7.5%). Headaches were reported by 4.5%. As will be described later, the VA has developed guidelines specifically to address back pain, since it is the most frequent type of chronic pain reported by veterans.

There is evidence that prevalence of chronic or persistent pain differs based upon several characteristics. Although there were no differences in the occurrence of chronic pain based upon the military service branch, Haskell et al. (2009) found that OEF/OIF officers had lower rates of persistent pain versus those who were enlisted. This may be due to differences in job responsibilities, combat exposure, and injury with those who were enlisted being more likely to be exposed to physical injuries in serving frontline combat roles versus those who were officers. Contrary to their expectations, female veterans had lower rates of persistent pain versus male veterans. Haskell et al. (2009) note that this pattern is the opposite of what is found among civilians, with female civilians having higher rates of persistent pain versus male civilians. They speculate that because female veterans are less likely to have served in combat mission roles, they may be less likely to have experienced combat-related physical injuries that produce persistent pain. They also note that attrition from military basic training might eliminate individuals who are otherwise predisposed to experience chronic pain and, thereby, equal out gender differences in chronic pain that are typically seen among civilians. Finally, they speculate that women may be less likely to seek out health care within the VA due to perceptions that the VA is less equipped to help female versus male veterans or due to mental health conditions that interfere with treatment engagement.

3 Comorbidity Between PTSD and Chronic Pain

Several studies have found a significant correlation between PTSD and chronic pain (Brennstuhl et al., 2014; Sareen et al., 2007; Shipherd et al., 2007; VonKorff et al., 2005). Brennstuhl et al. (2014) conducted a meta-analysis to examine the relationship between PTSD and chronic pain The meta-analysis found that a majority of the studies looked at chronic lower back pain and fibromyalgia. In 2005, the National Comorbidity Replication Survey stated that approximately 7.3% of individuals with chronic lower back pain also meet criteria for PTSD (VonKorff et al., 2005). Th Canadian Community Health Survey found a higher comorbidity rate of 46% between PTSD and chronic lower back pain (Sareen et al., 2007). The same study found a 7.7% comorbidity rate between PTSD and fibromyalgia. Another study was conducted specifically looking at veterans (Shipherd et al., 2007). The study found that 66% of veterans seeking PTSD treatment also had chronic pain.

There have also been studies that have looked at the co-occurrence between PTSD and chronic pain at different time periods. One study looked at the long-term relationship between PTSD and chronic pain following a motor vehicle accident (Mayou & Bryant, 2001). The findings indicated that the comorbidity rate is approximately 23% at 3 months after the accident, but dropped to 17% a year after the accident. A similar study conducted by Sterling et al. (2005) found, in a 36-month follow-up after the motor vehicle accident, 44% of individuals were suffering from pain. It was also noted that these individuals with co-occurring pain were found to have more symptoms of PTSD as compared to individuals who were no longer experiencing pain. This finding also shows the important connection between physical and psychological health, and indicates that physical and psychological symptoms often relate to each other in severity. The combination of these studies demonstrate that the comorbidity between PTSD and chronic pain are likely bidirectional, meaning that perceived strength of pain is related to the onset of PTSD, as well as the onset of PTSD symptoms often predicts chronic pain.

In addition to the comorbidity that exists between PTSD and chronic pain, there are also several other comorbidities that exist. Some of these studies were also highlighted within the meta-analysis (Brennstuhl et al., 2014). One study found that anxiety disorders, and PTSD were the most highly comorbid with chronic pain (McWilliams et al., 2003). Anxiety has been shown to be a predictive factor for PTSD and chronic pain comorbidity (Jakupcak et al., 2006). The same study also found that depression was also predictive of both PTSD and chronic pain specifically within the veteran population. An additional study reported that participants with comorbid PTSD and chronic pain demonstrated significantly worse affective distress than participants with only chronic pain alone (Otis et al., 2010). This finding held, even after controlling for the effects of depression. Research has indicated that both PTSD and major depression are strongly associated with chronic pain, and the presence of both PTSD and depression has increased the level of disability that a person experiences (Outcalt et al., 2015).

Another morbidity that has been found is a relationship with substance use concerns, PTSD, and chronic pain (Gros et al., 2015; Morasco et al., 2011). One study recruited veterans that were being treated for both PTSD and substance use disorder (SUD) (Gros et al., 2015). The study found that there was a significant relationship between PTSD severity and pain levels. However, this study found that there was no relationship between SUD and chronic pain. In contrast, Morasco et al. (2011) found that there were higher levels of substance use when chronic pain and PTSD were comorbid with each other, as compared to PTSD only or chronic pain only. More research is necessary to understand the relationship between the comorbidity of SUD, PTSD, and chronic pain, specifically. The need for this research is very important, due to the potential questions of SUD and medication that is often prescribed to treat chronic pain.

4 Risk Factors for PTSD and Chronic Pain

The high co-occurrence of PTSD and chronic pain may be explained, in part, by these conditions resulting from injuries that occur from exposure that military members and veterans have to psychologically and physically traumatizing situations. As noted previously, PTSD is, by definition, a condition that results from exposure to a psychological traumatic event (American Psychiatric Association, 2013). These psychological traumatizing events might also involve serious physical injuries that result in chronic pain. Although chronic pain can occur without a clearly defined event that produces physical injury, chronic pain can result from physical trauma or injury in the context of military members' jobs. For example, military members' duties may require them to carry heavy equipment, travel over rough terrain during missions, or experience impact from landing after parachuting or jumping out of helicopters. These physical demands may acutely produce significant injury or lead to military members and veterans to experience more subtle progressive injuries, such as disk or vertebrae displacements, which can then lead to chronic pain.

Although traumatic events are necessarily (in the case of PTSD) or commonly (in the case of chronic pain) a factor in producing these conditions, there can be a single traumatic event or multiple traumatic events that contribute to each condition. In some cases, a singular traumatic experience can produce both psychological and physical injuries. For example, a military member on a convoy might be exposed to blast from an improvised explosive device (IED) that produces both PTSD and chronic pain. However, it is common for military members and veterans to be exposed to multiple traumatic events during the context of their military service. In a national probability sample, Lehavot et al. (2018) found that 60.5% of female veterans experienced at least one lifetime traumatic event, and 36.2% experienced at least two lifetime traumatic events. Among male veterans, 66.2% experienced at least one lifetime traumatic event, and 40.6% experienced at least two lifetime traumatic events. Thus, the co-occurrence of PTSD and chronic pain can also be the result of events that are experienced at different points in time during a military member's career. An example is a military member who experiences chronic back pain due to physical injuries that result from repeated exposure to riding in convoys or rough terrain or the culmination of carrying heavy equipment during missions. However, in this case, the military member's PTSD is a result of witnessing deaths during a raid and not due to the same events that led to physical injuries underlying the chronic back pain. This example demonstrates how PTSD and chronic pain may co-occur yet also be due to separate events that occurred during the course of the military member's service.

In addition to exposure to traumatic events as a common risk factor for these conditions, other shared vulnerabilities may predispose individuals toward developing PTSD and chronic pain. There is evidence that genetic risk factors may contribute to alterations in neurotransmitter functioning involving neuropeptide Y, serotonin, and GABA, and these alterations may increase risk for the development of PTSD and chronic pain (Asmundson et al., 2002; Scioli-Sater et al., 2015). In addition, individuals exhibiting higher anxiety sensitivity appear to be at greater risk to develop PTSD and chronic pain. This may be due to a tendency for individuals with higher anxiety sensitivity to experience greater emotional reactivity to psychological trauma and physical injury (Asmundson et al., 2002). Higher anxiety sensitivity may also increase hyperresponsiveness to pain by producing attentional bias toward threatening stimuli. In contrast, dissociation, which is symptomatic of PTSD and can occur in response to trauma-related cues or other emotionally distressing triggers, appears to dampen the response time toward identifying increases in pain (Defrin et al., 2015). These factors may work in conjunction such that anxiety sensitivity predisposes individuals to be hyperreactive to painful stimuli, while dissociation undermines the ability to differentiate changes in pain levels (Defrin et al., 2015).

Once PTSD and chronic pain have developed, these conditions may become intertwined and mutually maintaining. This hypothesis has been referred to as the "mutual maintenance" model (Sharp & Harvey, 2001). According to this model, the previously discussed predisposing factors, including attentional bias toward threat and anxiety sensitivity are factors in producing and maintaining co-occurring PTSD and chronic pain. In addition, pain may serve as a reminder of the trauma and recurrently trigger or heighten PTSD symptoms (Sharp & Harvey, 2001). Pain can serve as a direct reminder of the trauma, particularly if the cause of the pain and PTSD are the same or similar events. An example is the case of a Military Member who experiences chronic back and limb pain as a result of a combat blast injury, which is also the event that led to PTSD. In this case, the chronic pain persistently reminds of the trauma and triggers PTSD-related intrusive memories and the constellation of PTSD symptoms that go along with these memories. In the opposite direction, PTSD might simultaneously increase pain by fixating attention toward threatening cues, including the sensations of pain (Defrin et al., 2015). The mutual maintenance model also proposes that avoidance coping also interferes with recovery from these conditions and perpetuates their occurrence (Sharp & Harvey, 2001). In this way, avoidant coping style may both be a predisposing risk factor for these co-occurring conditions and a learned reaction that is employed as a way of attempting to cope with noxious PTSD symptoms and experiences of pain. The role of avoidance was further advanced in the perpetual avoidance model (Liedl & Knaevelsrud, 2008), which proposes that PTSD-related dysfunctional cognitions lead to hyperarousal and, in turn, avoidance and increased pain sensations. Pain is then hypothesized to trigger additional dysfunctional thinking (e.g., catastrophizing about the experiences of pain) and, in turn, more avoidance.

Stratton et al. (2014) examined the association between PTSD and pain symptoms among 208 US military members and veterans who experienced combat-related blast exposure during their service in Afghanistan or Iraq. The sample was mostly male (97%) and White (79%). The study noted that 15% were African American and 6% were listed as "other" races. The association between PTSD and pain were assessed longitudinally at baseline, 6-month follow-up, and 12-month follow-up. As expected, the cross-lagged structural models showed autoregressive effects, such that prior PTSD predicted subsequent PTSD and prior pain predicted subsequent pain. The study found that age was positively related to PTSD and pain, and non-White participants had lower PTSD and pain versus White participants. The study also examined traumatic brain injury (TBI) status and found it to be positively associated with PTSD and pain. After accounting for the autoregressive effects of PTSD and pain along with the effects of age, race, and traumatic brain injury status, the model showed cross-lagged effects such that baseline PTSD predicted pain at 6 month follow-up, and baseline pain predicted PTSD at 6 month follow-up. However, the model showed that the cross-lagged effect from months 6 to 12 was present for PTSD (PTSD at 6-month predicted pain at 12-month) but not for pain (pain at 6-month did not predict PTSD at 12-month). These findings suggest that mutual maintenance between PTSD and pain may occur at more acute periods, whereas PTSD may exert a more sustained impact on pain as time progresses. This indicates that PTSD-focused treatment should be especially provided if these co-occurring conditions have become chronic, since PTSD symptoms were relatively stable and were robustly predictive of pain over time.

5 Treatment for PTSD

In aiding in the clinicians' treatment of veterans with PTSD the VA DoD guidelines begin by explaining that, "While these guidelines are broadly recommended, their implementation is intended to be patient centered. Thus, treatment and care should take into account a patient's needs and preferences.... and should be supported by evidence-based information tailored to the patient's needs" (VA DoD Clinical Practice Guidelines, 2017). When it came to recommending first-line treatment, the 2017 guidelines propose individual trauma-focused psychotherapy over pharmacotherapy. Furthermore, when individual trauma-focused psychotherapy is not available or not preferred, the next recommendation is non-trauma-focused psychotherapy or pharmacotherapy. These two are equally recommended as there was insufficient evidence to recommend one over the other (VA DoD Clinical Practice Guidelines, 2017).

Trauma-focused psychotherapy is defined as "therapy that uses cognitive, emotional, or behavioral techniques to facilitate processing a traumatic experience and in which the trauma focus is a central component of the therapeutic process" (VA DoD Clinical Practice Guidelines, 2017). The therapies for which there is the strongest evidence include: Prolonged Exposure (PE), Cognitive Processing Therapy (CPT), Eye Movement Desensitization and Reprocessing (EMDR), specific cognitive behavioral therapies for PTSD, Brief Eclectic Psychotherapy (BEP), Narrative Exposure Therapy (NET), and written narrative exposure. Regarding manualized non-trauma focused therapies, Stress Inoculation training (SIT), Present Centered therapy (PCT), and Interpersonal Psychotherapy (IPT) are recommended. Finally, there was insufficient evidence to recommend the use of Dialectical Behavior Therapy, Skills Training In Affect and Interpersonal Regulation, Acceptance and Commitment Therapy, Seeking Safety, hypnosis, brief psychodynamic therapy, and supportive counseling. Additionally, there was insufficient evidence to recommend for or against trauma-focus or non-trauma focused couples therapy for the primary treatment of PTSD. There was insufficient evidence to recommend using individual components of manualized psychotherapy protocols over or in addition to the full therapy protocol. And finally, the VA DoD guidelines suggest manualized group therapy treatment over no treatment, but were unable to recommend using one type of group therapy over another due to insufficient evidence (VA DoD Clinical Practice Guidelines, 2017).

When discussing using pharmacotherapy, for patients who are unable to or choose not to engage in one of the aforementioned recommended psychotherapies, four medications are recommended for monotherapy for PTSD: sertraline, paroxetine, fluoxetine, or venlafaxine. Additionally, there was weak evidence for nefazodone, imipramine, or phenelzine, but only if trauma-focus psychotherapy or non-trauma focused psychotherapy are ineffective, unavailable, or not agreeable for patient preference and tolerance (VA DoD Clinical Practice Guidelines, 2017). Finally, preliminary evidence that natural and synthetic cannabinoids could improve PTSD symptoms, particularly nightmares, is offset by the significant side effects, including tolerance, dependence, withdrawal syndrome, psychosis, cognitive deficits, and respiratory symptoms if smoked. A lack of well-designed randomized controlled trials (RCTs) evaluating the efficacy of cannabinoids in large samples of patients with PTSD, together with its serious side effects, does not support the use of natural or synthetic cannabinoids as a treatment for PTSD.

Although complementary and integrative health treatments have been shown to be helpful, the 2017 VA DoD guidelines recommend that, "There is insufficient evidence to recommend any complementary and integrative health (CIH) practice, such as meditation (including mindfulness), yoga, and mantram meditation, as a primary treatment for PTSD" (VA DoD Clinical Practice Guidelines, 2017). The VA DoD Guidelines (2017) acknowledge the widespread use of CIH practices as part of the treatment of individuals with PTSD in the DoD and VA health care systems. This recommendation does not argue against employing these treatments, but rather is stating that there is currently not sufficient evidence to recommend the use of any CIH practice for the primary treatment of PTSD.

Overall, the VA/DoD Guidelines recognize that CIH practices are increasingly offered as part of the treatment of PTSD. These practices hold promise as interventions to improve wellness and promote recovery. Meditation interventions in particular, when offered as augmentation to treatment-as-usual, were associated with a reduction in PTSD symptoms. The VA and DoD concluded that further research is needed to provide more information not only about meditation but other types of CIH as well for the primary and augmented treatment of PTSD (VA DoD Clinical Practice Guidelines, 2017).

6 Treatment for Chronic Pain

VA/DoD Guidelines for Opioid Therapy for Chronic Pain The VA/DoD Guideline for Opioid Therapy for Chronic Pain (2017) starts by explicitly stating that if there are alternatives that are available to opioid therapy (OT), these should first be utilized. The guidelines give examples of self-management strategies, other nonpharmacological treatments, and pharmacologic therapies utilizing non-opioid medication. Additionally, it is recommended that initiating long-term opioid therapy (LOT) be avoided, but specifically for individuals who have untreated SUD, simultaneous benzodiazepine use, and those individuals who are less than 30 years of age. When OT is being initiated, the guidelines continue into recommending less than 90-day dosage, the lowest dose that is clinically indicated. Additionally, it is recommended that random drug testing be utilized, evaluation of risk versus benefits of treatment every 3 months, tapering OT to reduced dose or discontinuation of OT when the risks outweigh the benefits, and interdisciplinary care for holistic treatment. There are additional factors to note when looking at continuing OT for chronic pain, including continuing to assess for risk of SUD and close monitoring of those who may be experiencing concerns regarding SUD. There are several specific flow charts that aid the clinician in deciding to initiate treatment of OT, ongoing treatment with OT, tapering or discontinuing OT, and for patients currently on OT.

VA/DoD Clinical Practice Guidelines for Diagnosis and Treatment of Lower Back Pain The VA/DoD Clinical Practice Guidelines for Diagnosis and Treatment of Lower Back Pain (2017) have similar guidelines for the treatment of lower back pain. Diagnosis of lower back pain begins with recommendations for clinicians to conduct a medical history interview, physical examination, diagnostic imaging, laboratory testing, and mental health screenings. It is also recommended that clinicians provide education about things that patients may be able to do in order to reduce lower back pain, such as remaining active. Cognitive-behavioral therapy is also recommended for individuals with chronic lower back pain, and techniques such as mindful-based stress reduction, and physical exercise programs such as yoga or pilates could also be utilized forms of treatment. For pharmacologic therapy, nonsteroidal anti-inflammatory drugs (NSAIDs) and duloxetine are recommended for chronic low back pain. Non-benzodiazepine muscle relaxants are suggested treatment regimes for acute lower back pain. The guidelines recommended against benzodiazepines, corticosteroids, LOT, and oral acetaminophen for chronic back pain.

Complementary and Alternative Medicine There are several studies that have looked into the effectiveness for complementary and alternative medicine (CAM) treatments for chronic pain (Baure et al., 2016; Kim et al., 2013; Sherman et al., 2004). There are multiple options for CAM treatment of chronic pain, including acupuncture, chiropractic care, massage therapy, self-help groups, spiritual healing, and yoga. One study found that within a sample of individuals with chronic lower back pain, 54% have utilized chiropractic treatment and 38% had utilized massage therapy (Sherman et al., 2004). Based on ratings from individuals who had tried both of these CAM treatments, massage therapy was rated as the most helpful. More recently, a study was compiled looking at the efficacy for many CAM treatments for chronic pain (Baure et al., 2016). Massage therapy was found to be one of the most effective forms of CAM treatment when conducted by a trained and experienced massage therapy. The risks with this type of CAM are relatively minor, with most complaints resulting in muscle soreness. The same article looked at the effectiveness of acupuncture, finding that its effectiveness was inconsistent among patients with lower back pain. However, there was another study that found significant improvement with overall pain intensity resulting from lumbar spinal stenosis (Kim et al., 2013). Dietary and herbal supplements were found to be ineffective in a standalone treatment for chronic pain (Baure et al., 2016). Finally, Yoga was recommended to be offered as an option to explore with patients, due to the relationship that exists between stress and chronic pain, and yoga may be effective in reducing overall stress levels.

7 Treatment of Comorbid PTSD and Chronic Pain

Studies have investigated the integration of various cognitive-behavioral therapy (CBT) protocols for the treatment of co-occurring PTSD and chronic pain. Otis et al. (2009) integrated CPT for PTSD with CBT for chronic pain and pilot-tested this protocol among 6 US Veterans. The protocol included 12 sessions and began with educating the client about PTSD and chronic pain. The protocol then taught clients how to apply skills that were drawn from CPT to address PTSD and chronic pain. These included using worksheets to guide clients in making meaning of the PTSD and pain and engaging in exercises to help clients to recognize and challenge dysfunctional thoughts that were related to PTSD and pain. In addition, the clients learned CBT-based skills to address pain. These included diaphragmatic breathing, progressive muscle relaxation, interoceptive cue exposure, pacing and activity scheduling, and ways to improve sleep hygiene. Three of the six participants did not complete the protocol and general challenges were noted in clients regularly attending therapy sessions and with homework completion. Several of the participants noted that the protocol seemed to be too long. Two of the three participants who completed treatment no longer met diagnosis for PTSD, and both reported reductions in chronic pain symptoms. These pilot study findings showed promise that this integrated treatment might benefit some veterans. However, there were also challenges with treatment engagement and dropout.

A more recent pilot study by Lacefield et al. (2020) investigated the feasibility of applying the Otis et al. (2009) protocol to female veterans with PTSD and fibromyalgia syndrome. The study included 11 participants. Five completed pretreatment assessment but then did not return to engage in the study intervention. Five of the six who engaged in the study intervention completed the full 12 sessions of the protocol. Four of the five who completed treatment reported a reduction in PTSD symptoms and negative impact of fibromyalgia. These findings are promising in suggesting that the protocol may have benefits for those who receive the intervention. However, initial engagement was challenging based upon 5 of the 11 participants that failed to return for treatment after completing the initial study assessment.

Plagge et al. (2013) investigated the implementation of behavioral activation (BA) for addressing PTSD and chronic pain in the context of a multidisciplinary clinic, including primary care, mental health, and physiatry. They noted that the model was built upon evidence suggesting that multidisciplinary clinics show benefits for treating patients with chronic pain. BA was chosen due to its promising benefits for addressing PTSD and helping patients to engage in rewarding activities that may be beneficial for reducing pain. Participants were 58 veterans, and 30 completed treatment. The multidisciplinary team recommended physical therapy for most (85%) of the veterans along with medication pain management (74%) and imaging or other workout (54%). Of the veterans who engaged in BA, 25 received the full 8 sessions. Participants reported medium-to-large effect size reductions in PTSD and medium-to-large reductions in pain severity and interference. This open trial suggested that BA implemented in a multidisciplinary team may be beneficial for veterans with PTSD and chronic pain. However, as with the other studies, attrition was high.

Chopin et al. (2020) completed an open trial pilot study of yoga for veterans with PTSD and chronic pain. The yoga intervention was modified over time and to shorten it from 12 to 8 weeks. The protocol was based upon Hatha Yoga, which involves a focus on breath and bodily alignment. The protocol was standardized with regard to the poses that were covered in each class. Each class began with an inspirational quote and ended with a relaxation exercise. The protocol was modified to be trauma-informed (e.g., no hands-on correction of poses). Eighty-seven veterans attended, and 49 completed the program. After statistically adjusting for multiple comparisons, there were no significant improvements found for PTSD or pain outcomes.

In one of the few randomized controlled trials examining integrated treatment for PTSD and chronic pain, Liedl et al. (2011) tested the efficacy of two active treatments: CBT with physical activity and CBT only. These were compared to a waitlist condition. Study participants were 36 traumatized refugees recruited from a treatment program in Germany. The CBT intervention was ten sessions and included psychoeducation about stress, pain, and PTSD, and use of multiple relaxation strategies such as diaphragmatic breathing, imagery, and progressive muscle relaxation. Cognitive strategies were taught in session 10 to address dysfunctional cognitions. The CBT plus exercise condition involved the aforementioned intervention plus an exercise plan developed with a physical therapist. Although effect size estimates favored the active treatment conditions, there were no significant differences on PTSD or pain outcomes. This may have been, in part, due to the study having a small sample size in each condition and being underpowered.

A randomized, controlled trial of somatic experiencing (SE) was conducted among 91 Danish individuals who exhibited PTSD or subthreshold PTSD along with chronic low back pain (Andersen et al., 2017). SE is based upon the premise of focusing attention on bodily sensations in a manner consistent with interoceptive cue exposure and mindfulness-based techniques. The idea is that learning these skills may help to shift focus away from dysfunctional cognitions and distressing emotions. The protocol was delivered in 6–12 h by a nurse. Participants either completed SE plus treatment as usual or treatment as usual only in the specialty care spine center. Assessors were blinded, and participants were followed for 12 months after completing treatment. The findings showed improvements in PTSD for the SE condition but not in the treatment as usual condition. Pain was unchanged, although the findings indicated reductions on a fear of pain scale for the SE condition but not for the treatment as usual condition.

In summary, studies have investigated integrated CBT-oriented treatments and yoga as an intervention for veterans with co-occurring PTSD and chronic pain. The findings suggest that the integrated CBT interventions may be promising as treatments for veterans with co-occurring PTSD and chronic pain. Pilot research on yoga for veterans did not find significant improvements on outcomes after correcting for multiple statistical comparisons. Each of these open trial studies showed substantial attrition and evidence that treatment engagement may be difficult for veterans with these co-occurring conditions. Two randomized, controlled trials in non-veteran samples also show promise for integrated interventions for PTSD that involve CBT, CBT plus physical activity, or SE. However, more research is needed to know if these findings are generalizable to veterans and military members.

8 Case Study 1

Alice is a 32-year-old, cisgender, White, female, bisexual army veteran. She served one tour in a combat support role in Iraq. She grew up in a lower middle-class family and was raised by her biological mother and stepfather along with her younger brother. She experienced emotional and physical abuse by her stepfather but not sexual abuse. While deployed to Iraq, Alice experienced multiple threats of sexual violence and repeated sexual harassment by several officers who outranked her. She was in constant fear for her safety but was not sexually assaulted. She was exposed to regular mortar rounds, and her convoy was hit by an IED while on a mission. Alice suffered blunt force trauma to her head and injuries to her left leg and back. She survived, but a fellow soldier in the vehicle died as a result of injuries that he suffered. After several months in a military hospital, Alice was discharged. However, she continued to have headaches, back, and leg pain. She also began experiencing nightmares related to her combat traumas and hypervigilance. She was not able to return to regular duty and received a medical discharge from the Army due to her injuries.

After her discharge from the military, Alice was initially seen in a female Veteran's clinic at a VA medical center. Although her headaches were less regular, she told her primary care doctor that she continued to experience sharp shooting pain in her back and leg. Her pain was worse when she sat for long periods, and she found that applying heat or cold would sometimes help with the pain. She was prescribed duloxetine and referred her for physical therapy to try to address her pain. She attended five sessions of physical therapy. She had some reduction in pain frequency and intensity, but the pain in her back and leg continued to persist.

She also screened positive for PTSD and was referred to the PTSD specialty clinic at the VA. She no-showed her first intake at the PTSD clinic. Her primary care provider saw her for a follow-up appointment, and was only after being referred a second time that she followed through with the intake in the PTSD clinic. The findings from her PTSD evaluation showed that she was exhibiting PTSD related to her military service. Most of her PTSD intrusive symptoms were related to the incident in which her convoy was hit by an IED and a fellow soldier in her vehicle was killed. She blamed herself for this incident and often thought that it should have been her who was killed instead of the other soldier. She also reported problems trusting men and people in authority, which became worse after her deployment. She had her fiancé drive her to her appointments and avoided going places during rush hour so that there would be less traffic.

Following the intake in the PTSD clinic, Alice met with a social worker in the PTSD program. They discussed treatment options and Alice's preferences for therapy. Alice selected CPT, citing a preference for writing and deciding that she did not want to have to regularly revisit the details of the traumatic memories in therapy. Alice began attending CPT sessions and noticed that her pain symptoms were becoming worse. She then began to cancel her CPT sessions. Alice spoke with her therapist and agreed to be seen in the VA specialty pain clinic, while also resuming

CPT. Alice's therapist also spoke with her about how avoidance can be a common barrier to completing PTSD treatment. Alice agreed to allow her therapist to speak with her fiancé so that her therapist could talk with her about how she could be supportive of Alice in keeping her appointments and completing the CPT homework. Alice began once again attending CPT and started a CBT pain management group through the multidisciplinary specialty pain clinic. Alice was able to complete the course of CPT and continued with the pain management group. Although she continued to experience some symptoms, she found that both her PTSD symptoms and difficulty in managing pain improved. The plan was for her to continue with less frequent follow-up visits in the PTSD clinic and to continue in seeing providers through the pain clinic.

9 Case Study 2

Julio is a 22-year-old, cisgendered, Mexican American, heterosexual male Marine. His family immigrated to the US when he was 4 years old. Growing up, he was close to his two younger brothers and his biological mother and father. He did not experience emotional, sexual, or physical abuse. Prior to Julio joining the Marines, one of his younger brothers was killed in a hit and run car accident. Julio joined the Marines at age 18 and was deployed to Afghanistan. He was involved in multiple combat missions and firefights. One of the missions involved house raids to locate Taliban, and during this mission, Julio witnessed a civilian being shot and killed. During his deployment, Julio began to experience recurrent lower back pain.

Upon returning from deployment, his back pain became more intense and frequent. He also began to experience occasional numbness in his right leg. He was referred to medical and imaging showed inflammation and compression on his spine. He was assigned to light duty and began to receive physical therapy and NSAIDs.

In addition to dealing with his back injury, he began having problems with sleep and started to drink more. He got into a fight at a local bar and was sent by command to see a psychologist on base. He initially denied being bothered by the combat traumas, but then, after learning to trust the psychologist, he admitted that he was having nightmares related to witnessing the civilian being killed in Afghanistan. He was further assessed and determined to have PTSD. He started to attend an alcohol treatment program that involved group counseling and agreed to see the psychologist for individual counseling. After discussing treatment options, he agreed to try a course of PE. After the first several sessions, he noticed that his back pain was worse and he was thinking more about the trauma. He considered quitting the treatment, but the psychologist advised him that it is common for military members to experience a temporary increase in some of these symptoms during the initial parts of PE. Julio agreed to stay with the treatment. After several more symptoms, he noticed that the intrusive memories and nightmares were becoming less frequent. He also felt less hypervigilant. He completed physical therapy and was able to return to a regular exercise routine, which further improved his lower back pain. After the course of PE was completed, he saw the psychologist for a follow-up visit and found that he was doing well in maintaining his treatment gains.

10 Conclusion and Future Directions

As noted in this chapter, PTSD and chronic pain are relatively common conditions that often co-occur among military members and veterans. The etiology of these conditions may be, in part, explained by the psychologically and physically demanding nature of military duty and traumas that can occur in the course of military service. Other shared underlying risk factors might also predispose some individuals to developing these conditions following exposure to trauma and injuries. Separate VA/DoD guidelines have been developed for assessment and PTSD, use of opioids in the context of chronic pain, and assessment and treatment of chronic lower back pain. These provide helpful information for diagnosing and treating each of these individual conditions. The current evidence suggests that multidisciplinary teams and multimodal forms of treatment may provide benefits to those with PTSD and chronic pain. However, there is limited research on the efficacy of integrated treatments to simultaneously treat this comorbidity. Findings to date suggest that treatment engagement and dropout may be challenges that are regularly encountered by providers and those with these co-occurring conditions. Future research is needed to improve treatment engagement and retention as well as examining the efficacy of multidisciplinary and multimodal approaches to treating PTSD and chronic pain among military members and veterans.

References

American Psychiatric Association. (2013). *Diagnostic and statistical manual of mental disorders: DSM-5* (5th ed.). Author.

Andersen, T. E., Lahav, Y., Ellegaard, H., & Manniche, C. (2017). A randomized controlled trial of brief Somatic Experiencing for chronic low back pain and comorbid post-traumatic stress disorder symptoms. *European Journal of Psychotraumatology, 8*(1). https://doi.org/10.1080/20008198.2017.1331108

Armed Forces Health Surveillance Branch. (2017). Mental health conditions among active component U.S. Armed Forces. Defense Medical Surveillance System (DMSS). *Public Health Division, Defense Health Agency.*

Asmundson, G. J. G., Coons, M. J., Taylor, S., & Katz, J. (2002). PTSD and the experience of pain: Research and clinical implications of shared vulnerability and mutual maintenance models. *The Canadian Journal of Psychiatry/La Revue Canadienne de Psychiatrie, 47*(10), 930–937.

Baure, B. A., Tilburt, J. C., Sood, A., Guang-Xi, L., & Shi-han, W. (2016). Complementary and alternative medicine therapies for chronic pain. *Chinese Journal of Integrative Medicine, 22,* 403–411.

Benedict, T. M., Singleton, M. D., Nitz, A. J., Shing, T. L., & Kardouni, J. R. (2019). Effect of chronic low back pain and post-traumatic stress disorder on the risk for separation from the US army. *Military Medicine, 184*(9–10), 431–439. https://doi.org/10.1093/milmed/usz020

Brennstuhl, M., Tarquinio, C., & Montel, S. (2014). Chronic pain and PTSD: Evolving views on their comorbidity. *Perspective is Psychiatric Care, 51*, 295–304.

Chopin, S. M., Sheerin, C. M., & Meyer, B. L. (2020). Yoga for warriors: An intervention for veterans with comorbid chronic pain and PTSD. *Psychological Trauma Theory Research Practice and Policy*. Advance online publication. https://doi.org/10.1037/tra0000649

Defrin, R., Schreiber, S., & Ginzburg, K. (2015). Paradoxical pain perception in posttraumatic stress disorder: The unique role of anxiety and dissociation. *The Journal of Pain, 16*(10), 961–970. https://doi.org/10.1016/j.jpain.2015.06.010

Eber, S., Barth, S., Kang, H., et al. (2013). The National Health Study for a New Generation of United States Veterans: Methods for a large-scale study on the health of recent veterans. *Military Medicine, 178*, 966–969.

Gironda, R. J., Clark, M. E., Massengale, J. P., & Walker, R. L. (2006). Pain among veterans of Operations Enduring Freedom and Iraqi Freedom. *Pain Medicine, 7*(4), 339–343.

Greenberg, G., & Hoff, R. (2016). *FY 2016 Veterans with PTSD data sheet: National, VISN, and VAMC tables*. Northeast Program Evaluation Center.

Gros, D. F., Szafranski, D. D., Brady, K. T., & Back, S. E. (2015). Relations between pain, PTSD symptoms, and substance use in veterans. *Psychiatry, 78*, 277–287.

Harpaz-Rotem, I., & Hoff, R. (2015). *FY 2015 overview of PTSD patient population data sheet*. VA Office of Mental Health Operations. Northeast Program Evaluation Center.

Haskell, S. G., Brandt, C. A., Krebs, E. E., Skanderson, M., Kerns, R. D., & Goulet, J. L. (2009). Pain among veterans of Operations Enduring Freedom and Iraqi Freedom: Do women and men differ? *Pain Medicine, 10*(7), 1167–1173. https://doi.org/10.1111/j.1526-4637.2009.00714.x

International Association for the Study of Pain. (1986). *Classification of chronic pain*. Author.

International Association for the Study of Pain. (2017). *IASP terminology*. Retrieved 28 Oct 2020 from https://www.iasp-pain.org/Education/Content.aspx?ItemNumber=1698

Jakupcak, M., Osborne, T., Michael, S., Cook, J., Albrizio, P., & McFall, M. (2006). Anxiety sensitivity and depression: Mechanisms for understanding somatic complaints in veterans with posttraumatic stress disorder. *Journal of Traumatic Stress, 19*, 471–479.

Kessler, R. C., Heeringa, S. G., Stein, M. B., et al. (2014). Thirty-day prevalence of DSM-IV mental disorders among nondeployed soldiers in the US Army: Results from the Army study to assess risk and resilience in Service Members (Army STARRS). *JAMA Psychiatry, 71*(5), 504–513.

Kim, K. H., Kim, T. H., Lee, B. R., Kim, J. K., Son, D. W., & Lee, S. W. (2013). Acupuncture for lumbar spinal stenosis: A systemic review and meta-analysis. *Complementary Therapy Medicine, 21*, 535–556.

Lacefield, K., Samph, S. P., Orbon, S., & Otis, J. (2020). Integrated intervention for comorbid posttraumatic stress disorder and fibromyalgia: A pilot study of women veterans. *Psychological Trauma Theory Research Practice and Policy, 12*(7), 725–729. https://doi.org/10.1037/tra0000635

Lehavot, K., Katon, J. G., Chen, J. A., Fortney, J. C., & Simpson, T. L. (2018). Post-traumatic stress disorder by gender and veteran status. *American Journal of Preventive Medicine, 54*(1), e1–e9. https://doi.org/10.1016/j.amepre.2017.09.008

Lew, H. L., Otis, J. D., Tun, C., Kerns, R. D., Clark, M. E., & Cifu, D. X. (2009). Prevalence of chronic pain, posttraumatic stress disorder, and persistent postconcussive symptoms in OIF/OEF veterans: Polytrauma clinical triad. *Journal of Rehabilitation Research and Development, 46*(6), 697–702. https://doi.org/10.1682/JRRD.2009.01.0006

Liedl, A., Müller, J., Morina, N., Karl, A., Denke, C., & Knaevelsrud, C. (2011). Physical activity within a CBT intervention improves coping with pain in traumatized refugees: Results of a randomized controlled design. *Pain Medicine, 12*(2), 234–245. https://doi.org/10.1111/j.1526-4637.2010.01040.x

Liedl, A., & Knaevelsrud, C. (2008). Chronic pain and PTSD: The perpetual avoidance model and its treatment implications. *Torture: Quarterly Journal on Rehabilitation of Torture Victims and Prevention of Torture, 18*(2), 69–76.

Magruder, K. M., & Yeager, D. E. (2019). The prevalence of PTSD across war eras and the effect of deployment on PTSD: A systematic review and meta-analysis. *Psychiatric Annals, 39*(8), 778–788.

Mayou, R., & Bryant, B. (2001). Outcome in consecutive emergency department attenders following a road traffic accident. *British Journal of Psychiatry, 179*, 528–534.

McWilliams, L. A., Cox, B. J., & Enns, M. W. (2003). Mood and anxiety disorders associated with chronic pain: An examination in a nationally representative sample. *Pain, 106*, 127–133.

Morasco, B., Gritzner, S., Lewis, L., Oldham, R., Turk, D. C., & Dobscha, S. K. (2011). Systematic review of prevalence, correlates, and treatment outcomes for chronic non-cancer pain in patients with comorbid substance use disorder. *Pain, 152*, 488–497.

Otis, J. D., Gregor, K., Hardway, C., Morrison, J., Scioli, E., & Sanderson, E. (2010). An examination of the co-morbidity between chronic pain and posttraumatic stress disorder on US veterans. *Psychological Services, 7*(3), 126–135.

Otis, J. D., Keane, T. M., Kerns, R. D., Monson, C., & Scioli, E. (2009). The development of an integrated treatment for veterans with comorbid chronic pain and posttraumatic stress disorder. *Pain Medicine, 10*(7), 1300–1311. https://doi.org/10.1111/j.1526-4637.2009.00715.x

Outcalt, S. D., Yu, Z., Hoen, H. M., Pennington, T. M., & Krebs, E. E. (2014). Health care utilization among veterans with pain and posttraumatic stress symptoms. *Pain Medicine, 15*(11), 1872–1879.

Outcalt, S. D., Kroenke, K., Krebs, E. E., Chumbler, N. R., Wu, J., Yu, Z., & Bair, M. J. (2015). Chronic pain and comorbid mental health conditions: Independent associations of posttraumatic stress disorder and depression with pain, disability, and quality of life. *Journal of Behavioral Medicine, 38*, 535–543.

Plagge, J. M., Lu, M. W., Lovejoy, T. I., Karl, A. I., & Dobscha, S. K. (2013). Treatment of comorbid pain and PTSD in returning veterans: A collaborative approach utilizing behavioral activation. *Pain Medicine, 14*(8), 1164–1172. https://doi.org/10.1111/pme.12155

Sareen, J., Cox, B., Stein, M., Afifi, T., Fleet, C., & Asmundson, G. (2007). Physical and mental co-morbidity, disability, and suicidal behavior associated with posttraumatic stress disorder in a large community sample. *Psychosomatic Medicine, 69*, 242–248.

Scioli-Salter, E. R., Forman, D. E., Otis, J. D., Gregor, K., Valovski, I., & Rasmusson, A. M. (2015). The shared neuroanatomy and neurobiology of comorbid chronic pain and PTSD. *Clinical Journal of Pain, 31*(4), 363–374. https://doi.org/10.1097/AJP.0000000000000115

Sharp, T. J., & Harvey, A. G. (2001). Chronic pain and posttraumatic stress disorder: Mutual maintenance? *Clinical Psychology Review, 21*(6), 857–877. https://doi.org/10.1016/S0272-7358(00)00071-4

Sherman, K. J., Cherkin, D. C., Connelly, M. T., Erro, J., Savetsky, J. B., Davis, R. B., & Eisenberg, D. M. (2004). Complementary and alternative medical therapies for chronic low back pain: What treatments are patients willing to try? *BMC Complementary and Alternative Medicine, 4*, 9.

Shipherd, J. C., Keyes, M., Jovanovic, T., Ready, D. J., Baltzell, D., Worley, V., Gordon-Brown, V., Hayslett, C., & Duncan, E. (2007). Veterans seeking treatment for posttraumatic stress disorder: What about comorbid chronic pain? *Journal of Rehabilitation Research and Development, 44*(2), 153–165. https://doi.org/10.1682/jrrd.2006.06.0065

Sterling, M., Jull, G., Vicenzio, B., Kenardy, J., & Darnell, R. (2005). Physical and psychological factors predict outcome following whiplash injury. *Pain, 114*, 141–148.

Stratton, K. J., Clark, S. L., Hawn, S. E., Amstadter, A. B., Cifu, D. X., & Walker, W. C. (2014). Longitudinal interactions of pain and posttraumatic stress disorder symptoms in US military service members following blast exposure. *The Journal of Pain, 15*(10), 1023–1032. https://doi.org/10.1016/j.jpain.2014.07.002

Tanielian, T., & Jaycox, L. H. (Eds.). (2008). *Invisible wounds of war: Psychological and cognitive injuries, their consequences, and services to assist recovery*. RAND Corporation.

U.S. Department of Veterans Affairs. (2015). *PTSD in Iraq and Afghanistan Veterans*. Available at www.publichealth.va.gov/epidemiology/studies/new-generation/ptsd.asp

VA/DoD Clinical Practice Guidelines for Diagnosis and Treatment of Lower Back Pain. (2017). Authors.

VA/DoD Guideline for Opioid Therapy for Chronic Pain. (2017). Authors.

VonKoff, M., Crane, P., Lane, M., Miglioretti, D. L., Simon, G., Saunders, K., & Kessler, R. (2005). Chronic spinal pain and physical-mental co-morbidity in the United States: Results from the national comorbidity survey replication. *Pain, 113*, 331–339.

Wisco, B. E., Marx, B. P., Wolf, E. J., Miller, M. W., Southwick, S. M., & Pietrzak, R. H. (2014). Posttraumatic stress disorder in the US Veteran population: Results from the national health and resilience in Veterans study. *Journal of Clinical Psychiatry, 75*(12), 1338–1346.

Chapter 11
Clinical Health Psychologists' Role in the COVID-19 Response in Veteran and Military Hospitals

Kelsey J. Pritchard and Larry C. James

The coronavirus disease 2019 (COVID-19) pandemic produced psychosocial stressors across the globe. Stressors that include social isolation, financial loss, and the disruption of daily routines were detrimental to long-term mental health as well for all populations affected (Gruber et al., 2020). In particular, the pandemic drastically altered the quality of life for military personnel and veterans. Psychologists in every sector of society, including in veteran and military hospitals, were faced with medical, psychological, and social challenges for both themselves and their patients. In the wake of the COVID-19 pandemic, health psychologists were called upon to better understand individuals' responses to the pandemic's effects on their daily lives, the public's transmission-related behaviors, and the potential psychosocial and physical impact of COVID-19 on frontline health care workers (Arden & Chilcot, 2020; Castelnuovo et al., 2020; Kazak, 2020). Health psychologists can apply their expertise to COVID-19-related health behaviors, including resistance to vaccine recommendations, mask wearing, and social isolation. Further, health psychologists can conduct essential public health research related to public health communication, health disparities, and the prolonged effects of the COVID-19 pandemic (Freedland et al., 2020).

This chapter describes how clinical health psychologists, the Veteran's Health Administration (VHA), and military hospitals adapted to address mental health service delivery in the face of the unique challenges posed by the COVID-19 pandemic. The sections that follow will summarize the impact of COVID-19 on military service members, veterans, military hospital administration, and frontline workers. Further, this chapter will discuss health psychology's role in the VHA's response to

K. J. Pritchard (✉)
Louis Stokes Cleveland Department of Veterans Affairs Medical Center, Cleveland, OH, USA
e-mail: kelsey.pritchard@rockets.utoledo.edu

L. C. James
Department of Behavioral Health, Tripler Army Medical Center, Honolulu, HI, USA

L. C. James et al. (eds.), *Clinical Health Psychology in Military and Veteran Settings*, https://doi.org/10.1007/978-3-031-12063-3_11

service delivery, will outline the factors that contributed to enabling access to services, and discuss the factors that impeded this progress. Finally, this chapter will discuss recommendations and will review areas for future work for health psychologists in veteran and military hospitals in future pandemics.

1 Impact of COVID-19 on Military and Veterans

Providing mental health treatment is essential during any global disaster. Pandemics and natural disasters are known to increase rates of depression, post-traumatic stress disorder (PTSD), and substance use disorders (SUD) in civilian populations (Galea et al., 2020). Symptoms of depression, anxiety, and substance abuse increased substantially in the United States population during the early phases of the COVID-19 pandemic (Czeisler et al., 2020; Holingue et al., 2020a, b; Holman et al., 2020). Military and veteran populations, however, held pre-existing vulnerabilities before the pandemic, including higher rates of suicide, psychiatric disorders, physical health conditions, and psychosocial stressors relative to nonveterans (Bruce, 2010; Levine & Sher, 2021). Veterans, as a vulnerable population, are at a higher risk of poor health because they experience barriers to vital resources (e.g., social, economic, political, and environmental) and limitations due to illness or disability. Veterans frequently report elevated rates of adverse childhood experiences (Katon et al., 2015), intimate partner violence, and military sexual trauma (Gerber, 2019). Thus, researchers posited that COVID-19 would place veterans and military service members at a unique risk for long-term mental health effects, given their pre-existing psychological vulnerabilities (Gerber, 2020; Ramchand et al., 2020).

Individuals with pre-existing mental illness are more likely to suffer worsened distress in response to pandemics (Egede et al., 2020; Panchal et al., 2020). While there is a dearth of research on the effects of pandemics on military and veteran populations, military personnel in humanitarian disasters have been shown to experience increased depressive and trauma symptoms (Cunha et al., 2018; West & Morganstein, 2016). Given evidence that the effects of the pandemic can contribute to the development and exacerbation of mental health symptoms, psychologists and clinicians must be aware of the impact of COVID-19 on veteran and military populations (Gerber, 2020; Ramchand et al., 2020). Indeed, preliminary studies have shown that veterans reported increased levels of depression, anxiety, and loneliness after the start of the COVID-19 pandemic, relative to pre-COVID-19 (Wynn et al., 2020a, b).

An estimated 30.9%, 12.1%, and 13.8% of Vietnam, Gulf War, and post-9/11 veterans meet criteria for a diagnosis of PTSD, respectively (Kang et al., 2003; Kulka et al., 1990; Tanielian et al., 2008). Acute stress disorder (ASD) and PTSD are likely to develop or worsen in military personnel and veterans due to several costly COVID-19 stressors, including significant life disruption, threats to safety, erosion of social supports, deaths of loved ones, and loss of financial supports

(Bonanno et al., 2010; Marini et al., 2020). Experiencing symptoms of PTSD also places individuals at risk for substance abuse and suicidal ideation (Sareen, 2014). The COVID-19 pandemic may also increase suicide rates among veterans (Gunnel et al., 2020; Levine & Sher, 2021; Sher, 2020). Indeed, a 2020 report by the Wounded Warriors Project concluded that "lack of social connection (loneliness) along with co-occurring mental health conditions (PTSD, depression, suicidal ideation) exacerbates and magnifies the burden warriors experience during adverse events like COVID-19" (Wounded Warrior Project, 2020). Conversely, the COVID-19 pandemic led to a decrease in VA psychiatric emergency room visits, suggesting that many veterans may have postponed necessary mental health and substance use treatment (Mitchell & Fuehrlein, 2021).

Those with PTSD are also at increased risk of developing physical health problems including obesity and sleep disturbances (Kubansky et al., 2014). In a cross-sectional analysis report of COVID-19 patient demographics, infection, mortality, and case-fatality rates in the veteran population, researchers found that 59.7% were 65-or-more years old, 92.5% were men, 68.7% were white, and 14.2% were black. Veterans over the age of 65 comprised 52.1% of cases and 89.9% of deaths (Luo et al., 2021). Veteran COVID-19 mortality was also associated with increased strains on VHA hospital capacity (Bravata et al., 2021).

1.1 Caregiver and Provider Stress

In addition to military and veterans, caregivers of individuals with mental illness are also at increased risk for developing mental illness (Ramchand et al., 2014). The mental health needs of healthcare workers should also not be neglected (Zaka et al., 2020). At present, there is little research that addresses the mental health needs of health care workers (Gruber et al., 2020). Health care workers are burdened by the task of managing the needs of their COVID-19 patients while putting themselves and coworkers at increased risk for transmission of the virus. From studies of prior pandemics, health care workers may suffer social isolation due to being perceived as having higher risk of infection (Williams et al., 2011). During prior pandemics, health care workers with a history of mental illness were more likely to report experiencing symptom relapse (Lai et al., 2020; Lancee et al., 2008).

2 Veteran Health Administration's Response to Service Provision During COVID-19

The Veterans Health Administration (VHA) is the nation's largest integrated health care system, providing annual services to over six million veterans at 1286 sites and mental health care to 1.7 million veterans alone in 2019 (Connolly et al., 2020a, b;

Harpaz-Rotem & Hoff, 2020; VHA Support Service Center, 2020). The VHA's initial response to COVID-19's challenges was driven by three priorities: (1) to continue providing mental health care to millions of patients; (2) to prevent the spread of COVID-19 in medical centers while balancing patient and staff safety; and (3) to expand access to mental health care in high-risk locations and states under "stay at home" orders (Heyworth et al., 2020). The VHA and psychologists were primarily able to address these priorities by delivering virtual care to patients.

2.1 VHA's Expansion of Virtual Care

As the nation's largest integrated healthcare system, the VHA has been a pioneer in implementing and developing telemental health for decades prior to the COVID-19 pandemic (Adams et al., 2019; Darkins, 2014; Perrin et al., 2020). In 2019 alone, VHA providers delivered nearly 786,000 video telemental health encounters to more than 230,000 veterans (Rosen et al., 2020). Thus, the VHA was well-prepared to expand telemental health by the onset of COVID-19. The rapid transition to telehealth psychotherapy services was spurred following COVID-19 restrictions of nonurgent in-person appointments. To address this challenge, the VHA specifically directed in-person psychotherapy visits to transition to telehealth appointments (Heyworth et al., 2020). Five key avenues were critical in rapidly shifting the VHA's virtual care initiative: (1) providing training to both staff and patients; (2) growing the VHA's technology infrastructure; (3) providing consistent messaging to diverse stakeholders; (4) meeting the needs of high-risk patients; and (5) as necessary, expanding support of the private sector (Heyworth et al., 2020). The US Department of Defense (DoD) published the DoD COVID-19 *Practice Management Guidelines: Clinical Management of COVID-19* (Matos & Chung, 2020), and, within these guidelines, the Department of Psychiatry at the Uniformed Services University in the DoD developed a Mental Health and Well-Being toolkit to support patients and medical providers (Uniformed Services University and Defense Health Agency, 2020). The VHA increased telemental health service delivery, which subsequently decreased in-person appointments by 80% (Rosen et al., 2020). In just the first six weeks following the World Health Organization's (WHO) pandemic declaration (March 11, 2020–April 22, 2020), daily telemental health encounters grew 556%, while in-person psychotherapy appointments dropped by 81% (Connolly et al., 2020a, b).

Other divisions of the VHA also quickly adapted to meet the unique needs of patients. Prior to COVID-19, the Cohen Veterans Network (CVN) was established to provide behavioral health care to veterans and their families. By late March 2020, CVN clinics converted more than 90% of their clinical services to telehealth (Shelton et al., 2020). The COVID-19 pandemic and stay-at-home orders put women veterans at a higher risk for interpersonal partner violence. As such, the VHA's existing Intimate Partner Violence Assistance Program (IPVAP) provided guidelines for screening and intervention through telehealth formats (Rossi et al.,

2020). In sum, not only was the VHA network prepared to manage the mental health of its broad veteran population, but also the unique needs of veteran subpopulations.

2.2 *Telemental Health*

Pre-pandemic teletherapy faced several barriers to its inception, including intrapsychic barriers (e.g., bias and low self-efficacy), environmental barriers (e.g., federal HIPAA security, Medicare regulations, state laws and regulations, and settings in which psychologists practice), and technical issues with clinicians or patients (Pierce et al., 2020). Nonetheless, the research shows great promise for the efficacy of virtual teletherapy. At least a decade of research supports the efficacy of psychological interventions delivered over the telephone, particularly in interventions targeting PTSD, depression, and anxiety (Varker et al., 2019). In several studies comparing teletherapy to traditional therapy, patients completed a higher number of sessions than those participating in face-to-face therapy (Hernandez-Tejada et al., 2014). In a systematic review, Turgoose et al. (2018) found that veterans with PTSD reported high levels of acceptability and satisfaction using teletherapy. Despite common misconceptions, evidence suggests that at least similar to strong therapeutic alliances can be established via telephone therapy (Irvine et al., 2020; Stiles-Shields et al., 2014). Telephone psychotherapy has also been shown to reduce suicidality (Rhee et al., 2005), as well as to successfully prevent relapse and improve health behaviors (Baker et al., 2018). Several treatment studies of veterans with PTSD found video teletherapy as effective as in-person psychotherapy (Acierno et al., 2016, 2017; Morland et al., 2010, 2014, 2015, 2019, 2020). Studies across a range of mental health conditions report high rates of patient satisfaction with video telemental health treatment (Campbell et al., 2015; Fletcher et al., 2018).

2.3 *Adjustment to Teletherapy During COVID-19*

Prior to the COVID-19 pandemic, psychologists working in Veterans Affairs medical centers performed 11.28% of their clinical work using telepsychology, which increased seven-fold to 80.65% during the pandemic (Pierce et al., 2020). The COVID-19 pandemic ameliorated much of psychologists' bias and barriers to teletherapy. During COVID-19, mental health practitioners reported positive experiences with telemental health that include treatment effectiveness, increased flexibility of services, lower threshold for contact, and a lack of travel time for delivering services (Feijt et al., 2020). In a recent review of clinicians' attitudes toward via videoconference telemental health, clinicians reported that video teletherapy was effective, they valued the improved access to care, they saved time and money, and experienced increased flexibility in their duties (Connolly et al., 2020a, b). Furthermore, most psychotherapists identified having a positive attitude toward online therapy, suggesting they are likely to keep using online therapy in the future (Bekes & Doorn, 2020).

Patient agreeableness and openness to telehealth and teletherapy also improved after the start of COVID-19. Relative to other types of care (e.g., primary care, rehabilitation care, specialty care), mental health care had the greatest percentage and number of video-based encounters provided in VA outpatient settings (Ferguson et al., 2020). One study found that veterans with a previous PTSD clinical diagnosis were more likely to get tested for COVID-19, and were less likely to test positive, than veterans without PTSD, which may indicate increased social isolation among veterans with PTSD (Haderlein et al., 2020). Outcomes for veterans during the COVID-19 pandemic may be promoted by encouraging veterans to engage in positive but safe social contact and by using existing coping skills that aided their resilience during past stressors (Fiori, 2020). Cornwell et al. (2021) compared Primary Care-Mental Health Integration (PC-MHI) service utilization in the VHA system before and after COVID-19 was declared a national emergency. While PCMHI services initially saw drastic increases of phone and home telemental health encounters (147% and 645%, respectively), overall encounters decreased to 82% of pre-pandemic volumes with some sites experiencing continual declines. Such increases suggest more acceptability of virtual care, while declines may be attributed to sites with limited to no access to remote care (Cornwell et al., 2021).

3 Post-pandemic Challenges and Future Directions for Health Psychologists in Military and Veteran Hospitals

Heyworth et al. (2020) reported several lessons learned from the VHA's expansion of virtual health in the initial months of the COVID-19 pandemic. First, clinicians' ability to conduct services across state lines was critical to the VHA's ability to marshal a national provision of telehealth services. Therefore, health psychologists and VHA administration should aim to promote service delivery across state lines in future pandemics to enhance military personnel and veterans' access and acceptability of services. Second, staff and patients displayed variable openness toward the adoption of telehealth, with many veterans opting to receive telehealth services by phone than by video-to-home methods. While the reasons for such are unknown, future research should aim to find the most ideal balance of in-person and virtual service delivery for patients. Third, many areas of the U.S. still have underdeveloped technological infrastructures. Thus, health psychologists and VHA administration should collaborate to expand internet and cellular access to military and veteran populations in rural or remote areas of the country to also provide access to telemental health in the future. Fourth, payment for clinical services was found to be both an incentive and barrier to virtual health care. Prior to COVID-19, the VHA was compensated three times more for video-to-home services than phone-only services, leading the VA to incentivize video-to-home services regardless of phone visits being both more accessible and preferred by patients. Health psychologists should advocate for the VHA to evaluate existing payment policies in order to balance the use of video and phone service delivery. Fifth, mental healthcare experienced the largest increase in video-to-home telehealth services relative to other specialties (e.g., primary care). Health psychologists may wish to further study the reasons for such differences, including patient preferences and clinicians' requirements for visual observation of their patients. Sixth, the adoption of a learning health organizational model was significant toward expanding the rapid transition to telehealth (Heyworth et al., 2020). The learning health model ensured that VHA hospitals could implement and monitor telehealth service delivery to provide continual improvement of services.

3.1 Maintaining Frontline Providers' Well-being

The relationship between provider and patient well-being is bidirectional. In future public health crises, health psychologists may prevent strain on military and veteran health care systems by promoting more self-awareness and self-care in their respective patient populations (Arora & Grey, 2020). Likewise, frontline responders who maintain basic self-care are likely to perform their best, while maintaining clear, concise, and consistent communication between team members, patients, and their families will facilitate the best outcomes. Thus, it is essential the frontline providers' mental and physical health are maintained during public health crises. Maintaining self-care and crisis communication are key elements to guide military mental healthcare provision (Wynn et al., 2020a, b). Interventions to improve frontline health care workers' mental health should initially target basic human needs, including promoting rest and health safety, followed by targeting more advanced psychological needs and other adaptive interventions (e.g., communication, problem-solving, and general coping skills; Zaka et al., 2020). Researchers have presented several basic guidelines for upkeeping medical provider well-being, some of which include connecting to a sense of unified purpose, recognizing burnout in self and others, focusing on what can be controlled, and accepting what cannot be controlled (Wynn et al., 2020a, b). For mental health providers, recommendations include providing proactive support to frontline workers (medical and support staff), tailoring support as much as possible, and facilitating additional mental health care for individuals in high need. Other approaches to maintaining health care workers' mental health include working with military and veteran hospitals to create supportive environments, developing systems for monitoring mental health concerns, increasing access to resources for reducing daily life stress, and assessing training needs of pandemic health care workers (Gruber et al., 2020).

3.2 Implementing and Improving Teletherapy Technology

Health psychologists may facilitate technological mental health treatment in veterans by increasing veterans' access to technology, promoting technology literacy, increasing patient buy-in, and familiarizing themselves with such tools (Gould & Hantke, 2020; Gould et al., 2020). Considering that many adults access the internet with smartphones, mental health apps may be beneficial for military serving members and veterans, and the U.S. Department of Veterans' Affairs already provides a library of free mental health apps (https://www.mobile.va.gov/; Torous & Keshavan, 2020). Though there is limited evidence for the efficacy and effectiveness of mental health apps (Marshall et al., 2020a, b), the VA provides at least one app to treat PTSD and has been the primary research base for the efficacy of mental health apps to treat PTSD (Kuhn et al., 2017; Owen et al., 2018).

Conflict of Interest Kelsey Pritchard is employed by the Department of Veterans Affairs. Larry James is employed by the Department of the Army. The views expressed here are those of the author(s) and do not necessarily represent the views, position, or policy of the Department of Veterans Affairs, Veterans Health Administration, or the United States Government.

References

Acierno, R., Gros, D. F., Ruggiero, K. J., Hernandez-Tejada, B. M., Knapp, R. G., Lejuez, C. W., Muzzy, M., Frueh, C. B., Egede, L. E., & Tuerk, P. W. (2016). Behavioral activation and therapeutic exposure for posttraumatic stress disorder: A noninferiority trial of treatment delivered in person versus home-based telehealth. *Depression & Anxiety, 33*(5), 415–423. https://doi.org/10.1002/da.22476

Acierno, R., Knapp, R., Tuerk, P., Gilmore, A. K., Lejuez, C., Ruggiero, K., Muzzy, W., Egede, L., Hernandez-Tejada, M. A., & Foa, E. B. (2017). A non-inferiority trial of prolonged exposure for posttraumatic stress disorder: In person versus home-based telehealth. *Behaviour Research and Therapy, 89*, 57–65. https://doi.org/10.1016/j.brat.2016.11.009

Adams, S. V., Mader, M. J., Bollinger, M. J., Wong, E. S., Hudson, T. J., & Littman, A. J. (2019). Utilization of interactive clinical video telemedicine by rural and urban veterans in the Veterans Health Administration health care system. *The Journal of Rural Health, 35*(3), 308–318. https://doi.org/10.1111/jrh.12343

Arden, M. A., & Chilcot, J. (2020). Health psychology and the coronavirus (COVID-19) global pandemic: A call for research. *British Journal of Health Psychology, 25*(2), 231–232. https://doi.org/10.1111/bjhp.12414

Arora, T., & Grey, I. (2020). Health behaviour changes during COVID-19 and the potential consequences: A mini-review. *Journal of Health Psychology, 25*(9), 1155–1163. https://doi.org/10.1177/1359105320937053

Baker, A. L., Turner, A., Beck, A., Berry, K., Haddock, G., Kelly, P. J., & Bucci, S. (2018). Telephone-delivered psychosocial interventions targeting key health priorities in adults with a psychotic disorder: Systematic review. *Psychological Medicine, 48*(16), 2637–2657. https://doi.org/10.1017/S0033291718001125

Békés, V., & Aafjes-van Doorn, K. (2020). Psychotherapists' attitudes toward online therapy during the COVID-19 pandemic. *Journal of Psychotherapy Integration, 30*(2), 238–247. https://psycnet.apa.org/doi/10.1037/int0000214

Bonanno, G. A., Brewin, C. R., Kaniasty, K., & La Greca, A. M. (2010). Weighing the costs of disaster: Consequences, risks, and resilience in individuals, families, and communities. *Psychological Science in the Public Interest, 11*(1), 1–49. https://doi.org/10.1177/1529100610387086
Bravata, D. M., Perkins, A. J., Myers, L. J., Arling, G., Zhang, Y., Zillich, A. J., Reese, L., Dysangco, A., Agarwal, R., Myers, J., Austin, C., Sexson, A., Leonard, S. J., Dev, S., & Keyhani, S. (2021). Association of intensive care unit patient load and demand with mortality rates in US Department of Veterans Affairs hospitals during the COVID-19 pandemic. *JAMA Network Open, 4*(1), e2034266. https://doi.org/10.1001/jamanetworkopen.2020.34266
Bruce, M. L. (2010). Suicide risk and prevention in veteran populations. *Annals of the New York Academy of Sciences, 1208*(1), 98–103. https://doi.org/10.1111/j.1749-6632.2010.05697.x
Campbell, R., O'Gorman, J., & Cernovsky, Z. Z. (2015). Reactions of psychiatric patients to telepsychiatry. *Mental Illness, 7*(2), 54–55. https://doi.org/10.1108/mi.2015.6101
Castelnuovo, G., De Giorgio, A., Manzoni, G. M., Treadway, D. C., & Mohiyeddini, C. (2020). Psychological, behavioral, and interpersonal effects and clinical implications for health systems of the coronavirus (COVID-19) pandemic: A call for research. *Frontiers in Psychology, 11*, 2146. https://doi.org/10.3389/fpsyg.2020.02146
Connolly, S. L., Miller, C. J., Lindsay, J. A., & Bauer, M. S. (2020a). A systematic review of providers' attitudes toward telemental health via videoconferencing. *Clinical Psychology: Science and Practice, 27*(2), e12311. https://doi.org/10.1111/cpsp.12311
Connolly, S. L., Stolzmann, K. L., Heyworth, L., Weaver, K. R., Bauer, M. S., & Miller, C. J. (2020b). Rapid increase in telemental health within the Department of Veterans Affairs during the COVID-19 pandemic. *Telemedicine and e-Health*. Advance online publication. https://doi.org/10.1089/tmj.2020.0233.
Cornwell, B. L., Szymanski, B. R., & McCarthy, J. F. (2021). Impact of the COVID-19 pandemic on primary care-mental health integration services in the VA health system. *Psychiatric Services*, appips202000607. Advance online publication. https://doi.org/10.1176/appi.ps.202000607.
Cunha, J. M., Shen, Y. C., & Burke, Z. R. (2018). Contrasting the impacts of combat and humanitarian assistance/disaster relief missions on the mental health of military service members. *Defence and Peace Economics, 29*(1), 62–77. https://doi.org/10.1080/10242694.2017.1349365
Czeisler, M. É., Lane, R. I., Petrosky, E., Wiley, J. F., Christensen, A., Njai, R., Weaver, M. D., Robbins, R., Facer-Childs, E. R., Barger, L. K., Czeisler, C. A., Howard, M. E., & Rajaratnam, S. (2020). Mental health, substance use, and suicidal ideation during the COVID-19 pandemic - United States, June 24–30, 2020. *MMWR. Morbidity and Mortality Weekly Report, 69*(32), 1049–1057. https://doi.org/10.15585/mmwr.mm6932a1.
Darkins, A. (2014). The growth of telehealth services in the Veterans Health Administration between 1994 and 2014: A study in the diffusion of innovation. *Telemedicine Journal and E-Health, 20*(9), 761–768. https://doi.org/10.1089/tmj.2014.0143
Egede, L. E., Ruggiero, K. J., & Frueh, B. C. (2020). Ensuring mental health access for vulnerable populations in COVID era. *Journal of Psychiatric Research, 129*, 147–148. https://doi.org/10.1016/j.jpsychires.2020.07.011
Feijt, M., de Kort, Y., Bongers, I., Bierbooms, J., Westerink, J., & IJsselsteijn, W. (2020). Mental health care goes online: Practitioners' experiences of providing mental health care during the COVID-19 pandemic. *Cyberpsychology, Behavior and Social Networking, 23*(12), 860–864. https://doi.org/10.1089/cyber.2020.0370
Ferguson, J. M., Jacobs, J., Yefimova, M., Greene, L., Heyworth, L., & Zulman, D. M. (2020). Virtual care expansion in the Veterans Health Administration during the COVID-19 pandemic: Clinical services and patient characteristics associated with utilization. *Journal of the American Medical Informatics Association*, ocaa284. Advance online publication. https://doi.org/10.1093/jamia/ocaa284.
Fletcher, T. L., Hogan, J. B., Keegan, F., Davis, M. L., Wassef, M., Day, S., & Lindsay, J. A. (2018). Recent advances in delivering mental health treatment via video to home. *Current Psychiatry Reports, 20*, 56. https://doi.org/10.1007/s11920-018-0922-y

Freedland, K. E., Dew, M. A., Sarwer, D. B., Burg, M. M., Hart, T. A., Ewing, S. W. F., . . . Kaufmann, P. G. (2020). Health psychology in the time of COVID-19. Health Psychology, 39(12), 1021–1025. https://doi.org/10.1037/hea0001049.

Galea, S., Merchant, R. M., & Lurie, N. (2020). The mental health consequences of COVID-19 and physical distancing: The need for prevention and early intervention. *JAMA Internal Medicine, 180*(6), 817–818. https://doi.org/10.1001/jamainternmed.2020.1562

Gerber, M. R. (2019). Trauma-informed care of veterans. In M. R. Gerber (Ed.), *Trauma-informed healthcare approaches* (pp. 107–122). Springer. https://doi.org/10.1007/978-3-030-04342-1_6

Gerber, M. R. (2020). The things they carry: Veterans and the COVID-19 pandemic. *Journal of General Internal Medicine, 35*(10), 3093–3094. https://doi.org/10.1007/s11606-020-06048-x

Gould, C. E., & Hantke, N. C. (2020). Promoting technology and virtual visits to improve older adult mental health in the face of COVID-19. *The American Journal of Geriatric Psychiatry, 28*(8), 889–890. https://doi.org/10.1016/j.jagp.2020.05.011

Gould, C. E., Loup, J. R., Scales, A. N., Juang, C., Carlson, C., Ma, F., & Sakai, E. Y. (2020). Development and refinement of educational materials to help older veterans use VA mental health mobile apps. *Professional Psychology: Research and Practice, 51*(4), 414–423. https://doi.org/10.1037/pro0000354

Gruber, J., Prinstein, M. J., Clark, L. A., Rottenberg, J., Abramowitz, J. S., Albano, A. M., Aldao, A., Borelli, J. L., Chung, T., Davila, J., Forbes, E. E., Gee, D. G., Nagayama Hall, G. C., Hallion, L. S., Hinshaw, S. P., Hofmann, S. G., Hollon, S. D., Joormann, J., Kazdin, A. E., Klein, D. N., La Greca, A. M., … Weinstock, L. M. (2020). Mental health and clinical psychological science in the time of COVID-19: Challenges, opportunities, and a call to action. *American Psychologist.* Advance online publication. https://psycnet.apa.org/doi/10.1037/amp0000707.

Gunnell, D., Appleby, L., Arensman, E., Hawton, K., John, A., Kapur, N., Khan, M., O'Connor, R. C., Pirkis, J., & COVID-19 Suicide Prevention Research Collaboration. (2020). Suicide risk and prevention during the COVID-19 pandemic. *The Lancet. Psychiatry, 7*(6), 468–471. https://doi.org/10.1016/S2215-0366(20)30171-1

Haderlein, T. P., Wong, M. S., Yuan, A., Llorente, M. D., & Washington, D. L. (2020). Association of PTSD with COVID-19 testing and infection in the Veterans Health Administration. *Journal of Psychiatric Research*, S0022-3956(20)31092-X. Advance online publication. https://doi.org/10.1016/j.jpsychires.2020.11.033

Harpaz-Rotem, I., & Hoff, R. (2020). *FY2019 overview of PTSD patient population data sheet. VA Office of Mental Health Operations*. Northeast Program Evaluation Center.

Hernandez-Tejada, M. A., Zoller, J. S., Ruggiero, K. J., Kazley, A. S., & Acierno, R. (2014). Early treatment withdrawal from evidence-based psychotherapy for PTSD: Telemedicine and in-person parameters. *The International Journal of Psychiatry in Medicine, 48*(1), 33–55. https://doi.org/10.2190%2FPM.48.1.d.

Heyworth, L., Kirsh, S., Zulman, D., Ferguson, J. M., & Kizer, K. W. (2020). Expanding access through virtual care: The VA's early experience with covid-19. *NEJM Catalyst Innovations in Care Delivery.* https://doi.org/10.1056/CAT.20.0327

Holingue, C., Badillo-Goicoechea, E., Riehm, K. E., Veldhuis, C. B., Thrul, J., Johnson, R. M., Fallin, M. D., Kreuter, F., Stuart, E. A., & Kalb, L. G. (2020a). Mental distress during the COVID-19 pandemic among US adults without a pre-existing mental health condition: Findings from American trend panel survey. *Preventive Medicine, 139*, 106231. https://doi.org/10.1016/j.ypmed.2020.106231

Holingue, C., Kalb, L. G., Riehm, K. E., Bennett, D., Kapteyn, A., Veldhuis, C. B., Johnson, R. M., Fallin, M. D., Kreuter, F., Stuart, E. A., & Thrul, J. (2020b). Mental distress in the United States at the beginning of the COVID-19 pandemic. *American Journal of Public Health, 110*(11), 1628–1634. https://doi.org/10.2105/AJPH.2020.305857

Holman, E. A., Thompson, R. R., Garfin, D. R., & Silver, R. C. (2020). The unfolding COVID-19 pandemic: A probability-based, nationally representative study of mental health in the United States. *Science. Advances, 6*(42), eabd5390. https://doi.org/10.1126/sciadv.abd5390

Irvine, A., Drew, P., Bower, P., Brooks, H., Gellatly, J., Armitage, C. J., Barkham, M., McMillan, D., & Bee, P. (2020). Are there interactional differences between telephone and face-to-face psychological therapy? A systematic review of comparative studies. *Journal of Affective Disorders, 265*(15), 120–131. https://doi.org/10.1016/j.jad.2020.01.057

Kang, H. K., Natelson, B. H., Mahan, C. M., Lee, K. Y., & Murphy, F. M. (2003). Post-traumatic stress disorder and chronic fatigue syndrome-like illness among Gulf War veterans: A population-based survey of 30,000 veterans. *American Journal of Epidemiology, 157*(2), 141–148. https://doi.org/10.1093/aje/kwf187

Katon, J. G., Lehavot, K., Simpson, T. L., Williams, E. C., Barnett, S. B., Grossbard, J. R., Schure, M. B., Gray, K. E., & Reiber, G. E. (2015). Adverse childhood experiences, military service, and adult health. *American Journal of Preventive Medicine, 49*(4), 573–582. https://doi.org/10.1016/j.amepre.2015.03.020

Kazak, A. E. (2020). Psychology is an essential science: American Psychologist highlights the role of psychology in understanding and addressing COVID-19. *American Psychologist, 75*(5), 605–606. https://doi.org/10.1037/amp0000682

Kuhn, E., Kanuri, N., Hoffman, J. E., Garvert, D. W., Ruzek, J. I., & Taylor, C. B. (2017). A randomized controlled trial of a smartphone app for posttraumatic stress disorder symptoms. *Journal of Consulting and Clinical Psychology, 85*(3), 267–273. https://doi.org/10.1037/ccp0000163

Kulka, R. A., Schlenger, W. E., Fairbank, J. A., Hough, R. L., Jordan, B. K., Marmar, C. R., & Weiss, D. S. (1990). *Brunner/Mazel psychosocial stress series, No. 18. Trauma and the Vietnam war generation: Report of findings from the National Vietnam Veterans Readjustment Study*. Brunner/Mazel. https://psycnet.apa.org/record/1990-97372-000

Lai, J., Ma, S., Wang, Y., Cai, Z., Hu, J., Wei, N., Wu, J., Du, H., Chen, T., Li, R., Tan, H., Kang, L., Yao, L., Huang, M., Wang, H., Wang, G., Liu, Z., & Hu, S. (2020). Factors associated with mental health outcomes among health care workers exposed to coronavirus disease 2019. *JAMA Network Open, 3*(3), e203976. https://doi.org/10.1001/jamanetworkopen.2020.3976

Lancee, W. J., Maunder, R. G., Goldbloom, D. S., & Coauthors for the Impact of SARS Study (2008). Prevalence of psychiatric disorders among Toronto hospital workers one to two years after the SARS outbreak. *Psychiatric Services (Washington, D.C.), 59*(1), 91–95. https://doi.org/10.1176/ps.2008.59.1.91.

Levine, J., & Sher, L. (2021). The prevention of suicide among military veterans during the COVID-19 pandemic. *European Archives of Psychiatry and Clinical Neuroscience*, 1–2. Advance online publication. https://doi.org/10.1007/s00406-020-01217-9

Kubzansky, L. D., Bordelois, P., Jun, H. J., Roberts, A. L., Cerda, M., Bluestone, N., & Koenen, K. C. (2014). The weight of traumatic stress: A prospective study of posttraumatic stress disorder symptoms and weight status in women. *JAMA Psychiatry, 71*(1), 44–51. https://doi.org/10.1001/jamapsychiatry.2013.2798

Luo, J., Jeyapalina, S., Stoddard, G. J., Kwok, A. C., & Agarwal, J. P. (2021). Coronavirus disease 2019 in veterans receiving care at veterans health administration facilities. *Annals of Epidemiology, 55*, 10–14. https://doi.org/10.1016/j.annepidem.2020.12.003

Marini, C. M., Pless Kaiser, A., Smith, B. N., & Fiori, K. L. (2020). Aging veterans' mental health and well-being in the context of COVID-19: The importance of social ties during physical distancing. *Psychological Trauma: Theory, Research, Practice and Policy, 12*(S1), S217–S219. https://doi.org/10.1037/tra0000736

Marshall, J. M., Dunstan, D. A., & Bartik, W. (2020a). Clinical or gimmickal: The use and effectiveness of mobile mental health apps for treating anxiety and depression. *The Australian and New Zealand Journal of Psychiatry, 54*(1), 20–28. https://doi.org/10.1177/0004867419876700

Marshall, J. M., Dunstan, D. A., & Bartik, W. (2020b). Treating psychological trauma in the midst of COVID-19: The role of smartphone apps. *Frontiers in Public Health, 8*, 402. https://doi.org/10.3389/fpubh.2020.00402

Matos, R. I., & Chung, K. K. (2020). DoD COVID-19 Practice Management Guide: Clinical Management of COVID-19. *Defense Health Agency Falls Church United States* . https://apps.dtic.mil/sti/pdfs/AD1097348.pdf.

Mitchell, L., & Fuehrlein, B. (2021). Patient volume and dispositions in a VA psychiatric emergency room during COVID-19. *Community Mental Health Journal*, 1–3. Advance online publication. https://doi.org/10.1007/s10597-021-00778-w.

Morland, L. A., Greene, C. J., Rosen, C. S., Foy, D., Reilly, P., Shore, J., He, Q., & Frueh, B. C. (2010). Telemedicine for anger management therapy in a rural population of combat veterans with posttraumatic stress disorder: A randomized noninferiority trial. *The Journal of Clinical Psychiatry, 71*(7), 855–863. https://doi.org/10.4088/JCP.09m05604blu

Morland, L. A., Mackintosh, M. A., Glassman, L. H., Wells, S. Y., Thorp, S. R., Rauch, S. A., Cunningham, P. B., Tuerk, P. W., Grubbs, K. M., Golshan, S., Sohn, M. J., & Acierno, R. (2020). Home-based delivery of variable length prolonged exposure therapy: A comparison of clinical efficacy between service modalities. *Depression & Anxiety, 37*(4), 346–355. https://doi.org/10.1002/da.22979

Morland, L. A., Mackintosh, M. A., Greene, C. J., Rosen, C. S., Chard, K. M., Resick, P., & Frueh, B. C. (2014). Cognitive processing therapy for posttraumatic stress disorder delivered to rural veterans via telemental health: A randomized noninferiority clinical trial. *The Journal of Clinical Psychiatry, 75*(5), 470–476. https://doi.org/10.4088/JCP.13m08842

Morland, L. A., Mackintosh, M. A., Rosen, C. S., Willis, E., Resick, P., Chard, K., & Frueh, B. C. (2015). Telemedicine versus in-person delivery of cognitive processing therapy for women with posttraumatic stress disorder: A randomized noninferiority trial. *Depression & Anxiety, 32*(11), 811–820. https://doi.org/10.1002/da.22397

Morland, L. A., Wells, S. Y., Glassman, L. H., Grubbs, K., Mackintosh, M. A., Golshan, S., Sohn, M. J., Thorp, S. R., Savage, U. C., & Acierno, R. (2019). What do veterans want? Veterans' preferences for PTSD treatment delivery modality. *Military Medicine, 184*(11–12), 686–692. https://doi.org/10.1093/milmed/usz035

Owen, J. E., Kuhn, E., Jaworski, B. K., McGee-Vincent, P., Juhasz, K., Hoffman, J. E., & Rosen, C. (2018). VA mobile apps for PTSD and related problems: Public health resources for veterans and those who care for them. *mHealth, 4*, 28. https://doi.org/10.21037/mhealth.2018.05.07.

Panchal, N., Kamal, R., Orgera, K., Cox, C., Garfield, R., Hamel, L., & Chidambaram, P. (2020). *The implications of COVID-19 for mental health and substance use*. Kaiser Family Foundation. https://abtcounseling.com/wp-content/uploads/2020/09/The-Implications-of-COVID-19-for-Mental-Health-and-Substance-Use-_-KFF.pdf.

Perrin, P. B., Pierce, B. S., & Elliott, T. R. (2020). COVID-19 and telemedicine: A revolution in healthcare delivery is at hand. *Health Science Reports, 3*(2), e166. https://doi.org/10.1002%2Fhsr2.166.

Pierce, B. S., Perrin, P. B., Tyler, C. M., McKee, G. B., & Watson, J. D. (2020). The COVID-19 telepsychology revolution: A national study of pandemic-based changes in U.S. mental health care delivery. *American Psychologist.* Advance online publication. https://doi.org/10.1037/amp0000722.

Ramchand, R., Harrell, M. C., Berglass, N., & Lauck, M. (2020). Veterans and COVID-19: Projecting the economic, social and mental health needs of America's veterans. The Bob Woodruff Foundation. https://bobwoodrufffoundation.org/wp-content/uploads/2020/04/BWF_WhitePaper-COVID19-5.0-Final.pdf

Ramchand, R., Tanielian, T., Fisher, M. P., Vaughan, C. A., Trail, T. E., Epley, C., Voorhies, P., Robbins, M., Robinson, E., & Ghosh-Dastidar, B. (2014). Hidden heroes: America's military caregivers – Executive summary. *Rand Health Quarterly*, *4*(2), 14 . https://www.ncbi.nlm.nih.gov/pmc/articles/PMC5052006/.

Rhee, W. K., Merbaum, M., Strube, M. J., & Self, S. M. (2005). Efficacy of brief telephone psychotherapy with callers to a suicide hotline. *Suicide and Life-threatening Behavior, 35*(3), 317–328. https://doi.org/10.1521/suli.2005.35.3.317

Rosen, C. S., Morland, L. A., Glassman, L. H., Marx, B. P., Weaver, K., Smith, C. A. Pollack, S., & Schnurr, P. P. (2020). Virtual mental health care in the Veterans Health Administration's immediate response to coronavirus disease-19. *American Psychologist*. Advance online publication. https://doi.org/10.1037/amp0000751.

Rossi, F. S., Shankar, M., Buckholdt, K., Bailey, Y., Israni, S. T., & Iverson, K. M. (2020). Trying times and trying out solutions: Intimate partner violence screening and support for women veterans during COVID-19. *Journal of General Internal Medicine, 35*(9), 2728–2731. https://doi.org/10.1007/s11606-020-05990-0

Sareen, J. (2014). Posttraumatic stress disorder in adults: Impact, comorbidity, risk factors, and treatment. *Canadian Journal of Psychiatry, 59*(9), 460–467. https://doi.org/10.1177/070674371405900902

Shelton, C. J., Kim, A., Hassan, A. M., Bhat, A., Barnello, J., & Castro, C. A. (2020). System-wide implementation of telehealth to support military veterans and their families in response to COVID-19: A paradigm shift. *Journal of Military, Veteran and Family Health, 6*(S2), 50–57. https://doi.org/10.3138/jmvfh-CO19-0003

Sher, L. (2020). An infectious disease pandemic and increased suicide risk. *Revista Brasileira de Psiquiatria (Sao Paulo, Brazil: 1999), 42*(3), 239–240. https://doi.org/10.1590/1516-4446-2020-0989

Stiles-Shields, C., Kwasny, M. J., Cai, X., & Mohr, D. C. (2014). Therapeutic alliance in face-to-face and telephone-administered cognitive behavioral therapy. *Journal of Consulting and Clinical Psychology, 82*(2), 349–354 . https://psycnet.apa.org/doi/10.1037/a0035554.

Tanielian, T. L., Tanielian, T., & Jaycox, L. (2008). *Invisible wounds of war: Psychological and cognitive injuries, their consequences, and services to assist recovery* (Vol. 1). Rand Corporation.

Torous, J., & Keshavan, M. (2020). COVID-19, mobile health and serious mental illness. *Schizophrenia Research, 218*, 36–37. https://doi.org/10.1016/j.schres.2020.04.013

Turgoose, D., Ashwick, R., & Murphy, D. (2018). Systematic review of lessons learned from delivering tele-therapy to veterans with post-traumatic stress disorder. *Journal of Telemedicine and Telecare, 24*(9), 575–585. https://doi.org/10.1177%2F1357633X17730443.

Uniformed Services University and Defense Health Agency (2020). DoD COVID-19 practice management guide: Clinical management of COVID-19 [technical document]. Bethesda: COVID-19 Practice Management Guidelines Work Group; 2020 [cited 2020 Aug 11]. 146 p. Available from: https://www.usuhs.edu/sites/default/files/media/vpe/pdf/dod_covid-19_pmg_v4_18jun20_acc.pdf

Varker, T., Brand, R. M., Ward, J., Terhaag, S., & Phelps, A. (2019). Efficacy of synchronous telepsychology interventions for people with anxiety, depression, posttraumatic stress disorder, and adjustment disorder: A rapid evidence assessment. *Psychological Services, 16*(4), 621–635. https://doi.org/10.1037/ser0000239

Veterans Health Administration Support Service Center. (2020). *Veterans Health Administration Support Service Center (VSSC) VHA Site Tracking (VAST) counts and changes report*. Department of Veterans Affairs.

West, J. C., & Morganstein, J. C. (2016). Psychological effects on military personnel assigned to humanitarian assistance and disaster response missions. In G. Christodoulou (Ed.), *Disasters: Mental health context and responses* (pp. 69–82). Cambridge Scholars Publishing.

Williams, J., & Gonzalez-Medina, D. (2011). Infectious diseases and social stigma. *Applied Innovations and Technologies, 4*(1), 58–70. https://academicpublishingplatforms.com/downloads/pdfs/ati/volume4/201105020547_07_ATI_V4_JoanWilliams_et_al_Social__Stigma.pdf.

Wounded Warrior Project. (2020). *Wounded Warrior Project (WWP) Annual Warrior Survey (2020). Invisible wounds and COVID-19: Heighted risk for wounded warriors*. https://www.woundedwarriorproject.org/media/wfbjwylf/wwp20_0135_exe_covid_wpaper.pdf

Wynn, G., Morganstein, J. C., Jetly, R., Ford, S. C., Vance, M. C., Meyer, E. G., West, J. C., Benedek, D. M., & Ursano, R. J. (2020a). Military mental health and COVID-19. *Journal of*

Military, Veteran and Family Health, 6(Suppl 2), 21–26. https://doi.org/10.3138/JMVFH-6.S2-2020-0048

Wynn, J. K., McCleery, A., Novacek, D., Reavis, E. A., Tsai, J., & Green, M. F. (2020b). *Clinical and functional effects of the COVID-19 pandemic and social distancing on veterans with psychotic disorders and recently-housed veterans*. https://psyarxiv.com/2saq5/download?format=pdf.

Zaka, A., Shamloo, S. E., Fiorente, P., & Tafuri, A. (2020). COVID-19 pandemic as a watershed moment: A call for systematic psychological health care for frontline medical staff. *Journal of Health Psychology, 25*(7), 883–887. https://doi.org/10.1177/1359105320925148

Chapter 12
Telehealth Applications in Military and Veteran Healthcare Settings

Larry C. James and Aina Katsikas

Telepsychology, also referred to as telehealth, is defined by the American Psychological Association as:

> the provision of psychological services using telecommunication technologies. Telecommunications is the preparation, transmission, communication, or related processing of information by electrical, electromagnetic, electromechanical, electro-optical, or electronic means (Committee on National Security Systems, 2010). Telecommunication technologies include, but are not limited to, telephone, mobile devices, interactive videoconferencing, email, chat, text, and Internet (e.g., self-help websites, blogs, and social media). The information that is transmitted may be in writing, or include images, sounds, or other data. These communications may be synchronous with multiple parties communicating in real time (e.g., interactive videoconferencing, telephone) or asynchronous (e.g., email, online bulletin boards, storing and forwarding information). Technologies may augment traditional in-person services (e.g., psychoeducational materials online after an in-person therapy session), or be used as standalone services (e.g., therapy or leadership development provided over videoconferencing). Different technologies may be used in various combinations and for different purposes during the provision of telepsychology services.

Since the mid-1950s, Telehealth applications have "waxed and waned" and come and gone. In the mid-1950s, at the Nebraska Psychiatric Institute, a collection of Psychologists, Psychiatrists and Nurses transformed old analog black and white televisions to connect therapists between the east and western borders of Nebraska. It was a successful outcome. However, amid all the excitement was the letdown of reality from two perspectives. First, would insurance companies reimburse for mental health services via tele health platforms in the 1950s? No! Behavioral Health interventions provided via technology was not a reimbursable clinical encounter.

L. C. James (✉)
Department of Behavioral Health, Tripler Army Medical Center, Honolulu, HI, USA

A. Katsikas
Department of Economics, College of Business, University of Nevada Reno, Reno, NV, USA

L. C. James et al. (eds.), *Clinical Health Psychology in Military and Veteran Settings*, https://doi.org/10.1007/978-3-031-12063-3_12

Second, very few medical centers throughout the world had the technological capacity to tele behavioral health in the mid-1950s.

Thus, telehealth enthusiasm across the United States whittered away. Behavioral Health practitioners returned to the face-to-face model of mental health delivery.

Then, in the mid-1990s, political pressure was placed upon military psychologists assigned to Tripler Army Medical Center in Honolulu, Hawaii by the US Congress. Military patients throughout the pacific region complained to their congressman and senators that they were deprived of tertiary medical care because they were assigned to South Korea or Japan rather than the Army Medical Center in Hawaii. The Health Psychology staff at Tripler Army Medical Center were "ordered" to pioneer technology to provide services via telehealth applications from the Army hospital in Honolulu, to South Korea and Japan.

To "jump start" the research into the feasibility of this project, Congress earmarked approximately $400,000.00 for Colonel (Dr.) Larry C. James and his colleagues to ascertain the possibility of service delivered thousands of miles apart via analog telephone technology. James and his colleagues (James et al., 1999, 2001, 2003).

1 Some Telehealth Applications

In 1999, James et al. published two papers describing tele-behavioral health clinical applications. In fact, James and his colleagues pioneered tele-behavioral health in the United States when very few, if any, large military Centers were engaged in tele-behavioral health applications.

Tele Biofeedback In 2001, Earles, Folen, and James published an article entitled "*Biofeedback Using Telemedicine: Clinical applications and case illustrations*." In this article the researchers developed technology whereby the provider was in his office in Honolulu and conducted biofeedback with chronic pain patients in Japan and South Korea. The researchers applied a software called "pcAnywhere" to control the computers between their office in Honolulu, Japan, and Korea. A behavioral science technician located at the clinics in Japan and Korea assisted in orienting the patient, equipment use, and assisting with any clinical emergencies. Figure 12.1 illustrates the equipment that was purchased "off the shelf" in the 1990s for the study.

Tele Biofeedback was applied to treat patients diagnosed with chronic pain, migraine headaches, and dental pain (such as TMJ).

Tele Health Applications in the Treatment of Obesity and Eating Disorders James et al. (2001) and Earles et al. (2001a, b) highlighted the use of telehealth applications in the treatment of obesity and eating disorders. In these studies, the researchers not only used video teleconferencing but interactive web-pages were applied for patients to track and log in their weight, food intake, exercise, and interact with

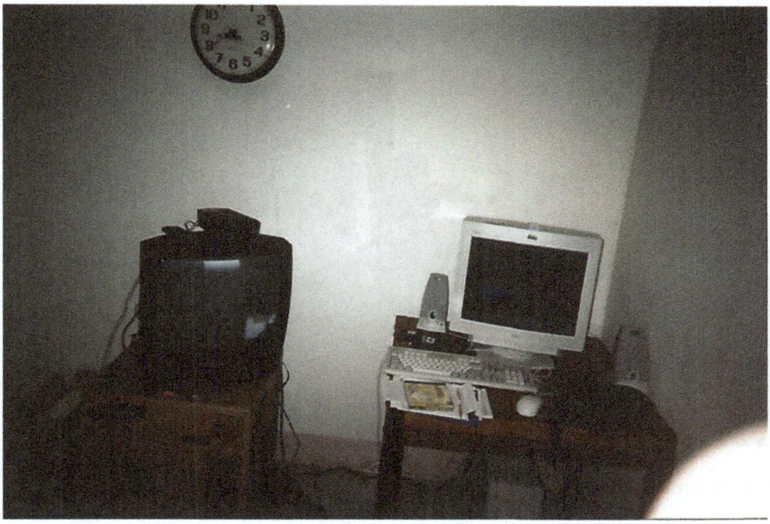

Fig. 12.1 Picture of telehealth equipment for health psychologists

counselors in real time. At the end of the project, the researchers found no significant differences in among variables and patients were very satisfied with the telehealth applications. Figure 12.2 illustrates a clinical health psychologist providing services to patients in Japan and Korea from the doctor's office in Honolulu.

Baggett et al. (2002) pushed the envelope to apply web-based evaluations to conduct neuropsychology assessments. Baggett and his team found no significant difference in conducting these evaluations either in person or via a web-based platform.

Telehealth Applications Post Covid-19 By the early- to mid-2000s, telehealth applications in behavioral health patients dramatically decreased. Perhaps one silver lining in the COVID-19 epidemic is the medical face-to-face clinic closures around the country championed in a new era in telehealth applications across the country. The United States Congress passing emergency legislation as well as numerous governors signing emergency authorizations forced insurance companies to reimburse providers for all medical services. As of this writing, it does appear that Telehealth is here to stay and will be a permanent and common platform for service delivery.

The US health and Human Services has approved several telehealth platforms that are HIPPA compliant and safe for not only patient care but also for behavioral telehealth services. Table 12.1 below provides a list of HIPPA approved and secure telehealth platforms.

Legal and Policy Telehealth Policy Changes Post COVID-19 In this section, the authors will discuss pre- and post-COVID19 legal and policy changes.

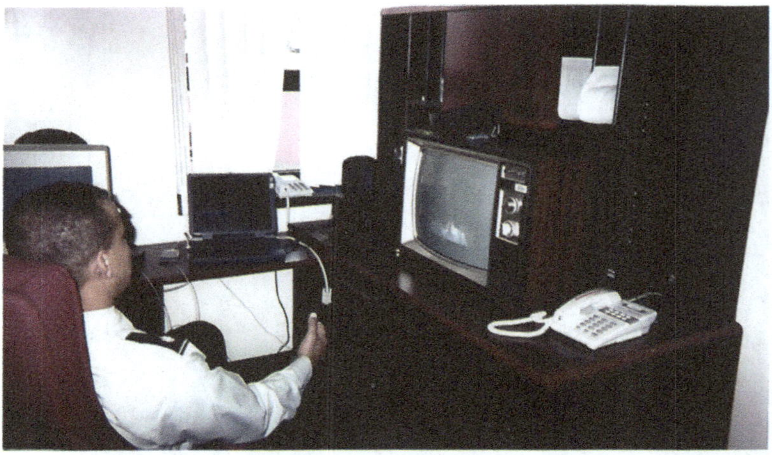

Fig. 12.2 Illustration of telehealth being performed by a health psychologist

Table 12.1 List of HIPPA approved telehealth platforms

Simple Practice	Doxy.Me
Vsee	Healthie
VtConnect	Thera-link
eVisit	Medici
TheraNest	

1.1 Before-COVID CMS Telehealth Policies

Prior to COVID-19, the Centers for Medicare and Medicaid Services (CMS) stipulated four requirements regarding reimbursement for telehealth services prior to March 6, 2020, the beginning of the COVID-19 pandemic (Congress, 2020). These included:

1. Patients must be located in an originating site to receive telehealth services, excluding their homes. Approved originating sites included physician offices, hospitals, rural health clinics, and federally qualified health centers (FQHCs). Only a few exceptions would permit a patient's home to be an originating site.
2. Telehealth services were only allowed for established patients. New patients must have had at least one in-person visit to be eligible for telehealth.
3. Telehealth services were only allowed for patients residing in rural areas. This included a county outside of a Metropolitan Statistical Area (MSA) or a rural Health Professional Shortage Area (HPSA) in a rural census tract.
4. Audio-only telephones did not meet the requirements for telehealth. There must be two-way real-time audio and visual communication capabilities.

All four of these policies were altered to address the COVID-19 Public Health Emergency (PHE) in March 2020.

After COVID-19 ravaged the nation during-COVID CMS Telehealth Policy, CMS expanded telehealth policies under the authority of the Coronavirus Preparedness and Response Supplemental Appropriations Act, effective March 6, 2020. This expansion worked to benefit both providers and their patients. CMS implemented Sect. 1135 Blanket Waivers that altered telehealth stipulations and adjusted billing policies for the COVID-19 Public Health Emergency (PHE) (Office of Health Care Financing, 2020). These changes were at the federal level. States implemented their own set of guidelines.

CMS uses Section 1135 Blanket Waivers to respond to disasters or emergencies. These waivers can modify stipulations such as pre-approval requirements, reporting requirements, and conditions of program participation. In the case of the COVID-19 PHE, two blanket waivers were initiated to expand flexibility for Medicare telehealth services.

The first waiver extended the list of healthcare practitioners that are eligible to provide telehealth services. For example, physical therapists, occupational therapists, speech language pathologists, and psychologists may now provide telehealth services. The second waiver allows for the use of audio-only technology to provide services. Only certain services are allowed to be delivered via audio-only. These allowable services are detailed in the table below.

The stipulations of furnishing telehealth services were altered for both providers and patients. This included:

- Providers are now eligible to provide telehealth services from their homes. The detailed list of services and billing codes are provided in the table below.
- Telehealth services are reimbursed for the same dollar amount as in-person visits, with the exception of a few services.
- Providers are able to serve both new and established Medicare patients as well as those living in both urban and rural areas.
- Providers can visit Skilled Nursing Facility patients via telehealth. Providers can deliver visits on the basis of need rather than once every 30 days.
- Penalties for HIPAA violations are waived against providers who employ non-HIPAA approved telecommunication platforms such as Skype or FaceTime, so long as they are used in good faith.
- Medicare patients are not required to be in an originating site but can now receive telehealth services in their own home.
- Providers may reduce or waive cost-sharing policies for telehealth visits. However, this does not apply to brief communications, known as E-Visits. E-Visits are patient-initiated forms of online communications via secure health platforms that require a professional patient assessment and subsequent health decision-making.
- Providers can deliver audio-only telephone assessment and management services. These are patient-initiated services. These are reimbursed at a lower rate than traditional psychotherapy because they are meant to be brief and direct.

They are not considered to be telehealth services and are not included in the table below.

- All states (excluding Oklahoma) have allowed some form of emergency licensure waiver for out-of-state providers to practice. However, many states require some form of registration and verification with local health departments. Oklahoma only allows out-of-state psychologists to practice for no more than 5 days in Oklahoma. Other states allow out-of-state providers to practice for much longer periods or for the entire duration of the PHE.

Telehealth Billing Billing policies for telehealth services are divided into three categories: (1) telehealth non-covered services; (2) traditional telehealth only; and (3) audio only and traditional telehealth.

The first category of telehealth services are allowed but not reimbursable by Medicare. The second category defines "Traditional Telehealth" to include telecommunication with audio and video functions that provide two-way real-time interactive communication. The third category includes both reimbursable audio only and traditional telehealth services.

The corresponding current procedural terminology (CPT) codes are in parentheses. All claims for traditional telehealth and audio-only telehealth services must include modifier 95. The Place of Service (POS) must be reported as if the service had been furnished in person. For example, a psychologist who would have seen a patient in a private office should use POS 11 rather than POS 02 (Table 12.2).

State telehealth guidelines mostly mirrored CMS' mandates. For example, every state (except for Wisconsin,) permitted coverage for telehealth services. Most states also allowed for some form of Emergency Out-of-State Licensure Waiver that would allow out-of-state licensed providers to practice in state. However, almost every state requires registration in the state that a provider intends to deliver services for a temporary permit.

Table 12.3 provides state guidelines for three stipulations: (1) state coverage of telehealth services under the PHE; (2) emergency out-of-state licensure waiver for providers; (3) supervised trainees can provide telehealth services. The last topic addresses if postdocs and interns can provide telehealth services and receive Medicaid reimbursement. It is important to note that these guidelines are only valid as part of the state's declared emergency. Each declaration is subject to end on the state's terms.

1.2 Interstate Medical Licensure Compact Relevant to Telehealth

The Federation of State Medical boards established The Interstate Medical Licensure Compact (IMLC) in 2014. Eligible physicians can practice medicine in multiple states that are involved in the IMLC. The licensing is still state-based, but the process is streamlined so physicians can easily qualify to practice in multiple states at once.

Table 12.2 Billing for telehealth services

Telehealth non-covered services	Traditional telehealth only	Audio only and traditional telehealth
Psychophysiological therapy (90875) Health behavior intervention, family without patient (96170, 96171)	Developmental screening and testing (96110, 96112, 96113) Adaptive behavior assessment (97151, 97152, 0362T) Adaptive behavior treatment (97153, 97154, 97155, 97156, 97157, 97158, 0373T)	Diagnostic interview (90791, 90792) Psychotherapy (90832, 90833, 90834, 90836, 90837, 90838) Psychoanalysis (90845) Group psychotherapy (90853) Family psychotherapy (90846, 90847) Crisis intervention and interactive complexity (90839, 90840, 90785) Neurobehavioral status exam (96116, 96121) Psychological evaluation (96130, 96131) Neuropsychological evaluation (96132, 96133) Psychological and neuropsychological test administration and scoring (96136, 96137, 96138, 96139) Health behavior assessment (96156) Health behavior intervention, individual (96158, 96159) Health behavior intervention, group (96164, 96165) Health behavior intervention, family with patient (96167, 96178) Behavioral screening (96127) Screening, brief intervention, and referral to treatment (G0396, G0397)

To be eligible, physicians must already have a full, unrestricted medical license in a member-state. This serves as the state of principal license (SPL). There are four stipulations for a physician to designate a state as an SPL:

1. The physician's SPL is his or her primary residence.
2. One quarter of the physician's practice occurs in the SPL.

Table 12.3 State guidelines for telehealth services under PHE

State	State coverage of telehealth services under PHE	Emergency out-of-state licensure waiver	Supervised trainee can provide telehealth services
AL	Yes	Yes	N/A
AK	Yes	Yes	No
AZ	Yes	Yes	Yes
AR	Yes	Yes	No
CA	Yes	Yes	Yes
CO	Yes	Yes	No
CT	Yes	Yes	No
DE	Yes	Yes	No
DC	Yes	Yes	No
FL	Yes	Yes	No
GA	Yes	No	Yes
HI	Yes	N/A	No
ID	Yes	No	No
IL	Yes	Yes	Yes
IN	Yes	Yes	Yes
IA	Yes	Yes	Yes
KS	Yes	Yes	No
KY	Yes	No	Postdocs only
LA	Yes	Yes	Yes
ME	Yes	Yes	No
MD	Yes	Yes	No
MA	Yes	Yes	Yes
MI	Yes	Yes	Yes
MN	Yes	Yes	N/A
MS	Yes	Yes	No
MO	Yes	Yes	Yes
MT	Yes	Yes	No
NE	Yes	Yes	No
NV	Yes	Yes	Yes
NH	Yes	Yes	No
NJ	Yes	Yes	Yes
NM	Yes	Yes	Yes
NY	Yes	Yes	No
NC	Yes	Yes	Postdocs only
ND	Yes	Yes	No
OH	Yes	Yes	Yes
OK	Yes	No	Yes
OR	Yes	Yes	Yes
PA	Yes	Yes	No
RI	Yes	Yes	No
SC	Yes	Yes	Yes

(continued)

Table 12.3 (continued)

State	State coverage of telehealth services under PHE	Emergency out-of-state licensure waiver	Supervised trainee can provide telehealth services
SD	Yes	Yes	No
TN	Yes	Yes	No
TX	Yes	N/A	Yes
UT	Yes	Yes	Yes
VT	Yes	Yes	Yes
VA	Yes	Yes	No
WA	Yes	Yes	No
WV	Yes	Yes	Postdocs only
WI	N/A	Yes	Yes
WY	Yes	Yes	Yes

3. The physician is employed to practice medicine by a person, business, or organization located in the SPL.
4. The physician's state of residence for US Federal Income Tax purposes is the SPL.

The use of the IMLC has grown significantly during the pandemic. Almost half of the issued licenses (8000) between 2017 and 2021 were issued between March 2020 and March 2021 (American Medical Association, n.d.). The Compact currently has 30 member states, as identified in the map below (Fig. 12.3).

1.3 After-COVID CMS Telehealth Policies

The COVID-19 Public Health Emergency (PHE) policies paved the way for the future of telehealth. Although the Department of Health and Human Services will most likely extend the duration of the PHE until the end of the year, some changes will surpass this calendar year.

CMS issued a final rule on Dec. 1, 2020, that updated the list of Medicare telehealth services. Services were added to either a Category 1 or Category 3 basis. Category 3 services will remain through the end of the calendar year of the PHE with the potential to become permanent at the end of the PHE. The table below outlines additions to these two categories with corresponding CPT codes. Audio-only services may not be reimbursable after the COVID-19 PHE (Table 12.4).

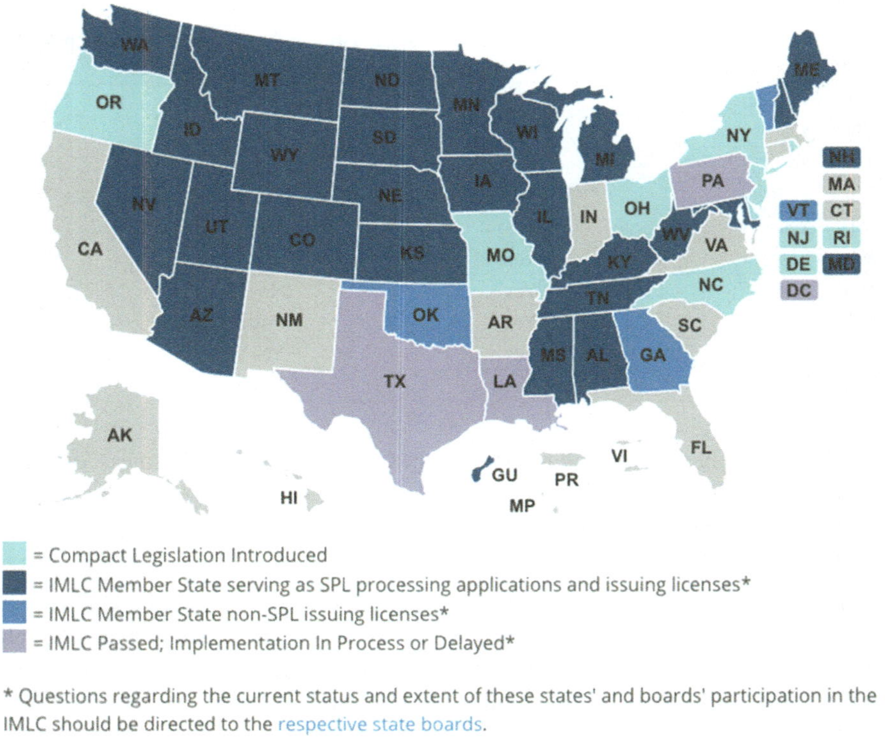

Fig. 12.3 Interstate medical licensure compact member states. (Source: https://www.imlcc.org/)

2 Discussion

In this chapter, the authors provided a discussion of the history of telehealth behavioral health and its development. Also, a review of the diseases that can benefit from behavioral interventions via telehealth platforms was discussed and important references were provided. Important information in regards to state telehealth policies and guidelines was offered. The benefits of Telehealth as a platform to deliver health psychology services are many.

Schoebel et al. (2021) provided an excellent article entitled "*Qualitative Analysis of Provider Experiences and Perspectives*." In this article, the researchers described updated advances in current telehealth outcome research as well as benefits and challenges. Telehealth has filled a terrible clinical void, particularly in military and Veteran hospitals, as many of these military treatment centers closed during the COVID outbreak. Through these telehealth applications, valuable patient needs will continue to be safely and efficaciously met.

Table 12.4 CMS list of telehealth services and CPT codes

Category 1	Category 3
Group psychotherapy (CPT code 90853)	Domiciliary, rest home, or custodial care services, established patients (99336–99337)
Psychological and neuropsychological testing (96121)	Home visits, established patient (99349–99350)
Domiciliary, rest home, or custodial care services, established patients (99334–99335)	Emergency department visits, levels 1–5 (99281–99285)
Home visits, established patient (99347–99348)	Nursing facilities discharge day management (99315–99316)
Cognitive assessment and care planning services (99483)	Psychological and neuropsychological testing (96130–96133; 96136–96139)
Visit complexity inherent to certain office/outpatient evaluation and management (E/M) (HCPCS code G2211)	Therapy services, physical and occupational therapy, all levels (97161–97168; 97110, 97112, 97116, 97535, 97750, 97755, 97760, 97761, 92521–92524, 92507)
Prolonged services (HCPCS code G2212)	Hospital discharge day management (99238–99239)
	Inpatient neonatal and pediatric critical care, subsequent (99469, 99472, 99476)
	Continuing neonatal intensive care services (99478–99480)
	Critical care services (99291–99292)
	End-stage renal disease monthly capitation payment codes (90952, 90953, 90956, 90959, 90962)
	Subsequent observation and observation discharge day management (99217; 99224–99226)

References

American Medical Association. (n.d.). *Cross-state licensing process now live in 30 states*. American Medical Association. Accessed 22 June 2021. https://www.ama-assn.org/practice-management/digital/cross-state-licensing-process-now-live-30-states

Baggett, M. R., Christensen, D. K., Korenman, L. M., Kelly, M. P., James, L. C., Leso, J. F., Goodlett, G., & Gahm, G. (2002, October). *Web-based neuropsychological assessment in the U.S. Army*. National Academy of Neuropsychology Conference in Miami, FL.

Congress, U. S. (2020). *HR 6074—Coronavirus preparedness and response supplemental appropriations act*.

Committee on National Security Systems Policy (CNSSP) No. 24, Policy on Assured Information Sharing (AIS) for National Security Systems (NSS), May 2010.

Earles, J., Folen, R. A., & James, L. C. (2001a). Biofeedback using telemedicine: Clinical applications and case illustrations. *Behavioral Medicine, 27*(2), 77–82.

Earles, J., James, L. C., Folen, R. A., & Verschell, M. (2001b). *Incorporating behavioral telehealth in the treatment of obesity*. A Poster Presented at The American Psychological Convention, August San Francisco.

James, L. C. (Chair)., Folen, R. A., Jerome, L. W., Earles, J, Cowings, P. (1999). *Telehealth: New applications in behavioral medicine*. A symposium presented at the Society of Behavioral Medicine Annual Convention, San Diego, Ca. March 5th. Proceedings of The Society of Behavioral Medicine.

James, L. C., Folen, R. A., & Earles, J. (2001). Behavioral telehealth applications in the treatment of obese soldiers. *Journal of Military Psychology, 13*(3), 177–186.

James, L. C., Korenman, L. M., & Baggett, M. (2003). *The walter reed virtual pain management clinic*. A Poster Presented at The American Telemedicine Association Convention, Orlando, Fl.

Office of Health Care Financing. (2020, December 22). *CMS addresses telehealth and supervision of testing in 2021 fee schedule final rule*. American Psychological Association Services, Inc. http://www.apaservices.org/practice/clinic/2021-telehealth-testing-supervision-fee-schedule-final-rule

Schoebel, V., Wayment, C., Gaiser, M., Cory-Page, J., & Beck, A. (2021, August 6). Telebehavioral health during the COVID-19 pandemic: A qualitative analysis of provider experiences and perspectives. *Telemedicine and e-Health, 27*(8). https://doi.org/10.1089/tmj.2021.0121

Chapter 13
The Health Psychologist Role in Providing Services to Transgender Veterans

Susan George, Seth Crocker, Amy Voltmer, and Larry C. James

1 General Overview of Population

Understanding the experience of transgender and gender-nonconforming (TGNC) veterans requires examining the fluctuating policies and work culture of the environment in which they serve. Internationally, openly transgender individuals' military service remains a rarity; as of 2017, only 19 nations allow transgender individuals to serve openly, including the United States (CBC, 2017). In the United States, transgender individuals were banned from serving openly until 2016, even though "Don't Ask, Don't Tell," which allowed lesbian, gay, bisexual service members to serve openly, was repealed in 2011 (The White House Office of the Press Secretary, 2011). Despite a long history of discrimination, transgender adults serve in the US military at significantly higher rates than their cisgender counterparts; research estimates that transgender adults comprise 22.9% of the veteran population, whereas prevalence rates in the general adult population are 4.3% (Blosnich et al., 2013).

S. George (✉)
School of Professional Psychology, Wright State University, Dayton, OH, USA

S. Crocker
Washington DC VA Medical Center, Washington, DC, USA
e-mail: sethcro@mail.regent.edu

A. Voltmer
VA North Florida/South Georgia, Gainesville, FL, USA
e-mail: amyvolt@mail.regent.edu

L. C. James
Department of Behavioral Health, Tripler Army Medical Center, Honolulu, HI, USA

L. C. James et al. (eds.), *Clinical Health Psychology in Military and Veteran Settings*, https://doi.org/10.1007/978-3-031-12063-3_13

1.1 Early Experiences of Transgender Veterans in the Military

During the Civil War, an estimated 250–400 women served in the military disguised as men, although the exact number is debated among scholars (Blanton & Cook, 2002). Fear of social repercussion led some of these soldiers to minimize the extent to which they presented as male while in the military, making estimates all the more difficult. In their extensive study on women in the Civil War, DeAnne Blanton and Lauren Cook describe this research area as "the best-kept historical secret of the Civil War" (2002, p. 7). Several of these soldiers continued to live as male even after completing their military service and were only discovered after undergoing emergency medical treatment or, in other cases, after their death. While some of these examples may simply reflect a desire to maintain a level of independence only offered to men, many scholars posit that at least some of these soldiers would be considered transgender. This period of history offers a fascinating and portentous glimpse into how gender normativity impacted early American soldiers' experiences. For the next century, there was no explicit ban against transgender military service. In the 1960s, however, formal prohibitions were enacted against LGBT service members (Somashekhar & Whitlock, 2015). In the 1980s, several lawsuits emerged in which the military successfully defended their ban on transgender service members (i.e., Doe v. Alexander, 510 F. Supp. 900, 1981).

1.2 Repeal of Transgender Ban

In 2014, the independent research program Palm Center, affiliated with Francisco State University, released its findings that the ban on transgender troops was both medically unsupported and inconsistent with military values (Palm Center, 2014). In 2015, the Pentagon announced that it would allow transgender individuals to openly serve in the military and formulate plans to allow open service (Somashekhar & Whitlock, 2015). With increased support from medical and mental health experts, the ban on transgender service members was officially lifted on June 30, 2016 (Directive-Type Memo 16-005; Secretary of Defense, 2016). This policy reverted when the Trump administration announced that with consultation from military experts, the US military would no longer allow transgender individuals to serve in the military. After the announcement via Twitter, several lawsuits challenged the policy change, and in January 2018, transgender individuals were allowed to serve again. Two months later, the Trump administration reinstated the military ban, and transgender individuals could no longer serve except under certain circumstances (Zucker, 2018). The order disqualified any individual with gender dysphoria, who had either completed a gender transition or was taking hormones to enlist in the military. Transgender military members diagnosed with gender dysphoria and gender non-conforming members were required to serve in their assigned sex at birth. They were not permitted to take hormones or receive gender reassignment surgery during their time in the military (Gomez, 2019).

1.3 Reinstatement of Transgender Ban

On March 12, 2019, the Department of Defense signed a memorandum that effectively banned most transgender individuals from service or enlistment in the United States Armed Forces (Office of the Deputy Secretary of Defense, 2019). This policy retracted many of the rights extended during the Obama administration; it did not retreat to the more restrictive policies of the past. Service members whose transition was completed before the ban could continue to serve, as could individuals who identified as transgender but were willing to continue serving in their biological sex. Recruiters were cautioned that "the new policy is NOT a ban on the accession of transgender persons" (United States Military Entrance Processing Command, 2019), and noted that individuals were not required to hide their gender identity. Despite framing the change as minimally impactful, the policy effectively stymied recruitment of openly transgender service members and prevented existing service members from engaging in any form of transition. For example, under this new policy, service members were held to the standards of their biological sex (Office of the Deputy Secretary of Defense, 2019). New recruits could not have undergone sex reassignment procedures or gender confirmation surgery (Office of the Deputy Secretary of Defense, 2019). This policy was met with protests from the transgender community. Legally, the policy was first challenged by a naval officer who faced discharge for seeking to transition (Richer, 2020). Other lawsuits followed, as well as proposed legislation to reject the ban on transgender military service. As of early 2020, there were four legal cases (Doe v. Trump, Stockman v. Trump, Stone v. Trump, Karnoski v. Trump) seeking to overturn the transgender ban. These lawsuits were first filed in 2017. A 2019 Gallup Poll found that over 70% of US Americans favored transgender persons serving in the military. Many states have also expressed their support of transgender military persons (Transgender, 2020).

As this review of US policy demonstrates, transgender service members have served under hostile and uncertain circumstances. Transgender veterans felt a sense of hope after the ban was lifted in 2016, such as Captain Sage Fox of the US Army Reserves, who stated, "It's going to go through and send a message to the rest of the world that the US isn't behind everyone, that we do care about human rights" (Rizzo & Cohen, 2016). The sudden reversal of these rights under President Trump continues the historical trend of utilizing transgender service members in service, without providing them the rights afforded their cisgender counterparts. Despite these challenges, some research indicates that transgender veterans experience lower rates of depression and greater health-related quality of life than their non-veteran counterparts, a finding which may reflect the resilience and post-traumatic growth of these veterans (Hoy-Ellis et al., 2017).

1.4 Transgender Care Within the Veterans Health Administration

The Veterans Health Administration (VHA) instructs staff to provide health care to transgender Veterans "in a manner that is consistent with their self-identified gender identity" (Department of Veterans Affairs, 2020). In addition to protection against discrimination during treatment, this directive provides veterans the right to change their name in the medical record to reflect their preferred name and pronouns. More recently, the VHA provided veterans the option to list their "birth sex" and "self-identified gender identity" in their medical records. Additionally, this directive protects the rights of transgender Veterans to utilize bathrooms consistent with their gender identity.

Regarding medical and mental health care, veterans are offered a range of specialty services, and each VA facility is required to have a local LGBT Veteran Care Coordinator to promote comprehensive, best-practice care (Department of Veterans Affairs, 2020). Veterans have access to hormone replacement therapy, pre-operative assessments, vocal coaching, and medical prosthetics. However, Veterans are still unable to receive gender-confirming surgery through the VA, nor will the VHA cover medical expenses for these procedures (Department of Veterans Affairs, 2020). Mental health treatment, including couples, individual, and group psychotherapy, and pre-operative psychological assessments, are also provided.

2 Transgender Health

TGNC veterans have historically faced health and social disparities, including financial challenges and reduced medical and mental health outcomes (Beckman et al., 2018; Carter et al., 2019). These discriminatory experiences extend beyond health care to employment and housing (Lehavot et al., 2016). Transgender veterans represent a highly marginalized subpopulation within the military and civilian populations. The US Department of Veteran Affairs (VA) reported a higher prevalence of transgender individuals than any other US general population (Beckman et al., 2018; Blosnich et al., 2016; Lehavot et al., 2016; Tucker et al., 2019). More specifically, VA records indicate that between 2000 and 2011, the number of individuals diagnosed with gender identity disorder was over five times higher for veterans than the general civilian population (Tucker et al., 2019). The Williams Institute at the University of California at Los Angeles (UCLA) conducted a study in 2014 and estimated almost 16,000 transgender individuals in either the active-duty military, Guard, or Reserves. Also, there were over 134,000 transgender veterans. Based on these large numbers, the Veterans Administration opened specialty transgender clinics in Cleveland, Ohio and Tucson, Arizona. There are large health disparities in the transgender population when compared to their cisgender counterparts, which has led to the National Academy of Medicine calling for increased research focused on the variables that contribute to the health differences found in transgender persons (Bukowski et al., 2017).

2.1 2015 US Transgender Survey

The National Center for Transgender Equality conducted an anonymous online survey for transgender adults (age 18 and older; English and Spanish versions). It was one of the most extensive surveys to take a more in-depth look into the lives and experiences of 27,715 transgender individuals from the United States, including the District of Columbia, Guam, Puerto Rico, American Samoa, and overseas US military bases. The US Transgender Survey (USTS) revealed extensive discrimination and disparities related to employment, housing, family/community support, and accessing health care (James & Herman, 2017).

2.2 Housing

In 2009, the United States Interagency Council on Homelessness declared efforts to eliminate homelessness among veterans by 2015. Consequently, according to the US Department of Housing and Urban Development (HUD), the overall veteran population's national rates of homelessness decreased by nearly 50% (Carter et al., 2019). Furthermore, the number of veterans who identified as transgender increased by almost 90% between 2015 and 2018. While homelessness was generally trending downward, transgender veterans experienced difficulties with housing at rates two times higher than others (Carter et al., 2019). Furthermore, Carter and colleagues found that transgender veterans were more likely to experience housing instability if they were White, unmarried, younger, and women (Carter et al., 2019). Overall, the transgender population is less likely to own a home, and up to one-third of the population has experienced homelessness during their lifetime (James & Herman, 2017).

2.3 Employment

Based on the 2015 US Transgender survey, another gap is economic hardship. At the time of the US Transgender survey, the transgender unemployment rate (15%) was three times larger than the general US population (5%). Transgender individuals with disabilities faced a higher unemployment rate of 24%, and approximately 45% lived below the poverty line. In a 2015 national survey, 15% of transgender respondents indicated harassment (verbally, physically, sexually) at their place of employment in the last year (Beckman et al., 2018). In the 2010 National Transgender

Discrimination Survey, 90% of respondents reported discrimination or harassment at their jobs across their lifetime (Beckman et al., 2018). Particular concerns arose from dealing with the stigma and distress in concealing their gender identity to maintain employment and retirement benefits. Other relevant employment issues include forcibly using a restroom that did not match their gender identity, denial of promotion, and private information shared with others without their consent (James & Herman, 2017). Of note, protective factors include living in a state with hate crimes and employment discrimination protections (Blosnich et al., 2016).

2.4 Health Care Utilization

Fears of discrimination and stigmatization related to their distress and disorder by health care professionals often deter individuals from seeking health services. Thus, health care utilization is often much lower in transgender populations (Aboussouan et al., 2019; Ruben et al., 2019). Reduced utilization tends to lead to an increase in serious health implications and lower life expectancy. Seelman et al. (2017) found that transgender individuals had worse overall health in the last month than those who immediately sought medical attention. The delay in seeking help was due primarily to fear surrounding how health care providers may see them and noninclusive care from medical staff. TGNC persons often have difficulty openly sharing their gender identity without being questioned or attacked or addressed with incorrect pronouns.

Furthermore, many transgender people expressed fear they would receive substandard care. They shared they were scared their health may be compromised, and that they may continue to be poorly treated.

Medical care settings are often perceived as more discriminatory than other settings and resources, such as employment or housing (Ruben et al., 2019; Seelman et al., 2017; Xavier et al., 2007). Transgender persons with disabilities reported higher mistreatment rates by their medical providers in the 2015 US Transgender Health Survey. Furthermore, individuals who sought gynecological care, hormone therapy, or surgery were at an increased likelihood to experience discrimination than transgender individuals who did not reveal their transgender status or those who were not pursuing gender reassignment surgery (Seelman et al., 2017). Thus, TGNC individuals tend to have a negative perception of health care providers, which leads to other concerns, such as non-engagement in health care screenings, lower or missed opportunities for health education, and overall poorer health (Ruben et al., 2019).

In a 2011 survey of 6000 transgender people, roughly one-fifth of the respondents indicated they were refused health care due to their transgender or gender non-conforming status. One-third postponed necessary medical care when they were either injured or sick (Legal, 2016). In another study conducted in 2010, 70% of transgender respondents shared they had one or more of the following experiences with providers who:

1. Refused to touch transgender patients or used excessive precautions
2. Used abusive or harsh language
3. Blamed the transgender patient for their health concern and
4. Were physically rough or abusive with the transgender patient

Furthermore, transgender respondents indicated rude and inappropriate behavior by health care professionals, which included laughing and mockery, HIPAA violations, unusually long waits for care, inappropriate questions and exams, and failure to follow established standards of care (Legal, 2016). Seeking medical care may be a daunting task, and when it is coupled with discriminatory experiences, transgender patients are deterred by fields of care that are designated to serve and help those in need.

2.5 *Suicide Risk*

Considering the impact of minority stress, transgender patients are much more likely than the general population to experience suicidal ideation and make suicide attempts. Of particular concern are those who engage in NSSI (non-suicidal self-injury) and other suicidal-related behaviors. According to Van Orden et al.' (2010) interpersonal theory of suicide, they discuss the concept of thwarted belongingness, which is a phenomenon in which an individual possesses unmet needs to belong. Thwarted belongingness, perceived burdensomeness, and associated hopelessness collectively increase an individual's suicidal ideation and behaviors. Transgender individuals experience an array of psychosocial vulnerabilities, which contribute to unmet needs, disheartenment, and hopelessness; thus, transgender veterans experience higher rates of suicidal ideation, attempts, and completion.

Research has found that veterans with gender-identity dysphoria are at increased likelihood of experiencing suicide-related events (20 times the rate of general VA population) (Blosnich et al., 2013). A national transgender study found that roughly 40% of transgender individuals indicated a past suicide attempt, which is significantly higher than the 3% that is reported among the general population (Blosnich et al., 2016; James et al., 2016; Lehavot et al., 2016). In a sample of 212 transgender veterans, 57% of veterans reported struggling with suicidal ideation within the last year, 34% reported having a suicide plan during their lifetime, and 32% had made a suicide attempt (Lehavot et al., 2016). Interestingly, while transgender veterans had lower rates of NSSI, they were more likely to be hospitalized than the transgender non-veteran population (Aboussouan et al., 2019). Furthermore, 41% of those who endorsed NSSI also indicated a history of suicide attempts, and 86.7% indicated suicidal ideation (Aboussouan et al., 2019). It is unclear why the rates are lower, but it may be attributed to military culture and resistance in disclosing mental health concerns.

- Transgender veterans are more likely to die by suicide (Blosnich et al., 2014).
- Transgender veterans are at 20 times higher risk of suicidal ideation (SI) and suicide attempt (SA) than the general veteran population (Blosnich et al., 2013).
- In a study sample, two-thirds of transgender veterans reported planning their death during their lifetime (Tucker et al., 2019).
- Transgender veterans die by suicide at an earlier age (49) than cisgender veterans (Blosnich et al., 2014).
- History of SI was reported by 61% of transgender veterans (57% reported in the last year; 11–32% reported one or more suicide attempts) (Lehavot et al., 2016; McDuffie & Brown, 2010).

2.6 *Mental Health*

Along with suicide risk, many indicated other mental health problems. The three most common diagnoses were mood disorders, substance use disorders, and post-traumatic stress disorder (PTSD) (Blosnich et al., 2016). In a study by Blosnich et al. (2016), transgender individuals who resided in states that enacted employment nondiscrimination protection had lower prevalence rates of mood disorder (54% vs. 46%) and lower rates of self-injurious behaviors. The researchers found that a history of homelessness, perceived military stigma, and current depression and PTSD symptoms were correlated with past year suicidal ideation and lifetime suicide plans and attempts.

Access to care has significantly improved in recent years. As of 2017, the VA reported that approximately 5000 transgender Veterans are engaged in VA health care (Cramer, 2017). The utilization of VA services by transgender Veterans increased dramatically in the 2 years following a 2011 VHA directive requiring the provision of medically necessary care (Kauth et al., 2014). While veterans generally report high levels of satisfaction with the VA, transgender veterans encounter unique risk factors that impact their VA experience. In a recent study on the experience of transgender veterans in the VA, 79% of respondents reported satisfaction with their medical care, whereas 69% reported satisfaction with their mental health care (Lehavot et al., 2017). Notably, this study found that dissatisfaction was associated with lower income and being a transgender male veteran.

2.7 *Sexual Assault and Associated Health Concerns*

Military sexual assault (MSA) encompasses penetrative acts of sexual assault, which does not include physical assault or sexual harassment. Military sexual trauma (MST) is a broader concept that includes physical assault and/or battery of a sexual nature and sexual harassment that occurred while on active duty (Beckman et al., 2018). Lindsay et al. (2016) found in a sample of 332 transgender veterans that nearly one in five transmen screened positive for military sexual trauma (MST) and one in seven transwomen. For transgender veterans, many experienced physical and sexual violence perpetrated by their peers (Beckman et al., 2018; Bukowski et al., 2017). Close to one-fourth of transgender people experience a form of violence motivated by gender bias and discrimination, and close to half were sexually assaulted during their lifetime (Beckman et al., 2018). Sexual assaults started as early as grade school (K-12) as these persons openly identified as transgender or appeared to others as transgender (13% of 2015 US Transgender Survey).

Studies have found that those with histories of MST had a higher prevalence of mental health disorders, especially depression, anxiety, and PTSD. Older transgender individuals are more likely to suffer from poorer health than cisgender individuals of the same age and report more significant perceived stress (Fredriksen-Goldsen et al., 2014). Transgender and gender non-conforming (TGNC) individuals may also struggle with body image concerns and eating disorders as transwomen may seek a slimmer figure or transmen may try to reduce their hip to shoulder ratio (Goldberg & Ashbee, 2006).

HIV/AIDS is another factor to consider as the TGNC population, mainly transwomen have high rates of the disease (De Santis, 2009). According to the 2015 US Transgender Survey, respondents were five times more likely than the general US population to be living with HIV (1.4% vs. 0.3%). HIV rates were much higher for transgender women, especially Black transgender women (19%). These findings are consistent with the 2008 study conducted by Herbst and colleagues, who found that 27.7% of male-to-female individuals acquired HIV/AIDS across a meta-analysis of four studies, with the highest rates being found among African American transwomen at 56.3%. Researchers wrote that these numbers could be explained by higher rates of unprotected sex, sex work, and substance use, which may be used to cope with minority stress or reflect efforts to survive.

2.8 *Support*

The 2015 US Transgender Survey explored family and community support among the transgender population. They found that 60% of respondents reported their immediate family was generally supportive, 22% indicated their family was neither supportive or unsupportive, and 18% shared their family was unsupportive of their transgender status. One-tenth of the respondents reported they experienced violence from a family member because they are transgender, and 8% stated they were forced to leave their home. Almost one-fifth of the survey participants left their spiritual/religious community due to the rejection of their transgender status. However, almost half of those respondents indicated they later found another spiritual/religious community where they felt welcomed and accepted. Overall, they found that transgender persons with supportive family members were less likely to be homeless, attempt suicide, and experience significant psychological distress.

3 Male to Female (MTF) and Female to Male (FTM) Transgender Veterans

The transgender population consists of male to female (MTF) and female to male (FTM) persons. Studies have shown that there are qualitative differences between these two subpopulations. The following are general distinctions between MTFs and FTMs:

- MTF group tended to transition at a later age than FTMs. The average age of transition for FTMs was 23 years.
- While MTFs were less educated than FTMs, they indicated higher yearly incomes.
- Due to transgender discrimination, MTFs are more likely to be fired from their employment.
- While FTMs experienced less job discrimination, they were more likely to lose housing and become homeless.
- FTMs are more likely to have children living with them and less likely to have biological or adopted children.

Regarding health and sexual practices:

- MTFs were more likely to receive transgender hormonal therapy and, most likely, from someone other than a medical doctor.
- MTFs are more likely to undergo genital sex reassignment surgery and cosmetic surgery.
- FTMs are more likely to be either uncomfortable or very uncomfortable revealing their transgender status and engaging in discussion with their health care provider when compared to MTFs.
- Approximately half of MTFs with primary partners never used condoms or other forms (protective barriers), whereas almost one-quarter of MTFs tend to use a form of protection consistently.
- Slightly over half of FTMs with primary partners tend not to use condoms or other protective barriers, whereas one-fifth tend to use a form of protection consistently.
- One-tenth of MTFs with other partners outside their primary partner rarely use protection.
- MTFs who shared they were HIV positive also indicated that the primary source of infection was unprotected sex with a non-transgender man (nearly 90%).
- FTMs strongly indicate they need transgender-sensitive gynecological care, but only one-third reported actually receiving transgender-sensitive gynecological care.
- FTMs rate the quality of transgender care services and provider sensitivity consistently lower than MTFs.

Mental health needs and concerns:

- FTMs are more likely to be physically attacked and sexually assaulted than MTFs.
- FTMs experienced higher rates of SI. Of note, there were little difference in rates of suicide attempts between MTFs and FTMs.
- FTMs reported higher rates of drug use and tobacco use and earlier age of first drug use.

3.1 Veteran MTFs and FTMs

When explicitly examining transgender veterans, military transgender men were more likely to experience military sexual assault than transgender women (30% MTF vs. 15.2% FTM), with an overall rate for transgender veterans at 17.2% (Beckman et al., 2018). Upon further examination, it was found that transgender men were more likely to be diagnosed with post-traumatic stress disorder and a personality disorder, specifically for those who have experienced military sexual trauma (MST). On the other hand, transgender women who have experienced MST were more likely to be diagnosed with PTSD, personality disorder, depressive disorder, and bipolar disorder. Additionally, when military transgender individuals were divided by ethnicity (white, non-Hispanic, or ethnic minority), they found that 50% of transgender men and nearly 20% of transgender women identified as an ethnic minority (Beckman et al., 2018; Lindsay et al., 2016). Thus, treatment and assessment need to include cultural sensitivity alongside inclusive, transgender-sensitive care.

4 Treatment Considerations

4.1 Minority Stress Model

The Minority Stress Model (MSM) identifies various types of stressors unique to an individual's minority identity. There are *distal minority* stressors, which are discriminatory and prejudicial events that occur in one's environment. *Proximal minority* stressors are characterized as internal processes. For transgender individuals in the military, distal minority stressors may include events such as losing housing or employment, being interrogated about their gender identity, or being forced into psychological treatment. Proximal minority stressors for this population take into account their stress, anxiety, and concern about how others may perceive them, or the immense amount of energy consumed in concealing their gender identity. This model suggests that overarching, general life stressors may influence both distal and proximal stressors. Thus, as transgender veterans not only navigate specific stressors related to their gender identity, they also face daily life stressors, which create unique vulnerabilities and predispositions to illness, disease, and mental health disorders (Beckman et al., 2018). For example, these stressors contribute to the increased likelihood of suicidal ideation and military sexual trauma. The Minority Stress Model may help practitioners identify and understand existing health, housing, and employment disparities among the transgender population. As mental health practitioners actively engage with this population, it is imperative also to recognize their internalized stigmatizing beliefs and shame (Lehavot et al., 2016; Tucker et al., 2019). The Minority Stress Model also suggests that social support and an influential community connection act as a protective factor to a variety of problems.

4.2 Responding to Transgender Clients

The discrimination against transgender clients by providers violates human rights and the law. Mental health professionals are expected to uphold high standards of care and excellence and to do no harm (APA ethics). This means implementing and following standards of care that are respectful, sensitive, and inclusive. It is essential to be aware of workplace policies and procedures and to keep your eyes open. If you witness acts of discrimination, it is crucial to speak up or report the incident to your supervisor, employer, or human resources department. If you are unsure, seek guidance and consultation with another professional, your supervisor, human resources, licensing board, or a lawyer. Additionally, mental health providers should examine their own biases and seek avenues to challenge their personal and professional beliefs and educate themselves on culturally sensitive practice. Learning and discussing anti-discriminatory practices are a part of a lifelong journey that will positively serve both yourself and patients.

5 Intake and Clinical Interview

Transgender and gender-nonconforming (TGNC) patients may seek psychological services for various reasons, whether to address concerns that any patient may bring to treatment, such as depression or anxiety, or more specific problems, like discrimination or identity questions. They may also seek more specific expertise for transition-related services, such as readiness evaluations for hormone replacement therapy or gender affirmative surgeries. When assessing transgender patients, it is vital to consider the impact of minority stress (Meyer, 2003) on symptom presentation to avoid over-pathologizing patients. This means that practitioners should consider how the impact of familial, societal, economic, and political stressors can create collective trauma for transgender individuals as they navigate their day-to-day lives and how these cumulative experiences can create psychological distress. This approach can help clinicians avoid assumptions that patient distress is due to gender dysphoria when it may be better explained by oppressive societal factors (American Psychological Association [APA], 2015).

6 Considerations for Clinical Interviews with Transgender Patients

Clinicians should ask all their patients about gender identity when assessing for cultural identities and experiences. This can be done verbally in the clinical interview or in the history and symptom paperwork completed prior to the intake (Trittschuh et al., 2018). When asking about gender identity in paperwork, it is advisable to leave the question open-ended, or provide options such as Cisgender (meaning that one's biological sex matches their gender identity) Male and Female, Transman/transgender man/female-to-male, Transwoman/transgender woman/ male-to-female, Other, or Choose not to answer (Kauth, 2017). When patients disclose having a transgender identity, several factors are helpful to consider. TGNC patients may identify with a binary perspective of sex as either male or female, but many TGNC individuals also identify as gender nonbinary, such as androgynous genderqueer, gender-fluid, or two-spirit (Hendricks & Testa, 2012).

Terms	Definitions
Androgynous	Identify/present as neither masculine or feminine
Asexual	Lack of sexual attraction or desire for other people
Bisexual	Emotionally, romantically, or sexually attracted to more than one sex, gender, or gender identity
Cisgender	Gender identity aligns with the sex assigned to the individual at birth
Gender Non-Conforming	Gender expression does not conform to the traditional expectations of that specific gender
Genderqueer/Third Gender/Gender Fluid	A general rejection of gender categories and embraces a fluidity of gender identity; may see themselves as both male and female, neither male or female, or they may see themselves completely outside of these categories
Non-binary	Adjective used to describe a person who does not exclusively identify as a man or a woman
Queer	Term often used to express fluid identities and orientations; often used interchangeably with LGBTQ
Transgender	Term for individuals whose gender identity and/or expression is different from the cultural expectations based on the sex they were assigned at birth.
Two-Spirit	Individual who identifies with the Native American tradition of characterizing members of the community as having the spirit of both the male and female genders.

Asking patients about their preferred pronouns offers another affirmative approach in working with TGNC patients. TGNC patients may be gender binary or nonbinary (i.e., patients may use they/them pronouns). It is essential to ask if the patient has a preference for the name and pronouns used in clinical notes and assessment reports, depending on whether the patient has publicly come out as transgender. Trittschuh et al. (2018) noted this could impact the gendered forms of address that clinicians should use (such as Mr., Ms., Mrs.). It can also be helpful to refer to TGNC individuals without a gendered title, such as "Veteran Smith" or "Smith" as opposed to "Mr. Smith." The authors also recommended giving ticket numbers as another approach to avoid assuming and misgendering individuals. These considerations demonstrate respect and can assist clinicians in building rapport with their TGNC patients.

Determining the history and development of gender dysphoric feelings is an important step in the assessment process, along with ensuring that gender dysphoria is not better explained by another diagnosis (WPATH, 2012). Clinicians should assess if the patient has received any medical procedures related to transitioning, such as hormone replacement therapy or gender affirmative surgeries. Additionally, Trittschuh et al. (2018) wrote that conceptualizing patients from a developmental model can help gather information to track the progression from birth gender to where the patient currently experiences authenticity. The authors recommended Lev's (2004) model of transgender identity development, which includes the stages of Awareness, Seeking information/Reaching out, Disclosure to significant others, Exploration-Identity and self-labeling, Exploration-Transition issues/Possible body modification, and Integration-Acceptance and post-transition issues. However, identity does not always develop in a linear progression, so caution should be exercised when utilizing any model (Bockting et al., 2016). Trittschuh et al. (2018) wrote that developmental models could provide clinicians with a heuristic to conceptualize a patient's background and direct services for the patient.

Clinicians should also remember that sexual orientation and gender identity are two separate constructs (APA, 2015). A TGNC individual may identify as heterosexual or as a sexual minority. Sherman et al. (2014) found that 24% of sexual and gender minority veterans ($n = 58$) had never disclosed their sexual orientation to a Veterans Affairs (VA) provider, while 33% had disclosed this information to all their providers, leaving 43% of veterans who had shared with some number of their providers. Over 60% of veterans reported none of their providers asked about their sexual orientation, and 81% reported that none of their providers had asked about their gender identity. Not all veterans believe they are safe to share this information with their health care providers, so clinicians should take the initiative to ask about sexual orientation and gender identity and facilitate safety during the intake interview. Fifty-nine percent of the sample expressed being quite or very comfortable talking about their sexual and/or gender identity with their providers. Yet, there may be a gap in understanding how these constructs connect to veterans' physical and mental health.

Hendricks and Testa (2012) recommended that clinicians consider Meyer's (2003) minority stress theory when assessing transgender patients. These factors include "prior discrimination or victimization, expectations of future victimization or rejection, internalized transphobia, and resilience" (p. 465). Discrimination toward TGNC individuals comes in many forms, including difficulty obtaining housing, access to health care, finding and maintaining employment, barriers in education, and difficulties receiving social services (APA, 2015). TGNC patients have likely had experiences of being misgendered (referring to a TGNC person by the wrong pronouns) or deadnamed (calling a TGNC person by their birth or former name), along with potentially dealing with inappropriate questions about their bodies (APA, 2015). Psychologists should also consider an intersectional approach for transgender and gender-nonconforming patients of color who may have unique experiences of trauma and discrimination, even perpetrated by those within the larger LGBTQ+ community targeting their racial/ethnic or transgender identities (APA, 2015; Chang & Singh, 2016). TGNC women, especially those of color, are particularly vulnerable to violence and homicide, including violence from police officers (APA, 2015). Thus, it is important to consider other diversity variables and the potential impact on one's overall development and experiences as the clinical interview is conducted and during the process in which one is determining the assessment battery.

TGNC patients also present a variety of protective factors that should be considered beyond symptom complaints and risk factors that can help patients achieve treatment goals or direct recommendations (Chang & Singh, 2016). Family support can be an especially salient protective factor for TGNC individuals (Bockting et al., 2013; Moody & Smith, 2013; Ryan et al., 2010). Instruments like the Gender Minority Stress and Resilience measure (Testa et al., 2015) can help provide information about not only stressors but strengths like community connectedness and transgender pride.

7 Holistic Treatment of Transgender Veterans

As clearly indicated, this population is poorly connected with inclusive health care services. Considering the multiple layers of risk and problems, a multi-level intervention approach is warranted to engage and treat the transgender veteran population. As a psychologist, it begins with the field addressing one's own biases, beliefs, and competencies. It is strongly suggested that psychologists and other mental health professionals complete cultural competence and humility training and training on sexual identities and the transgender population specifically. As one builds their expertise and gains valuable experience, one may even consider providing training to mental health clinicians and other fields, such as medicine, social work, shelters, substance use programs, transitional housing, and employment programs. An area to consider focusing on is how to engage in relationship-building and apply a culturally humble, inclusive, on-going discussion about the veteran's transgender status and health care needs. It is imperative the treating clinician foster openness, trust, sensitivity, and relational repair if there is a rupture in the relationship. This will likely increase the likelihood of seeking help and meaningful engagement in services. Practitioners may employ their diversity training by honing their sensitivity and awareness of the population, including risk and protective factors. Another focus may include assisting transgender clients with navigating systems and advocating for care, including transgender-sensitive gynecological care to FTMs or housing or providing education on the client's needs (Xavier et al., 2007).

As a mental health clinician and advocate, thinking holistically and systemically about the needs of the transgender veteran includes the following:

- Medication.
- Hormones.
- Financial costs.
- Individual, family, couples, group therapy.
- Substance use treatment.
- Case management.
- Sexual health (testing and protective methods).
- Housing.
- Employment.
- Transportation.
- Psychiatric services.
- Health concerns.
- Surgery.
- Food banks.
- School/academic.
- Parenting.
- Spirituality.
- Legal.
- Changing ID documents.
- Telehealth.

Psychological services may consider implementing prevention and outreach programs and workshops, which promote transgender-specific materials. This may include educational programs for transgender veterans about transgender care. A study involving both urban and rural VA providers utilized a VA Transgender e-consult program to assist medical professions with care plans, hormone therapy recommendations and sexual, reproductive health education, surgery treatment education, patient-provider communication, and consultation. This VA program permits transgender veterans to seek local health care providers, who receive consultation and support from others with expertise in transgender health. The four main consultation topics were: psychotherapy, mental health evaluation and hormone readiness, prescription of hormone therapy, and primary medical care. The providers reported time constraints, unrealistic recommendations for under-resourced VA sites, communication problems, and misunderstanding the purpose of the e-consult platform created barriers in treatment. The study found that providers and patients were not using the program because they were unaware of the program (over half), received assistance elsewhere, or did not feel a need for the program. Participants shared the program would be further utilized if they were given information on where to locate the program, utilization guidance, discussion points to address with patients, and email announcements to improve awareness of the e-consult program (Blosnich et al., 2016). As a treating clinician, it may be beneficial to create one's own personal network of other expert practitioners for consultation purposes, especially as unexpected needs and concerns arise with transgender clients.

8 Psychological Assessment Considerations with Transgender Patients

TGNC patients may pursue psychological assessments like other patients to seek answers for different questions, such as differential diagnosis, treatment recommendations, or specific questions like memory concerns. TGNC may also seek specialized assessment services, such as readiness evaluations to obtain access to hormone treatment and gender affirmative surgeries. Mental health providers should consider what the literature states on working with TGNC individuals to provide competent care.

8.1 Psychological Testing

8.1.1 Norms and Test Selection

A major problem in testing psychology for the transgender population is the lack of norms (Keo-Meier & Fitzgerald, 2017; Trittschuh et al., 2018). When psychologists do not consider factors such as Meyer's (2003) minority stress theory, there is potential for over-pathologizing transgender and gender-nonconforming patients. Keo-Meier and Fitzgerald (2017) recommended either using gender-stratified tests that incorporate norms from both cisgender men and women or tests with non-gendered norms. Specific tests like the MMPI-2 have been found to have significant scale elevations for transgender patients compared to their cisgender counterparts and should be used with caution. Trittschuh et al. (2018) suggested that it can also be helpful to examine both male and female norms to examine whether there are significant differences in the results.

Clinicians should also consider the length of time their patient has been on exogenous hormones that may affect brain structures, though the research remains unclear how this may impact testing (Trittschuh et al., 2018). Postmortem data have shown differences in the brain's overall size and different regions of the brain, such as the hypothalamus (Hulsho Pol et al., 2006; Seiger et al., 2016). The research revealed mixed findings about how transgender participants compared to cisgender individuals in control groups. Some found that transgender participant scores fell between cisgender male and female scores (Smith et al., 2015), nearer to the scores of controls from their birth sex (Luders et al., 2009), and neared to those of their gender identity (Rametti et al., 2011a, b). Studies have also indicated that hormone treatment may increase spatial intelligence in transmen on testosterone (Slabbekoorn et al., 1999) and may increase verbal intelligence in transwomen on estrogen (Van Goozen et al., 1994, 1995). However, the research remains inconsistent and unclear. Trittschuh et al. (2018) wrote that given the conflicting data from the research, clinicians should consider results from norms of both sexes and weigh the findings in light of the referral question, the individual, and the background information of the patient to determine which norms are most appropriate to determine test interpretation.

8.1.2 Interpretation and Report Writing

While clinicians desire expectations for performance in psychological testing, Trittschuh et al. (2018) warned against using instruments with gendered norms to determine premorbid abilities because of the increased risk of bias and skewing interpretations. Additionally, the researchers expressed that clinicians should exercise great caution when any subjective or objective performance validity concerns manifest themselves in test interpretation, given the difficulties and health disparities the TGNC population encounter. The authors also suggested discussing the limitations uncovered during the testing process and making looser diagnostic conclusions than might be typical in an assessment report.

As psychologists create recommendations for TGNC patients, they should explore what resources are available in the client's specific community that could be beneficial for the patient. This could include affirming health care and mental health providers, housing services, religious and spiritual communities, or local LGBTQ+ centers, LGBTQ+ care providers, and/or services offered by the provider's facility or practice (APA, 2015).

8.1.3 Providing Feedback to Transgender Patients

The feedback session is one of the most crucial parts of assessment as the provider communicates the patient's findings in a way that the patient can understand. This is especially important for TGNC patients given the complexity of their cases. Trittschuh et al. (2018) provided several suggestions for managing feedback sessions well with TGNC patients. First, they remind clinicians to remain relaxed. Providers tend to be more anxious than their patients. The researchers recommended having a clear rationale and transparent discussion with the patient, along with having an open attitude on the subject of gender identity and willingness to be corrected when wrong. Second, framing the feedback session with the referral question can help the provider and patient stay on track and help the patient form questions to discuss. Third, reminding the patient of discussions in the clinical interview, such as the impact of sex and hormones on cognition can help direct the conversation. Fourth, asking permission to discuss gender identity and the patient's transition process can help build a spirit of collaboration between the clinician and patient. Fifth, clinicians should be transparent in dialoguing about the normative differences by sex in testing. The researchers note it can be helpful to discuss with patients when there are interpretive differences by sex, and also show the patients when there are discrepancies between male and female scores to have a collaborative conversation. Having these discussions in the feedback session can minimize future questions about written implications about gender in the report. Lastly, clinicians should also express positive contributions of the transition for the TGNC patient. The authors provide examples of cognitive congruence that can occur after transitioning and improved mental health benefits. This strength-based approach can help foster hope in the feedback session.

8.2 Readiness Evaluations

The WPATH (2012) established multiple guidelines for ensuring competent care of TGNC individuals, especially those seeking gender affirmative medical interventions. Providers discuss the various options and roles that TGNC patients can pursue to find an identity that best fits their experience. Providers should screen for other diagnoses that could be associated with gender dysphoria and minority stress or could be unrelated to these experiences, such as “anxiety, depression, self-harm, a history of abuse and neglect, compulsivity, substance abuse, sexual concerns, personality disorders, eating disorders, psychotic disorders, and autistic spectrum disorders” (WPATH, 2012, p. 24). When these conditions remain unaddressed, they can complicate identity exploration and create barriers to resolving gender dysphoria. The WPATH guidelines note that while these conditions may not mean a TGNC patient would be disqualified from receiving medical services, these clinical concerns should be addressed and managed well before beginning hormone treatment or surgical procedures.

Mental health clinicians play an essential role in the health care of TGNC patients, especially in readiness evaluations. They ensure that the patient is fully informed and prepared for the major changes ahead. Family and community provide important support for navigating hormonal changes or healing from surgical procedures. Patients should also know the impacts that hormone replacement therapy and surgical interventions have on fertility and reproductive health, allowing them to consider options before proceeding.

8.2.1 Guidelines for Referrals to Feminizing/Masculinizing Hormone Therapy

Within the Veterans Health Administration (VHA), mental health providers evaluate TGNC veterans for the presence of the DSM diagnosis of Gender Dysphoria must be given to initiate a referral for hormone treatment (VHA, 2020). Providers should create a referral letter or document in the patient’s chart and include the patient’s personal and treatment history, progress, and eligibility for the procedure (WPATH, 2012). This would include identifying the patient’s characteristics, the results of the patient’s psychological evaluation and any diagnoses given, dates for how long the provider has worked with the patient, including the type of evaluation and/or therapy conducted. The provider must also explain what criteria have been met for hormone therapy and a clinical rationale that supports the patient’s request for hormones. Clinicians should also write that informed consent has been obtained from the patient and that the provider is available to coordinate care and welcomes phone calls to begin this process.

WPATH (2012) criteria for hormone treatment include persistent and well-documented gender dysphoria, the ability to make informed decisions, consent to treatment, and be of age of majority in the given country. If there are any physical or mental disorders present, they must be relatively managed. If the patient has been taking illicit hormones, this may be a rationale for bypassing the criteria to ensure the patient is properly monitored by a licensed professional. It is also unethical to deny hormone treatment for patients with HIV/AIDS or hepatitis B or C. However, certain health conditions may be contraindicated for hormone treatment, and other options should be considered.

When obtaining informed consent, WPATH (2012) recommends that the provider discuss the irreversible changes from hormone treatment with the patient. It should be documented that the patient is legally able to give informed consent, which can include those declared by the court to be emancipated minors, incarcerated individuals, and cognitively impaired patients who have been deemed competent to participate in their medical decisions. Providers should discuss all the relevant considerations of hormone therapy with the patient that includes the benefits and risks of the intervention and the impact on reproductive health, which should be all documented.

Physical changes that can be expected for female-to-male patients include an enlarged clitoris, deepened voice, increased facial and body hair, cessation of menses, atrophy of breast tissue, and lowered body fat percentage compared to muscle mass. In male-to-female patients, this can include breast growth, lowered erectile functioning, smaller testicular size, and increased body fat percentage compared to muscle mass. These physical changes tend to occur over 2 years and will be variable in each patient. This can depend on the dose received, how the hormones are administered, the medications used, and the medical risk profile (WPATH, 2012).

WPATH (2012) lists several categories of risks for hormone replacement therapy that vary in level of likelihood. Likely increased risks include "venous thromboembolic disease," "gallstones," "elevated liver enzymes," "weight gain," and "hypertriglyceridemia" for feminizing hormones and "polycythemia," "weight gain," "acne," "androgenic alopecia (balding)," and "sleep apnea" for masculinizing hormones (p. 40). Additional risk factors will likely increase the cardiovascular risk for those taking feminizing hormones. Possible risks include "hypertension" and "hyperprolactinemia or prolactinoma" for feminizing hormones and "elevated liver enzymes" and "hyperlipidemia" for masculinizing hormones (p. 40). With additional health risk factors, additional risks can include "Type 2 diabetes" for feminizing hormones and "destabilization of certain psychiatric disorders," "cardiovascular disease," "hypertension," and "Type 2 diabetes" with masculinizing hormones (p. 40). Lastly, there is not a risk or the evidence is inconclusive for the following conditions: "breast cancer" for feminizing hormones and "loss of bone density", "breast cancer," "cervical cancer," "ovarian cancer," and "uterine cancer" for masculinizing hormones (p. 40).

Additionally, reproductive options should be discussed with patients, such as sperm-preservation options and sperm-banks for male-to-female patients and oocyte or embryo freezing for female-to-male patients. These options are not available in all locations and can be expensive. However, TGNC individuals should never be refused reproductive options, and this should be discussed as part of the evaluation process.

8.2.2 Guidelines for Referrals to Surgery

Mental health professionals would follow similar guidelines for making surgical referrals as they would for hormone treatment. Providers create a referral letter or document in the patient's chart that includes the patient's personal and treatment history, treatment progress, and eligibility. The provider recognizes that they share in the ethical and legal responsibility in this decision with the surgeon. A major difference for gender affirmative surgical interventions is that two letters of reference are required from mental health professionals for some of these procedures, which will likely be written by the patient's therapist and an evaluating mental health provider (WPATH, 2012).

Again, the letter from providers should cover identifying characteristics of the patient, the assessment results and any diagnoses given to the patient, the history of the relationship between the provider and patient and what types of services have been utilized such as assessment or therapy. Providers should specify what criteria the patient has met for the surgery and the clinical rationale that supports the patient's request. The provider must document that informed consent was obtained from the patient and the provider must state that they are available for coordination of care and to take calls to begin this process.

The WPATH (2012) criteria is similar for gender affirmative surgical procedures, yet some considerations are depending on the type of surgery. For chest surgeries, only one referral is typically needed. For mastectomies in female-to-male patients to create a male chest, hormone treatment is not a prerequisite. Breast augmentation in male-to-female patients includes a recommendation of feminizing hormones for 12 months to maximize breast growth and ensure better surgical results. Genital surgeries require two referral letters from mental health providers. In addition to the criteria for hormone treatment, a fifth criterion is included for hysterectomies and salpingo-oophorectomies in female-to-male patients and orchiectomies in male-to-female patients. This additional criterion includes 12 months of continuous hormone therapy tailored to the patient's goals unless hormone treatment is contraindicated for the patient. A sixth criterion is included for metaoidioplasty or phalloplasties in female-to-male patients and vaginoplasties in male-to-female patients. This criterion involves living 12 months in the gender role that is congruent with one's gender identity.

If the patient has been diagnosed with a severe psychiatric disorder and suffers from impaired reality testing, the WPATH (2012) recommends that efforts must be made to utilize psychotropic medication and psychotherapy prior to surgery. These disorders can include psychotic episodes, bipolar disorder, dissociative identity disorder, and borderline personality disorder. The patient should be reexamined by a mental health professional who has competency with severe and persistent mental illness. The provider should assess the patient's current condition, mental status, and readiness for surgical procedures. In addition, surgery should not be performed on actively psychotic patients.

8.2.3 Additional Considerations

Providers should also consider several factors when conducting readiness evaluations. Hendricks and Testa (2012) wrote that transgender patients may be reticent to share about their experiences of trauma, transphobia, or psychological distress because their own research revealed that divulging a certain level of psychopathology can create barriers in their ability to obtain a letter of recommendation for gender-affirming medical procedures. Providers should recognize that they are not gatekeepers but function to assist transgender patients with preparedness for the changes that will come with hormone therapy or gender-affirmative surgical interventions. Spending time clarifying the provider's role, the purpose of the evaluation, and any concerns of the patient can help create more transparency in the assessment along with helping the patient determine the steps that will ensure a smooth transition process that will set up the patient for success.

9 Conclusion

Working with TGNC patients can be a complicated yet rewarding experience. Mental health providers should be aware of the pertinent literature on conducting clinical intakes and avoiding bias in test administration. Maintaining competency can assist clinicians with facilitating an affirmative and meaningful experience for their TGNC patients who encounter prejudice and discrimination in many other domains of their lives, even in their health care. Mental health providers can create emotionally corrective experiences in the assessment experience and advocate for their TGNC patients to receive the services they need.

General Recommendations for Mental Health Providers

- Recognize and attend to personal and professional biases toward transgender persons and other diversity variables.
- Seek and attend specific training regarding best standards of practice and care of transgender persons.
- Ask clients about their gender identity and preferred pronouns; inquire about their preference for the name and pronouns they wished to use in clinical notes and assessment reports.
- Instead of referring to TGNC individuals by a gendered title (e.g., Mr., Ms., Mrs.), you may consider referring to them as "Veteran Smith" or "Smith."
- Explore barriers to accessing other systems of care (e.g., employment, housing, education).
- Explore current support systems and collaborate with the TGNC individual to discover other avenues to obtain and receive support.
- Provide inclusive and transgender-sensitive care via an open, trusting, genuine relationship with the TGNC patient.
- Consult with expert professionals in the field.
- Connect with other service providers on the treatment team to foster continuity of care.
- For psychological assessment batteries, use gender-stratified tests that incorporate norms from cisgender men and women or measures with non-gendered norms.
- Discuss limitations in the testing process and, consequently, make looser diagnostic conclusions.

Resources

- Camouflaged Identity: How Trans Veterans Survive Military Culture: https://time.com/camouflaged-identity/
- Identity Documents: https://www.lambdalegal.org/know-your-rights/article/trans-identity-document-faq
- Summary of VHA Care for Transgender Veterans: https://transequality.org/issues/resources/veterans-health-administration-care-for-transgender-veterans
- Transgender American Veterans Association: http://transveteran.org/
- Transgender Law & Policy Institute: http://www.transgenderlaw.org/
- Transgender Resources: https://www.glaad.org/transgender/resources
- Transgender Rights Toolkit: https://www.lambdalegal.org/publications/trans-toolkit

References

Aboussouan, A., Snow, A., Cerel, J., & Tucker, R. P. (2019). Non-suicidal self-injury, suicide ideation, and past suicide attempts: Comparison between transgender and gender diverse veterans and non-veterans. *Journal of Affective Disorders, 259*, 186–194. https://doi-org.ezproxy.libraries.wright.edu/10.1016/j.jad.2019.08.046

American Psychological Association. (2015). Guidelines for psychological practice with transgender and gender nonconforming people. *American Psychologist, 70*(9), 832–864.

Beckman, K., Shipherd, J., Simpson, T., & Lehavot, K. (2018). Military sexual assault in transgender veterans: Results from a nationwide survey. *Journal of Traumatic Stress, 31*(2), 181–190. https://doi-org.ezproxy.libraries.wright.edu/10.1002/jts.22280

Blanton, D., & Cook, L. M. (2002). *They fought like demons: Women soldiers in the American Civil War*. Louisiana State University Press.

Bloscnich, J. R., Marsiglio, M. C., Gao, S., Gordon, A. J., Shipherd, J. C., Kauth, M., Brown, G. R., & Fine, M. J. (2016). Mental health of transgender veterans in U.S. states with and without discrimination and hate crime legal protection. *American Journal of Public Health, 106*(3), 534–540.

Blosnich, J. R., Brown, G. R., Shipherd, J. D., Michael Kauth, R., Piegari, R. M., & Bossarte, R. M. (2013). Prevalence of gender identity disorder and suicide risk among transgender veterans utilizing veterans health administration care. *American Journal of Public Health, 103*(10), 27–32.

Blosnich, J. R., Brown, G. R., Wojcio, S., Jones, K. T., & Bossarte, R. M. (2014). Mortality among veterans with transgender-related diagnoses in the veterans health administration, FY2000-2009. *LGBT Health, 1*, 269–276. https://doi.org/10.1089/lgbt.2014.0050

Blosnich, J. R., Marsiglio, M. C., Gao, S., Gordon, A. J., Shipherd, J. C., Kauth, M., Brown, G. R., & Fine, M. J. (2016). Mental health of transgender veterans in U.S. states with and without discrimination and hate crime legal protection. *American Journal of Public Health, 106*(3), 534–540. https://doi-org.ezproxy.libraries.wright.edu/10.2105/AJPH.2015.302981

Bockting, W. O., Miner, M. H., Swinburne Romine, R. E., Hamilton, A., & Coleman, E. (2013). Stigma, mental health, and resilience in an online sample of the U.S. transgender population. *American Journal of Public Health, 103*, 943–951.

Bockting, W., Coleman, E., Deutsch, M. B., Guillamon, A., Meyer, I., Meyer, W., 3rd, … Ettner, R. (2016). Adult development and quality of life of transgender and gender non-conforming people. *Current Opinion in Endocrinology, Diabetes, and Obesity, 23*(2), 188–197.

Bukowski, L. A., Blosnich, J., Shipherd, J. C., Kauth, M. R., Brown, G. R., & Gordon, A. J. (2017). Exploring rural disparities in medical diagnoses among veterans with transgender-related diagnoses utilizing veterans health administration care. *Medical Care, 55*, S97–S103.

Carter, S. P., Montgomery, A. E., Henderson, E. R., Ketterer, B., Dichter, M., Gordon, A. J., Shipherd, J. C., Kauth, M. R., & Blosnich, J. R. (2019). Housing instability characteristics among transgender veterans cared for in the veterans health administration, 2013–2016. *American Journal of Public Health, 109*(10), 1413–1418.

CBC. (2017, July 26). *Countries that allow transgender members in the military*. http://www.cbc.ca/news/world/countries-that-allow-transgender-members-in-the-military1.4222205

Chang, S. C., & Singh, A. A. (2016). Affirming psychological practice with transgender and gender nonconforming people of color. *Psychology of Sexual Orientation and Gender Diversity, 3*(2), 140.

Cramer, T. (2017, January 3). *Transgender vets, the V.A., and respect*. Veterans Health Administration. https://www.va.gov/health/NewsFeatures/2017/January/Transgender-Vets-the-VA-and-Respect.asp

De Santis, J. P. (2009). HIV infection risk factors among male-to-female transgender persons: A review of the literature. *Journal of the Association of Nurses in AIDS Care, 20*(5), 362–372.

Department of Veterans Affairs. (2020, June 26). *VHA directive 1341(2): Providing health care for transgender and intersex veterans*. Retrieved from www.va.gov/vhapublications

Doe v. Alexander, 510 F. Supp. 900. (1981, March 27). Retrieved from law.justia.com

Fredriksen-Goldsen, K. I., Cook-Daniels, L., Kim, H.-J., Erosheva, E. A., Emlet, C. A., Hoy-Ellis, C. P., & Muraco, A. (2014). Physical and mental health of transgender older adults: An at-risk and underserved population. *The Gerontologist, 54*, 488–500.

Goldberg, J. M., & Ashbee, O. (2006). *Fit or fatphobic: Trans people, weight and health*. Vancouver Coastal Health. Retrieved 30 Apr 2012 from http://transhealth.vch.ca/resources/careguidelines.html

Gomez, M. (2019). Timeline: Transgender service members and the military. *Los Angeles Times*. Retrieved from https://www.latimes.com/politics/la-na-col1-transgender-military-timeline-20190528-story.html

Hendricks, M. L., & Testa, R. J. (2012). A conceptual framework for clinical work with transgender and gender non-conforming clients: An adaptation of the minority stress model. *Professional Psychology: Research and Practice, 43*, 460–467.

Herbst, J. H., Jacobs, E. D., Finlayson, T. J., McKleroy, V. S., Neumann, M. S., Crepaz, N., & HIV/AIDS Prevention Research Synthesis Team. (2008). Estimating HIV prevalence and risk behaviors of transgender persons in the United States: A systematic review. *AIDS and Behavior, 12*(1), 1–17.

Hoy-Ellis, C. P., Shiu, C., Sullivan, K. M., Kim, H., Sturges, A. M., & Fredriksen-Goldsen, K. I. (2017). Prior military service, identity stigma, and mental health among transgender older adults. *The Gerontologist, 57*(1), S63–S71. https://doi.org/10.1093/geront/gnw173

Hulsho Pol, H. E., Cohen-Kettenis, P. T., Van Haren, N. E. M., Peper, J. S., Brans, R. G. H., Cahn, W., … Kahn, R. S. (2006). Changing your sex changes your brain: In uences of testosterone and estrogen on adult human brain structure. *European Journal of Endocrinology, 155*, 107–114.

James, S. E., & Herman, J. (2017). *The report of the 2015 U.S. transgender survey: Executive summary*. National Center for Transgender Equality.

James, S. E., Herman, J. L., Rankin, S., Keisling, M., Mottet, L., & Ana, M. (2016). *The report of the 2015 U.S. transgender survey*. National Center for Transgender Equality.

Kauth, M. R. (2017, March 3). *An overview of LGBT veteran health*. Presented at the V.A. Physician Assistant Association Conference.

Kauth, M. R., Shipherd, J. C., Lindsay, J., Blosnich, J. R., Brown, G. R., & Jones, K. T. (2014). Access to care for transgender veterans in the Veterans Health Administration: 2006–2013. *American Journal of Public Health, 104*(S4), S532–S534.

Keo-Meier, C. L., & Fitzgerald, K. M. (2017). Affirmative psychological testing and neurocognitive assessment with transgender adults. *The Psychiatric Clinics of North America, 40*, 51–64.

Lehavot, K., Simpson, T. L., & Shipherd, J. C. (2016). Factors associated with suicidality among a national sample of transgender veterans. *Suicide & Life-Threatening Behavior, 46*(5), 507–524. https://doi-org.ezproxy.libraries.wright.edu/10.1111/sltb.12233

Legal, L. (2016). *Creating equal access to quality health care for transgender patients: transgender-affirming hospital policies*. New York: Lambda Legal.

Lehavot, K., Katon, J. G., Simpson, T. L., & Shipherd, J. C. (2017). Transgender veterans' satisfaction with care and unmet health needs. *Medical Care, 55*(9), 90–96.

Lev, A. I. (2004). *Transgender emergence: Therapeutic guidelines for working for gender-variant people and their families*. Haworth Press.

Lindsay, J. A., Keo-Meier, C., Hudson, S., Walder, A., Martin, L. A., & Kauth, M. R. (2016). Mental health of transgender veterans of the Iraq and Afghanistan conflicts who experienced military sexual trauma. *Journal of Traumatic Stress, 29*, 563–567.

Luders, E., Sánchez, F. J., Gaser, C., Toga, A. W., Narr, K. L., Hamilton, L. S., & Vilain, E. (2009). Regional gray matter variation in male-to-female transsexualism. *NeuroImage, 46*(4), 904–907.

McDuffie, E., & Brown, G. R. (2010). 70 U.S. veterans with gender identity disturbances: A descriptive study. *International Journal of Transgender Health, 12*, 21–30.

Meyer, I. H. (2003). Prejudice, social stress, and mental health in lesbian, gay, and bisexual populations: Conceptual issues and research evidence. *Psychological Bulletin, 129*, 674–697.

Military Sexual Trauma. *Journal of Traumatic Stress, 29*(6), 563–567. https://doi-org.ezproxy.libraries.wright.edu/10.1002/jts.22146

Moody, C. L., & Smith, N. G. (2013). Suicide protective factors among trans adults. *Archives of Sexual Behavior, 42*, 739–752.

National Center for Transgender Equality. (2019, May 17). *Veterans health administration care for transgender veterans*. https://transequality.org/issues/resources/veterans-health-administration-care-for-transgender-veterans

Office of the Deputy Secretary of Defense. (2019, March 12). *Directive-type Memorandum (DTM)-19-004 – Military service by transgender persons and persons with gender dysphoria.* https://drive.google.com/file/d/1tQugAtmmg-cDrhwQVRPtCGNBA6c7b3x2/view

Palm Center. (2014). *Report of the planning commission on transgender military service.* https://www.palmcenter.org/wp-content/uploads/2014/08/Report-of-Planning-Commission-on-Transgender-Military-Service_0–2.pdf

Rametti, G., Carrillo, B., Gómez-Gil, E., Junque, C., Segovia, S., Gomez, Á., & Guillamon, A. (2011a). White matter microstructure in female to male transsexuals before cross-sex hormonal treatment. A di usion tensor imaging study. *Journal of Psychiatric Research, 45*(2), 199–204.

Rametti, G., Carrillo, B., Gómez-Gil, E., Junque, C., Zubiarre-Elorza, L., Segovia, S., & Gomez, Á. (2011b). The microstructure of white matter in male to female transsexuals before cross-sex hormonal treatment. A DTI study. *Journal of Psychiatric Research, 45*(7), 949–954.

Richer, A. (2020, March 18). *U.S. naval officer sues over military transgender ban.* Retrieved from https://www.navytimes.com/news/your-navy/2020/03/19/us-naval-officer-sues-over-military-transgender-ban/

Rizzo, J., & Cohen, Z. (2016, June 30). *Pentagon ends transgender ban.* https://www.cnn.com/2016/06/30/politics/transgender-ban-lifted-us-military/index.html

Ruben, M. A., Livingston, N. A., Berke, D. S., Matza, A. R., & Shipherd, J. C. (2019). Lesbian, gay, bisexual, and transgender veterans' experiences of discrimination in health care and their relation to health outcomes: A pilot study examining the moderating role of provider communication. *Health Equity, 3*(1), 480–488. https://doi-org.ezproxy.libraries.wright.edu/10.1089/HEQ.2019.0069

Ryan, C., Russell, S. T., Huebner, D., Diaz, R., & Sanchez, J. (2010). Family acceptance in adolescence and the health of LGBT young adults. *Journal of Child and Adolescence and the Health of LGBT Young Adults, 23*, 205–213.

Secretary of Defense. (2016, June 30). *Directive-Type Memo 16-005 (DTM 16-005) – Military service of transgender service members.* https://dod.defense.gov/Portals/1/features/2016/0616_policy/DTM-16-005.pdf

Seelman, K. L., Colon-Diaz, M. J. P., LeCroix, R. H., Xavier-Brier, M., & Kattari, L. (2017). Transgender noninclusive healthcare and delaying care because of fear: Connections to general health and mental health among transgender adults. *Transgender Health, 2*, 17–28. https://doi.org/10.1089/trgh.2016.0024

Seiger, R., Hahn, A., Hummer, A., Kranz, G. S., Ganger, S., Woletz, M., … Lanzenberger, R. (2016). Subcortical gray matter changes in transgender subjects after long-term cross-sex hormone administration. *Psychoneuroendocrinology, 74*, 371–379.

Sherman, M. D., Kauth, M. R., Shipherd, J. C., & Street, R. L., Jr. (2014). Communication between VA providers and sexual and gender minority veterans: A pilot study. *Psychological Services.* Advance online publication. https://doi.org/10.1037/a0035840

Slabbekoorn, D., van Goozen, S. H. M., Megens, J., Gooren, L. J. G., & Cohen-Kettenis, P. T. (1999). Activating e ects of cross-sex hormones on cognitive functioning: A study of short-term and long- term hormone e ects in transsexuals. *Psychoneuroendocrinology, 24*, 423–447.

Smith, E. S., Junger, J., Derntl, B., & Habel, U. (2015). The transsexual brain – A review of ndings on the neural basis of transsexualism. *Neuroscience and Biobehavioral Reviews, 59*, 251–266.

Somashekhar, S., & Whitlock, C. (2015, July 13). *Military to allow transgender members to serve openly*. https://www.washingtonpost.com/politics/pentagon-to-allow-transgender-members-to-serve-openly/2015/07/13/fe9b054a-298d-11e5-a5ea-cf74396e59ec_story.html

Testa, R. J., Habarth, J., Peta, J., Balsam, K., & Bockting, W. (2015). Development of the gender minority stress and resilience measure. *Psychology of Sexual Orientation and Gender Diversity, 2*(1), 65–77.

The White House Office of the Press Secretary. (2011, September 20). *Statement by the president on the repeal of don't ask don't tell*. https://obamawhitehouse.archives.gov/the-press-office/2011/09/20/statement-president-repeal-dont-ask-dont-tell

Transgender Military Ban FAQ. (2020). Retrieved July 12, 2020 from https://notransmilitaryban.org/wp-content/uploads/2020/03/Transgender-Military-Ban-FAQ-Updated-3.17.20.pdf

Trittschuh, E. H., Parmenter, B. A., Clausell, E. R., Mariano, M. J., & Reger, M. A. (2018). Conducting neuropsychological assessment with transgender individuals. *The Clinical Neuropsychologist, 32*(8), 1393–1410. https://doi.org/10.1080/13854046.2018.1440632

Tucker, R. P., Testa, R. J., Reger, M. A., Simpson, T. L., Shipherd, J. C., & Lehavot, K. (2019). Current and military-specific gender minority stress factors and their relationship with suicide ideation in transgender veterans. *Suicide and Life-threatening Behavior, 49*(1), 155–166. https://doi-org.ezproxy.libraries.wright.edu/10.1111/sltb.12432

United States Military Entrance Processing Command. (2019, April 7). *Military service by transgender persons and persons with gender identity disorder: Fact sheet for Military recruiters*. https://www.mepcom.army.mil/Portals/112/FactSheet_ApplicantsForMilitaryService_ForRecruiters_7Apr19.pdf

Van Goozen, S. H. M., Cohen-Kettenis, P. T., Gooren, L. J. G., Frijda, N. H., & Van de Poll, N. E. (1994). Activating effects of androgens on cognitive performance: Causal evidence in a group of female-to-male transsexuals. *Neuropsychologia, 32*(10), 1153–1157.

Van Goozen, S. H. M., Cohen-Kettenis, P. T., Gooren, L. J. G., Frijda, N. H., & Van De Poll, N. E. (1995). Gender differences in behaviour: Activating effects of cross-sex hormones. *Psychoneuroendocrinology, 20*(4), 343–363.

Van Orden, K. A., Witte, T. K., Cukrowicz, K. C., Braithwaite, S. R., Selby, E. A., & Joiner, T. E. (2010). The interpersonal theory of suicide. *Psychological Review, 117*, 575.

Veterans Cared for in the Veterans Health Administration, 2013–2016. *American Journal of Public Health, 109*(10), 1413–1418. Retrieved from https://doi-org.ezproxy.libraries.wright.edu/10.2105/AJPH.2019.305219

Veterans Health Administration. (2020, June 26). *Providing health care for transgender and intersex veterans*. Retrieved from https://www.albuquerque.va.gov/docs/ProvidingHealthCareforTransgenderandIntersexVeterans.pdf

World Professional Association for Gender Health (WPATH). (2012). Standards of care for the health of transsexual, transgender, and gender non-conforming people, version 7. *International Journal of Transgenderism, 13*(4), 165–232. https://doi.org/10.1080/15532739.2011.700873

Xavier, J., Honnold, J. A., & Bradford, J. (2007). *The Health, health-related needs, and life course experiences of transgender virginians*. Retrieved from www.vdh.virginia.gov/epidemiology/DiseasePrevention/documents/pdf/THISFINALREPORTVol1.pdf

Zucker, B. (2018). Transcending limitations: Obstacles to benefits for transgender veterans. *27 Fed Circuit BJ, 321*.

Chapter 14
The Health Psychologist Role in Providing Services to the Military Families and Parenting

Susan George, Walter Garcia Hernandez, and Larry James

1 Military Parenting

The US Military offers opportunities and benefits, such as job security, a sense of purpose, community, and several challenges (Kritikos et al., 2019). Military members face a barrage of threats during their deployment. Most service members have shared their most significant source of stress is not related to combat, but instead the separation from their family (Sories et al., 2015). During the wars in Iraq and Afghanistan, approximately three million military families were affected (Gewirtz et al., 2017; Nolan et al., 2019). After the draft ended in 1973 and the US military became completely voluntary, the number of military service members declined from 1.9 million to 1.3 million in 2018. However, the number of women serving in the military increased from 2% of enlisted forces and 8% active duty commissioned officers corps to 16% and 19%, respectively ("Demographics," 2020). In 2010, it was estimated that 44% of military service members were parents. Of the two million American children with a parent in the military, about 37% were under the age of 6, many of whom have experienced their parents leaving for several deployments (Walsh et al., 2014). While military families tend to function generally well, there are unique service-related vulnerabilities that may contribute to an increased risk for mental health concerns and maladjustment (Kritikos et al., 2019; O'Grady et al., 2018). Furthermore, the active and extensive engagement of the military in Iraq and Afghanistan for over

S. George (✉) · W. G. Hernandez
School of Professional Psychology, Wright State University, Dayton, OH, USA
e-mail: garciahernandez.2@wright.edu

L. James
Department of Behavioral Health, Tripler Army Medical Center, Honolulu, HI, USA

L. C. James et al. (eds.), *Clinical Health Psychology in Military and Veteran Settings*, https://doi.org/10.1007/978-3-031-12063-3_14

15 years has shed light on the health and adjustment variables during post-deployment for both military members and their families (Kritikos et al., 2019). This chapter will focus on such concerns and provide recommendations on how clinicians may help military members and veterans.

1.1 Military Families

According to the US Department of Defense (2015), about 2.7 million American troops were deployed to Iraq or Afghanistan, and roughly 48% had children under the age of 6. Many military members who return to the United States after deployment do not meet cutoff criteria for the diagnosis of post-traumatic stress disorder (PTSD) but instead exhibit subclinical levels of the disorder. Parents who have been deployed indicated high levels of stress associated with their ability to adapt to family expectations after being trained to adapt to military expectations. High-stress levels are also associated with being separated from their families and the strong desire to be reunited with them (Walsh et al., 2014).

Huebner (2019) stated that the military workforce is highly comprised of younger individuals who marry and have children at a young age. Individuals in the military tend to have a higher income than their civilian counterparts, but this higher rate of pay comes with more stressors and demands than a civilian job. Military families are often separated or have to relocate to different locations in the world due to deployments. These relocations may result in a lack of employment opportunities for the partners of military personnel.

According to Padden and Agazio (2013), there are four significant stressors for children who are members of military families: frequent relocation, family separation, adaptation to danger, and adaptation to the military "institution." The family's ability to adapt to these factors may have a substantial effect on morale and job performance. Each deployment is its own unique experience in what the military member encounters while away from their family. The deployed family member may be exposed to unsuspected dangers, changes in location, and demanding tasks as a result of their deployment. Consequently, their family members may be stressed out of concern for their loved one and because of a lack of information. The stress the family withstands increases when the parent is fighting in a war zone as communication may be limited or non-existent. Thus, they may solely rely on the media. With the dearth of information, family members continuously struggle between hope and despair when it comes to their deployed family members' safety. Unfortunately, family members may nervously anticipate information, such as the death of the deployed family member, which often significantly influences their current stress levels and emotional state (Padden & Agazio, 2013).

1.2 Parenting Cycle of Deployment

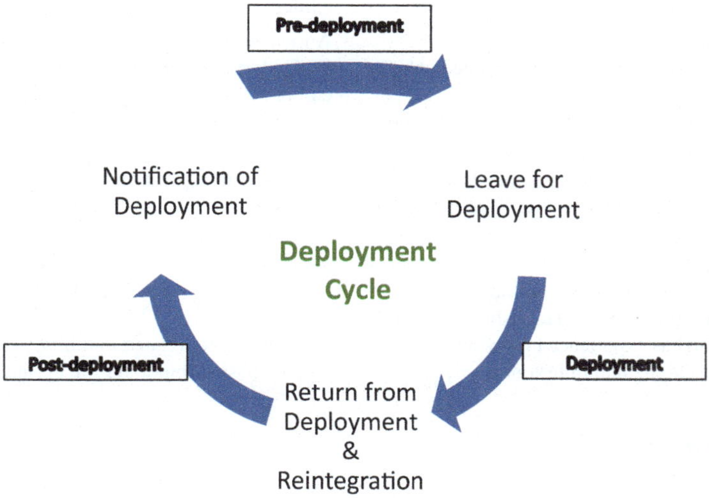

Active duty military personnel and their family members experience an array of emotions as they move through the deployment cycle, which may exacerbate their overall health and wellness. The cycle begins when a service member is notified of their future deployment. This event begins the pre-deployment phase, which ends the moment they leave for their assigned destination. After completion of their deployment, they return to their lives stateside, in which a host of new challenges may arise. Hence, it is essential to understand the needs of the military parent and their child(ren) as they navigate the deployment cycle, which may occur several times during the family's involvement with the military (O'Grady et al., 2018) (Table 14.1).

1.2.1 Pre-deployment Phase

Partners and spouses of the military parent often feel their life is stalled once they are notified of their future deployment. Upon notification, the family begins thinking and planning for when the service member is away. It may be hard for families with young children to prepare their kids for what is to come. Due to their age and cognitive development, young children often have difficulty understanding why the parent is leaving and have a hard time sharing their feelings (O'Grady et al., 2018). During this phase, service members must attend to the needs of their family if possible, as they may not be given ample time to process and plan before their departure.

Table 14.1 Challenges associated with each phase

Phase of deployment	Parents	Children
Pre-deployment	Life is "on-hold" Preparing and making arrangements for deployment Hardest phase for parents with younger children	Anticipation of separation Difficulties understanding why parent is deploying, especially young children
Deployment	Increased parenting demands and household responsibilities of the at-home parent	Dealing with separation Increased anxiety and concern Grief reactions
Post-deployment	Re-negotiating roles, Changes in family routines Re-establishing relationship with child who has experienced growth/developmental milestones	Readjustment Re-establishing relationships, roles, routines Grief and anger related to military parent missing important life events

1.2.2 Deployment Phase

After the parent is deployed, additional stress is placed on the at-home parent as they are now solely responsible for caring for their family and household. The at-home parent has increased parenting and domestic responsibilities and is attending to their child(ren) who are experiencing their own reactions and grief due to their parent's deployment (O'Grady et al., 2018; Walsh et al., 2014). Consequently, at-home parents may feel worried, anxious, depressed, and experience an increase in sleep difficulties and overall adjustment difficulties (O'Grady et al., 2018; Walsh et al., 2014). Children may also experience anxiety and worry. Typically, children turn to their at-home parents for support, comfort, reassurance, stability, and warmth. Older children may feel a sense of obligation and responsibility to share the burden of managing the household and assisting the at-home parent. Child adjustment is influenced by factors, such as age, cognitive ability, family expectations, and prior experience with deployment (Nolan et al., 2019; O'Grady et al., 2018). The youth's adjustment is also affected by their parent's mental health and the parent's sensitivity and responsiveness toward their children (O'Grady et al., 2018). Children are likely to experience elevated stress and anxiety when their caregivers are less responsive versus when parents are more attentive. As parents become attuned to their children's needs, children learn to depend on their parents for support and nurturance, which fosters a sense of stability and security (Walsh et al., 2014).

1.2.3 Post-deployment Phase

While the service member is away from their family, their children continue to grow and develop and reach various developmental milestones. Thus, their emotional and relational needs also change, which creates a unique reunification experience once the service member returns (Walsh et al., 2014). These struggles are often private, and many military members do not receive adequate support in this area. There may be a mix of relief, joy, and stress as the service member returns and assimilates back into family routines. Reintegration involves re-establishing relationships with their partner and children. Household responsibilities and parent roles are re-negotiated and re-instated (O'Grady et al., 2018; Walsh et al., 2014). Studies have found that factors such as duration of deployment and missed life events contribute to the increased depression of family members (Nolan et al. 2019). In a study conducted by Walsh and colleagues (2014), military service members, who were also fathers, reported in their interviews that they felt regret over missing portions of their child's life due to deployment. More specifically, the fathers shared they needed help and support with expressing emotions, managing their anger, and nurturing their children.

2 Risk Factors

Military families reside in a unique subculture that is distinct from their civilian counterparts. For example, military families lead nomadic lifestyles consisting of frequent moves and changing school districts. These continuous shifts in geographic location make it difficult to settle and establish long-term friendships and community, which may add to the stress of the family (Walsh et al., 2014).

2.1 Children

2.1.1 Effects of Deployment

Military family members are subject to risk factors that engender vulnerabilities in this population. Children of military parents often have similar life experiences. Military families are sent to various parts of the USA and the world; therefore, their children must relocate and attend different schools, be separated from their parents for prolonged periods, and become accustomed to new cultures. Interestingly, children from military parents often form bonds with other military kids with the same lived experiences, and they may be more likely to enlist in the military in the future than their civilian counterparts (Huebner, 2019). Frequent family relocation exacerbated negative responses to parental deployment in children (Nolan et al., 2019). Children of service members are influenced by the number, length, and frequency of deployments, especially with the subsequent shifts in the family's routine, parental roles, and associated concerns about deployments. Furthermore, these factors tend to increase levels of depression, anxiety, and isolation within the child (Gewirtz et al., 2011; Sories et al., 2015).

According to the Office of the Deputy Under Secretary of Defense for Military Community and Family Policy (2012), children who depend on military service members surpassed one million, with more than 750,000 around the ages of birth to 10. Julian and colleagues (2018) found that children of military parents are at a higher risk of having mental health struggles as they rely on their parents to help them cope with difficult emotions and look to obtain guidance when it comes to certain behaviors. However, due to the nature of military life and the stress that comes with it, their parents may not be as physically or emotionally available for their children. Children of military parents (ages 4–17) who were deployed exhibited higher levels of depression and stress than those in families where a parent was not deployed (Jensen et al., 1996). Studies found approximately a 19% increase in behavioral and stress disorders and increased numbers of outpatient psychiatric or behavioral care visits in children between the ages of 3 and 8 who were affected by military deployments (Gorman & Hisle-Gorman, 2010).

2.1.2 Younger Children

The accumulation of risks beginning in childhood may have long-lasting consequences for children regarding depression and anxiety (Wadsworth et al., 2016). Younger children appear most vulnerable. Considering that the first five years is essential for attachment, socio-emotional development, and learning, these early years also create the template for behavioral responses, social skills, adaptation to changes in the environment, and regulation of emotions and stress. Young children may be most reactive to deployments, which may be attributed to their lack of coping skills and resources.

The impact on younger children is important to consider as many military families have children under the age of 6. Service members will be hesitant to re-enlist if their children are having behavioral problems and are negatively affected (Stepka & Callahan, 2016). Younger children experience an increase in tantrums, attention-seeking behaviors, and problems with sleeping and eating from the deployment phase to the reintegration phase. Accordingly, there was an 11% increase in the use of mental and behavioral health visits, an increase in ADHD symptoms, and a higher rate of utilization of medications during the deployment period. Parents shared that the pre-deployment phase was the most painful because they found it challenging to discuss and prepare young children because of their limited understanding (Stepka & Callahan, 2016).

2.1.3 Older Children and Teenagers

Consistent with the literature, children of deployed parents experience increased feelings of sadness and depression and fear. Between the ages of 5 and 12, children who had a deployed parent with mental health concerns experience higher rates of child maltreatment by their parents. Children of deployed parents are also at risk for attention problems, behavioral problems at school, and social difficulties (Chandra, 2016). In an analysis of parenting style based on Baumrind's framework of authoritative, authoritarian, and permissive parenting, military parents were more likely to be classified as authoritarian than their civilian counterparts. Furthermore, military mothers tended to be less nurturing and more restrictive.

Children and adolescents typically observe and model the behavior of their parents. This is particularly important during times of transition and high stress as problem-solving techniques and communication can significantly affect overall stress and emotion management (Chandra, 2016). Parental deployment also adds stress to the relational dynamics of the family, particularly the parent-child relationship and the absence of the military parent. In a study in which the researchers implemented focus groups, teens of military parents reported a sense of loss and uncertainty. They expressed specific concern regarding if they will ever see their parent again (Chandra, 2016). The teenagers also indicated a climate of greater emotional intensity and conflicted parent-child interactions during deployment, which is likely influenced by both parent and child anxiety.

2.1.4 Relocation

Relocation is a part of military life, and many families experience it. Padden and Agazio (2013) found that military families move at a rate of 2.4 times more frequently than civilian families. During this process, children may transition to new educational institutions up to nine times before they turn 18-years-old. Millegan et al. (2014) found that increased mental health encounters may be more common for military youth after a geographic move within 12 months of the relocation. They also discovered an increase in emergency room visits and that psychiatric hospitalizations often occurred after relocation. However, while deployments are transitions that may increase stress levels in families, they are also related to increased resilience in military children. Such optimistic outcomes also include reductions in school problems and increased positivity regarding the move for some children (Clever & Segal, 2013).

2.1.5 Separation from Parent

Children experiencing the separation and absence of their parents due to deployment are at a higher risk for internalizing (e.g., anxiety and depression) and externalizing behaviors (e.g., defiant and aggressive behaviors). Regarding family separation, one study found an 11% increase in the number of behavioral and mental outpatient visits of children ages 3–8 years old (Gorman & Hisle-Gorman, 2010). Infants, toddlers, and preschool-aged children who have one parent deployed are more prone to anticipate and worry about potential future separation from their caretaker, which may increase symptoms of separation anxiety (Lester et al., 2010). Additionally, due to these deployments' unexpected nature, parents may lack the time and ability to prepare the child to say goodbye to the military parent being deployed. There may be limited time to properly prepare the child to adapt to new care routines. As a result of these unanticipated transitions, the child's perception and worry about their parent's safety and welfare may be intensified (Lieberman & Van Horn, 2011). Mustillo et al. (2015) found that kids between the ages of 3 and 5 years had increased levels of anxiety. An increase in peer and behavioral problems was observed in children between the ages of 6 and 10 years old. Children between 6 and 12 years old compared to civilian children were found to have increased levels of depression, anxiety, and externalizing symptoms, which were highly associated with their parent's risk of endangerment (Lester et al., 2010). Additionally, the researchers observed an increase in antidepressant and anxiolytic use and a rise in well-child visits (Gorman & Hisle-Gorman, 2010).

2.1.6 Mental Health

Problems adapting to transitions requiring a child to be separated from their parents, such as starting a new daycare or school, may present a more significant challenge for children who have previously experienced the deployment of a caregiver (Lester et al., 2010). Due to the lack of coping skills when it comes to separations related to deployment, children in military families may struggle to adapt to changes in family structure or routines. These struggles may continue even after the deployed parent has returned home (Hodges & Bloom, 1984).

Overall, there is a higher susceptibility to developing anxiety, depression, and substance use disorders in youth related to their maladaptive response to deployment (Gewirtz et al., 2017; Wadsworth et al., 2016). Consistent with research previously mentioned, children exposed to a separation from their parent due to combat-related deployment are at elevated risk for a variety of negative consequences including both internalizing and externalizing behaviors (Wadsworth et al., 2016), and higher rates of anxiety, depression, and substance use disorders (Cederbaum et al., 2014; Gewirtz et al., 2017, Kelly et al., 2001). Studies found that younger children are at higher risk of increased social and emotional adjustment problems when their parents have been deployed (Gorman et al., 2010). Deployment is also associated with a variety of challenges for children, related to the changes in roles and relationships in the family, and behavioral and mental health problems of the parent who stays at home (Lester et al., 2016).

2.1.7 Parents

Throughout the deployment cycle, the at-home parent is likely to be stressed and feel the impact of the partner leaving, especially with parenting and household responsibilities. The at-home parent's ability to adjust to the separation may be either a risk or a protective factor for the children. The military parent faces heightened challenges, particularly in the reintegration phase, as they return to their family system. The reintegration phase places the family and couple dynamics at risk for impaired marital and familial functioning, financial stress, problems with intimacy, co-parenting difficulties, altered parent-child alliances, conflicts with new roles and responsibilities, and the children having difficulties adjusting to the return of the parent. The child may perhaps not respond as warmly or are fearful of the military parent (Gewirtz et al., 2011; Nolan et al., 2019). Moreover, there may also be marital disturbances that may indirectly affect the child. The result of these marital conflicts may be that parents are not emotionally available or responsive when needed by their children (Paley et al., 2013).

Furthermore, military parents' health and mental health are also critical factors that are influenced by war-related trauma, physical and mental health issues, and readjustment concerns. The military parent is at higher risk for drug and alcohol abuse (Gewirtz et al., 2017; Lipari et al., 2017). Cumulatively, these risk factors may lead to impaired parenting practices and poor child adjustment (Gewirtz et al., 2017). Research has shown that depression, trauma-related disorders, and emotional numbing from PTSD may skew the veteran's perception of their children and engender adjustment problems (Lipari et al., 2017). Inconsistent parent involvement is connected to a higher risk of substance abuse, tobacco use, and nonmedical use of psychotherapeutic drugs among adolescents (Lipari et al., 2017).

2.1.8 Parental Traumatic Stress

It is meaningful to take a closer look at military members and their trauma exposure. Overall, PTSD symptoms are connected with the development of maladaptive responses to deployment as the related stress and severity of symptoms depletes the family's resources to cope (Kritikos et al., 2019). Of note, combat-related PTSD versus PTSD from other traumatic events has shown to be less resolved and longer-lasting in military members. PTSD symptoms, such as hyperarousal and marked changes in sleep and mood, may lower parental engagement, consistency, and responsiveness and affect children's overall psychosocial functioning during deployment (Kritikos et al., 2019). There are mixed findings as to how parental PTSD may influence family functioning. Some studies found an increase in family dysfunction, and other studies demonstrated that parental PTSD was negatively associated with family problems reported by the children (Kritikos et al., 2019). Additional studies indicate that fathers with low inhibitory control skills are more likely to have PTSD symptoms and associated maladaptive parenting behaviors (Monn et al., 2018).

Furthermore, while it has been noted that children with deployed parents are more likely to exhibit internalizing and externalizing behaviors, if these same children have a parent diagnosed with PTSD, they then have a higher risk of engaging in problematic behaviors (Monn et al., 2018). These risks may likely be due to fewer displays of sensitivity, warmth, and social responsiveness and increased verbal aggression, demeaning statements, coercive parent-child dynamics, and dismissive actions by the parent (Monn et al., 2018). The parent's PTSD symptoms of avoidance, hypervigilance, and intrusive thoughts may interfere with their ability to regulate their emotions and hinder positive relational dynamics. Other areas of parenting that may be affected are child supervision and consistency of discipline. In another study, 42% of military parents reported parenting stress classified in the clinically significant range, and 29% of service members reported trouble with reconnecting with their children upon returning from their deployment. High parenting stress and stress of deployment are also associated with divorce, higher suicide rates, and child maltreatment (Walsh et al., 2014).

2.1.9 Protective Factors

Military life brings many challenges to families, and simultaneously strengthens familial bonds. According to Easterbrooks et al. (2013), several studies found positive outcomes related to being a part of a military family and community, such as strengthening the family bonds while a member is deployed and enhanced social connections due to shared experiences. Meadows and associates (2016) found that improved functioning was related to socialization with other military children during the deployment process; this socialization was also viewed as a protective factor.

The US Military provides resources for families to assist them with coping for deployment, but access to these services may vary. National Guard family members tend to live in civilian communities, whereas active-duty families often live on or near a military base, which offers easy access to services and support (Gewirtz et al., 2017; O'Grady et al., 2018). Research indicates that positive relationships improve the reintegration of the military parent (Nolan et al., 2019). Military parents that engage in relationship-building activities (e.g., helping with homework and problems and spending time with their children) also tend to have open communication, offer warmth, and are emotionally responsive. Overall, intentional engagement with their children promotes healthy child development. These activities and attitudes are also reflective of an authoritative parenting style (Lipari et al., 2017).

3 Clinical Recommendations for Deployment Cycle

3.1 Pre-deployment

Individuals who provide support to these families may find it important to recognize the different parts of the emotional cycle of deployment to provide better services. Understanding the deployment cycle assists clinicians with meeting the needs of these families and providing psychoeducation about what they are experiencing (Padden & Agazio, 2013). These stages may last 6 months or longer and may bring up different emotional challenges. The pre-deployment stage is where families are first notified about the upcoming deployment of the family member. Thus, families may experience feelings of denial and may anticipate the worst outcomes (death of the individual being deployed). The individual being deployed must also begin to prepare themselves to be separated from their family for a period perhaps ranging from 4 months to many years. This stage may bring high levels of stress. Families would benefit from finding other supportive adults who may assist with an array of responsibilities, such as caring for the children, helping with matters related to schooling, finding new employment for the at-home parent, cancelling leases, or finding storage for their belongings. Notably, one of the most challenging parts of this process is for the parent who is being deployed to pull back from the day-to-day care of their children because they will not be able to accomplish these tasks once they are deployed (Gewirtz et al., 2011; Padden & Agazio, 2013).

3.1.1 Recommendations

Health care providers allow and encourage families experiencing the pre-deployment stage to discuss fears that may arise as a result of deployment. They may benefit from providing emotional support by actively listening and providing guidance on how to access resources and additional community supports. Consider encouraging the military parent to spend time with their children and assisting them with articulating an age-appropriate explanation as to why they will be gone for an extended time. It is suggested to provide children with the prospective deployment location, if possible (Padden & Agazio, 2013). Clinicians may consider assisting the family with creating realistic expectations during deployment and having open conversations with the child about what changes they can expect.

Tip: Create a list of household rules, rewards, and consequences so that parents and children understand their expectations and responsibilities.

Clinicians may consider building on the military family's strengths and resilience by eliciting and processing the following information (Gewirtz et al., 2011):

- As a parent, what are your strengths?
- As a parent/family, what are your core values?
- What are your children's strengths?
- What are your parenting goals?
- Connect the parent's values and strengths to their goals.
- How has the family persevered, successfully confronted, and grown from previous significant life events (military and/or general stressors)?
- Connect existing, useful practices and skills the family utilizes in times of stress to create a plan on how they will address and navigate the upcoming deployment.
- During a family therapy session, facilitate family goal planning so parents and children are on the same page and may identify avenues of support both within and outside the family system.

3.2 *Deployment Recommendations*

As the military parent leaves, the deployment stage begins. The partners/spouses become stressed in response to being the sole provider and now managing the numerous responsibilities they have inherited. Spouses may experience a mix of emotions, including feeling empty, alone, sad, or abandoned. Heightened levels of anxiety and issues with sleep have been reported along with feeling overwhelmed with worry and concern for the deployed member. Hence, these intense emotions further escalate their emotional dysregulation (Padden & Agazio, 2013).

3.2.1 Recommendations

It is beneficial for health care providers to validate the range of emotions each family member is experiencing. Clinicians may take time to understand how each person feels and processes. Each member of the family will have their personalized ways of coping with the flood of emotions that arise once the parent is deployed. The family members would benefit from reminders and reassurance that they are not going through this process alone. Identifying and correcting underlying misconceptions and unhelpful thoughts may be necessary for children. Some children (depending on age) may feel guilty because they believe they are the reason their parents left. Like the pre-deployment phase, it is vital to provide the family with a safe space to express and discuss their emotions and guide them to the proper resources (Padden & Agazio, 2013).

Tip: Parents and children will benefit from receiving validation as well as learning how to validate each other's emotions. This will especially help parents acknowledge and reflect the emotional state of their child. The child will then feel heard, seen, and understood.

3.3 *Sustainment of Military Parent and Family Members*

During this period, the parent who is deployed must distance themselves from the daily lives of their family, as too much involvement may distract them from their current mission, which may put them or members of their squad in danger. The deployed parent navigates managing their feelings and concerns regarding their children. During sustainment, families will eventually become accustomed to their "new normal." However, this does not minimize their concern, which may be further aggravated by how the media portrays the military or the lack of support by community members. Spouses may be affected by this stage the most. Studies have indicated they may begin to develop psychological symptoms such as depression, anxiety, nightmares, irritability, acute stress reaction, adjustment disorder, or increased alcohol use. Some of these symptoms may also manifest physically through sleep disturbances, fatigue, headaches, appetite changes, weight changes, or back pain (Padden & Agazio, 2013).

According to Wexler and McGrath (1991), over 50% of military spouses reported adverse emotional reactions such as anxiety, loneliness, sadness, and worry. The symptoms reported by these military spouses are often associated with the deployment of their significant other; it has also been found that these spouses are at a higher risk of developing a mental health disorder during the deployment of their husbands. Mansfield et al. (2010) found that compared to nondeployed spouses, wives with deployed husbands were 18–24% more likely to develop a depressive disorder, 21–40% more likely to develop a sleep disorder, 25–29% more likely to develop an anxiety disorder, and 23–39% more likely to have an acute stress reaction and adjustment disorder. Military families may face economic challenges that include periods of food insecurity (Huebner, 2019).

3.3.1 Recommendations

Due to the nature of the demands of deployment, members of the military may feel they have to limit their exposure to their family and their typical, day-to-day happenings, as it may distract them from their mission. It is recommended that members who are deployed should maintain a constant line of communication with their families. This is done to keep a sense of normalcy and connection for service members. It is important to note that family members should not overwhelm services members with problems they cannot solve from a distance because these may overwhelm or frustrate them (Padden & Agazio, 2013).

It is suggested for mental health professionals to encourage families to develop and maintain routines as much as possible, which is especially emphasized for families who have young children. This is a stage where creativity can be a great resource. It is recommended that parents empower their children to find innovative ways to keep the deployed parent up-to-date with their lives. This may be done through drawings, pictures, video recordings, and apps. It is also encouraged to provide younger children with adult companionship that matches the gender of the deployed member, such as uncles, aunts, grandparents, or other close relatives and friends.

> Tip: Consider recommending an app that helps facilitate connection between the family and the deployed parent.

Social support becomes imperative during this stage, and there may be times where caretakers need a break from childcare and parenting, but do not know what resources are available to them that may allow them respite. During these times, it is recommended that parents seek out military-specific services such as Family Readiness Groups in the Army, Fleet and Family in the Navy, and Family Support Centers in the Air Force (Padden & Agazio, 2013). These services are most knowledgeable about issues that arise during deployment and can readily assist family members with any issues that are specific to their branch of the military. Furthermore, according to the social theory of action and change (SOAC), connections with both informal (e.g., friends, neighbors, extended family members, colleagues) and formal networks (e.g., professionals, organizations, agencies) create a community around the family that provides acceptance, reciprocity of help and support, and close relationships with others in which the family can draw strength and support from during times of transition and crises (O'Neal et al., 2018).

Tip: If the military family has an under-developed community, it may be beneficial to assist the family with expanding their network over time. Consider associations, agencies, faith-based organizations, interest groups and other avenues for added support.

Health care professionals are also recommended to encourage families to develop and maintain routines. The at-home parent and family would benefit from accepting they do not have total control of the deployment process, and their focus should be on the things they can control such as themselves, the well-being of their family, and their employment (if they are employed). Social support should be heavily emphasized by the professional and encourage families to seek out support from members of their support system such as friends, and family. If these are not available, they should be provided with different support groups and service organizations. Lastly, it should be emphasized that the family keeps an open line of communication with the deployed member (Padden & Agazio, 2013).

3.4 *Notification of Return from Deployment*

This is a period where the at-home parent is notified that the deployed member is returning back home. This period may provide a sense of relief to the family member as it signals an end to the deployment. In the midst of the exciting news, partners may also feel conflicted. On the one hand, they may be enthusiastic that their significant other is returning home. They may also feel apprehensive about re-establishing a new routine that involves the deployed family member. They may need to become accustomed to losing their newly gained independence and role as sole decisionmaker (Padden & Agazio, 2013).

3.4.1 Recommendations

The mental health professional may first explore the range of feelings the at-home partner is experiencing. Normalization and validation of their thoughts and feelings will set the at-home parent at ease and also prepare them to engage in purposeful discussion about how to navigate the return of the military parent. Mental health professionals may validate and commend family members for their ability to adapt to the different changes that deployment has brought to their family, as well as their ability to cope with the separation. The strengths-based approach will also highlight their willingness to be autonomous and taking on added responsibilities for the overall well-being of the family. The clinician may consider engaging the family in mentally and emotionally preparing and focus on communication skills that will enhance the reintegration of the service member. The family member must acknowledge their apprehension and expectations while also embracing their partner's expectations about returning home. Fostering open discussions will help the family transition more smoothly (Padden & Agazio, 2013).

3.5 *Post-deployment*

The clinician may find it beneficial to prepare the family for some of the physical and emotional symptoms the service member may present with upon their arrival to the United States. Military members may experience post-combat fatigue or stress reactions. Sleep struggles are common, and members may become extremely sensitive to loud noise, have difficulties transitioning back into their home culture, and quickly become irritable. In severe cases, the service member may present with symptomatology that is parallel to long term stress reactions or post-traumatic stress disorder (PTSD). Service members may need additional space to mentally process, as they may become overwhelmed with adapting to the demands of their household. They may need added flexibility and more extended periods to reintegrate to family life and responsibilities fully. Clinicians should be alert as to how these symptoms and transition difficulties may affect spouses. Spouses are likely to observe these changes and not understand how or why their military partner seems different.

The family members at home will now experience another transition. While they are excited to welcome back the military parent, they may also experience some grief over having to change their role from single parent and sole decisionmaker to co-parenting and shared responsibilities. Padden and Agazio (2013) recommend that this is a time where families need to work together to establish a "new family normal," which may require vast amounts of effort and time. Families should expect younger children to experience a more extended period of adaptation to this transition, as the child may have been too young to have any memories of the deployed member. Deployed parents often have to form a new bond with their child when they return from deployment, as the child may be in a different developmental stage. Adding to these difficulties, the child may be cautious or even fearful of approaching their parent. As the parent patiently re-establishes their connection and becomes attuned to this child, they may also need to acquire age-appropriate parenting skills and techniques to manage the child's behaviors (Julian et al., 2018). Clinicians may consider validating the military parent and providing support through psychoeducation and parenting skills.

4 General Clinical Recommendations and Tips During the Deployment Cycle (Gewirtz et al., 2011)

- "The Three R's" during times of uncertainty: maintaining predictable Routines, clear Rules or limits, and family Rituals, also create a cohesive and shared family narrative that supports family stability.
- Assist the parent in establishing a daily routine.
- Assist the parent with establishing rules, consequences, and limit-setting that are age-appropriate.
- Support the parent with consistent implementation of a predictable routine and rules to improve the child's sense of security. The parent will likely benefit from psychoeducation, skill-building, practice, and regular feedback.
- Build emotional regulation skills of parents to address family stressors during deployment. Consider implementing mindfulness and DBT skills to promote stress management and reduction techniques.
- Teach and foster problem-solving skills and effective means of communication between all family members.
- Facilitate and teach parents to become more attuned with their children. Parents will benefit from learning how to recognize, understand, and sensitively respond to their child's intense emotions.
- Encourage parents to maintain a united parenting front and facilitate dialogue about roles, responsibilities, expectations, and transition planning.
- Implement and practice positive and neutral approaches to interacting with children.
- Assist parents with intentionally spending quality time with children that promotes attunement and building stronger relationships.
- Create balance between encouragement and discipline through the use of token systems, tangible rewards, praise, incentive charts. It is suggested to provide psychoeducation on the effectiveness of the 5:1 ratio (five positive, encouraging statements for every one correction and/or consequence given to the child). This will equip parents with creating a nurturing environment versus a coercive climate.

5 Recommendations, Interventions, and Resources

The following are various parent–child and family-based interventions. In a needs assessment conducted with National Guard Soldiers who returned from deployment, there was a strong preference for family-based services over individual therapy (Gewirtz et al., 2011). Given the extensive research on deployment and reintegration of military members and the large number of risk factors and family stressors, a crucial component that has been identified is an emphasis on parenting practices (Palmer, 2008). The Social Interaction Learning model suggests that parenting practices, associated child behaviors, and overall health are influenced by stressful life events. The impact of stress on parenting practices leads to high levels of coercive parent–child interactions and infrequent positive communication (Gewirtz et al., 2011). Hence the need to provide military members and veterans with parenting practices that are positive and provide increased attunement between the parent and child. Of note, the following considerations should be taken into account before starting treatment:

- If a military parent/veteran is experiencing significant distress, they may need individual therapy first.
- Military member/veteran has clinically significant PTSD, depression, or substance use concerns and may primarily need individual therapy first before engaging in other services.
- Families with injured or ill military members may require more intensive individual and/or family treatment.
- Families who have lost a parent in combat may first need grief-focused/trauma-focused individual and family-based treatment.
- If deemed appropriate, parenting strategies can serve as an adjunct to the above conditions and treatment when the individual's symptoms lower in intensity.

5.1 FOCUS

The Families Over Coming Under Stress (FOCUS) provides families with resilience training, which is geared to strengthen families and couples to better face obstacles brought by military life such as deployments, stress, injury, and other transitions. It was originally developed by the University of California, Los Angeles and Harvard Medical School. The FOCUS program is provided for active duty military families and couples. During sessions, families will learn skills to help them cope with different feelings, improve communication, and help with problem-solving and goal setting. Consultations with professionals regarding how military life may impact the family are also available; the main goal is to better understand behavioral changes in children during deployment or reintegration and trauma, grief, or loss issues. FOCUS incorporates skill-building groups and educational workshops that deal with stress management, developmental reactions to deployment, and other transitions. The main core components of FOCUS include psychoeducation, problem-solving, family communication, and emotional regulation skills (DiNallo et al., 2016).

5.2 PMTO

The Parent Management Training-Oregon Model (PMTO™) is informed by the social interaction learning model with well-supported parenting interventions. There are five specific parenting practices that are actively promoted by PMTO: effective family problem-solving, positive involvement, contingent skill encouragement, limit-setting, and monitoring children's activities. The practitioner engages the parents in these five principles through teaching, continuous practice, and support regarding implementation. Numerous longitudinal studies have demonstrated strong evidence of improved parent–child relationships and adjustment as well as family functioning. Notably, PMTO has extensive research on fathers. This is vitally important as most military parents that are deployed are men (Gewirtz et al., 2011).

5.3 ADAPT

The After Deployment: Adaptive Parenting Tools (ADAPT) Intervention is a 14-week parenting program focused on teaching six core-parenting skills: "teaching through encouragement, discipline, problem-solving, monitoring, positive involvement with children, and emotional socialization" (Gewirtz et al., 2017). ADAPT is an extension of PMTO and was created by Dr. Abigail Gewirtz to address adjustment concerns in children (ages 5–12) of families in the National Guard and Reserve. ADAPT strengthens parents' capacities to regulate their children's emotions (DiNallo et al., 2016). The ADAPT program had moderately positive effects on observed parenting six months after the program; these positive effects resulted in improved child adjustment (Gewirtz et al., 2017). Additionally, the curriculum and materials, including role-play exercises and audio-visual materials, are relevant and appropriate to military culture. ADAPT focuses on post-deployment trauma symptoms of irritability, avoidance, and hypervigilance (Gewirtz et al., 2011).

5.4 Strong Military Families Intervention

The Strong Military Families (SMF) program (Rosenblum & Muzik, 2014) was created to aid families in reducing problems related to mental health in military families with young children (birth to age 6). The program is mainly geared toward families who often experience geographic isolation and have fewer opportunities to connect with other military families (National Guard and Reserve Families). The main goals of MSF are to promote parent resilience and to enhance parenting skills during the Post-Deployment phase (Dodge et al., 2018). The SMF program comprises 13 sessions that are broken down to three individual family sessions and ten multifamily sessions. The five core components are attachment-based parenting, positive parent–child interactions, self-care, social supports, and developing community resource (Dodge et al., 2018; Rosenblum & Muzik, 2014).

5.5 *Sesame Street for Military Families*

The Sesame Street for Military Families Initiatives is a bilingual (English/Spanish) multimedia experience that helps military families cope with the challenges that military deployments pose. The program focuses on building resilience when children are separated from their parent. Additionally, the program has workshops geared toward multiple deployments, homecomings, injuries, self-expression, and grief. Sesame Street for Military Families is an initiative that is under the Sesame Workshop, a leading expert in developing programs and materials for building resilience in children and families. Another program under Sesame Workshop is the Talk, Listen, Connect (TLC) program. TLC addresses deployment, military parent injury, and parental death. The program was found to be beneficial for military families and their children (Gewirtz et al., 2011; Sherman et al., 2018).

5.6 *Child–Parent Psychotherapy*

Child–Parent Psychotherapy (CPP) is a form of treatment used when young children go through behavioral, attachment, or mental health problems as a result of experiencing a traumatic event such as being separated from a primary caregiver (Osofsky & Chartrand, 2013). This form of treatment emphasizes the relationship between the child and parent/caregiver and aims to strengthen it. The goals of the treatment are to restore the child's sense of safety, to support the attachment relationship, and to improve the child's cognitive, emotional, and social functioning. CPP has been found to help military parents respond in a more sensitive manner to emotional cues presented by their children, as well as anticipating situations that may bring distress to both the parent and child while building empathy in the process (Osofsky & Chartrand, 2013). CPP significantly reduced stigma related to seeking mental health resources, as the program is provided at military bases.

5.7 *Family Advocacy Program*

The Family Advocacy Program (FAP) (Military OneSource, 2017) provides families with resources to prevent abuse and assist families if abuse has occurred. FAP consists of professionals who assist with families in many ways, including workshops and support programs for parents. FAP conducts investigations when abuse is alleged. New Parent Support Program uses licensed clinicians, nurses, and home-visit specialists who assist families with young children and provide them with resources (home visits, parenting classes, and community and department of defense resource information) to help with the parenting process and to lower the risk of abuse in the future.

6 Mobile Apps

Military deployments and the long distance can now be addressed through the use of mobile apps. Technology offers various components, such as messages, pictures, and video features that may enhance communication between the military members and their families.

6.1 Babies on the Homefront

This is an educational tool to assist parents with considering the age and developmental stage of the child and how they may be responding to their parent's deployment. The app also provides recommendations on how to respond to various behaviors the child may be exhibiting. Since younger children generally have a harder time than others, the caregiver can hone their attunement skills by watching and appropriately responding to their child's emotional state. The information presented in the app is based on the child's age and the deployment status of the military member. The app allows the at-home parent to share photos, videos, and messages with the deployed parent (Nolan et al., 2019).

6.2 The Big Moving Adventure

This app focuses on the relocation aspect of military life, which may cause significant stress for certain children and teens. The app offers a cognitive reframe for moving: an adventure. The app allows users to build an avatar and work through the process of identifying and exploring feelings, saying goodbye, and making new friends. The child chooses an emotion the avatar may be feeling and is then able to explore the other interpretations related to moving. This mechanism acts to bring balance to the child's negative cognitions. Additionally, this app offers psychoeducation to parents and incorporates discussion points related to informing the child about the move, moving, starting a new school, and managing emotions. This app may be helpful to enhance treatment and to promote practice and application outside of the therapy sessions (Nolan et al., 2019).

6.3 Sandboxx

One of the challenges of the military parent being away is that family members feel disconnected from their loved ones. Studies have shown that contact with the deployed parent reduces stress, supports healthy coping, and lowers the risk of the military member from developing PTSD and other mental health disorders. The app was developed by a team of civilians, military members, and veterans. Users are able to:

- Communicate with the military member
- Securely send messages and pictures between each other
- Scroll through news feeds with military news, articles, and other materials
- Print letters, track and overnight the letter with a return envelope to any recruiting base via Sandboxx
- Receive updates and milestones as recruits progress through basic training

It is recommended that the military member and family practice using the app as they prepare for deployment (Nolan et al., 2019).

There are a number of other apps, YouTube videos, and other resources available for military families. The clinician would benefit from exploring the resources and adding it to treatment to not only to enhance clinical services but to also provide a broad range of psychoeducation, tools, and skills. Parenting is a difficult task. Parenting in the midst of deployment and relocation is even more grueling and complicated. As military families face these encounters, they can use technology coupled with therapy and community resources to navigate and facilitate these unpredictable transitions. The mental health professional and other health care providers may also rise to this challenge by coming alongside these families with compassion, guidance, and wisdom as they traverse these challenges together.

References

Chandra, A. (2016). Parenting school-age children and adolescents through military deployments. In A. H. In Gewirtz & A. M. Youssef (Eds.), *Risk and resilience in military and veteran families* (1st ed., pp. 27–45). Springer. https://doi.org/10.1007/978-3-319-12556-5

Cederbaum, J. A., Gilreath, T. D., Benbenishty, R., Astor, R. A., Pineda, D., DePedro, K. T., Esqueda, M. C., & Atuel, H. (2014). Well-being and suicidal ideation of secondary school students from military families. *Journal of Adolescent Health, 54*(6), 672–677. https://doi.org/10.1016/j.jadohealth.2013.09.006

Clever, M., & Segal, D. R. (2013). The demographics of military children and families. *The Future of Children, 23*(2), 13–39. https://doi.org/10.1353/foc.2013.0018

"Demographics of the U.S. military". (2020). *Council on Foreign Relations*. Retrieved from https://www.cfr.org/backgrounder/demographics-us-military

DiNallo, J., Kuhl, M., Borden, L. M., & Perkins, D. (2016). Interventions to support and strengthen parenting in military families: State of the evidence. In A. H. In Gewirtz & A. M. Youssef (Eds.), *Rise and resilience in military and veteran families* (1st ed., pp. 195–212). Springer. https://doi.org/10.1007/978-3-319-12556-5

Dodge, J., Gonzalez, M., Muzik, M., & Rosenblum, K. (2018). Fathers' perspectives on strengthening military families: A mixed method evaluation of a 10-week resiliency building program. *Clinical Social Work Journal, 46*(2), 145–155. https://doi.org/10.1007/s10615-017-0641-6

Easterbrooks, M., Ginsburg, K., & Lerner, R. M. (2013). Resilience among military youth. *The Future of Children, 23*(2), 99–120. https://doi.org/10.1353/foc.2013.0014

Gewirtz, A. H., Erbes, C. R., Polusny, M. A., Forgatch, M. S., & DeGarmo, D. S. (2011). Helping military families through the deployment process: Strategies to support parenting. *Professional Psychology, Research, and Practice, 42*(1), 36–62.

Gewirtz, A. H., Degarmo, D. S., & Zamir, O. (2017). After deployment, adaptive parenting tools: 1-year outcomes of an evidence-based parenting program for military families following deployment. *Prevention Science, 19*(4), 589–599. https://doi.org/10.1007/s11121-017-0839-4

Gorman, G. H., Eide, M., & Hisle-Gorman, E. (2010). Wartime military deployment and increased pediatric mental and behavioral health complaints. *Pediatrics, 126*(6), 1058–1066. https://doi.org/10.1542/peds.2009-2856

Gorman, G., & Hisle-Gorman, M. (2010). Wartime military deployment and increased pediatric mental and behavioral health complaints. *Pediatrics, 127*(2). https://doi.org/10.1542/peds.2009-2856d

Hodges, D. W. F., & Bloom, D. B. L. (1984). Parent's report of children's adjustment to marital separation. *Journal of Divorce, 8*(1), 33–50. https://doi.org/10.1300/j279v08n01_03

Huebner, C. R. (2019). Health and mental health needs of children in US military families. *Pediatrics, 143*(1), e20183258. https://doi-org.ezproxy.libraries.wright.edu/10.1542/peds.2018-3258

Jensen, P. S., Hoagwood, K., & Petti, T. (1996). Outcomes of mental health care for children and adolescents: II. Literature review and application of a comprehensive model. *Journal of the American Academy of Child & Adolescent Psychiatry, 35*(8), 1064–1077. https://doi.org/10.1097/00004583-199608000-00018

Julian, M.M., Muzik, M., Kees, M., Valenstein, M., Dexter, C., Rosenblum. (2018). Intervention effects on reflectivity explain change in positive parenting in military families with young children. *Journal of Family Psychology, 32*(6), 804–815. http://dx.doi.org/10.1037/fam0000431

Kelly, Y. J., Nazroo, J. Y., McMunn, A., Boreham, R., & Marmot, M. (2001). Birthweight and behavioural problems in children: a modifiable effect? *International Journal of Epidemiology, 30*(1), 88–94. https://doi.org/10.1093/ije/30.1.88

Kritikos, T. K., Comer, J. S., He, M., Curren, L. C., & Tompson, M. C. (2019). Combat experience and posttraumatic stress symptoms among military-serving parents: A meta-analytic examination of associated offspring and family outcomes. *Journal of Abnormal Child Psychology, 47*, 131–148. https://doi.org/10.1007/s10802-018-0427-5

Lester, P., Aralis, H., Sinclair, M., Kiff, C., Kyung-Hee, L., Mustillo, S., Wadsworth, S. (2016). The impact of deployment on parental, family, and child adjustment in military families. *Child Psychiatry & Human Development, 47*, 938–949. https://doi.org/10.1007/s10578-016-0624-9

Lester, P., Peterson, K., Reeves, J., Knauss, L., Glover, D., Mogil, C., & Beardslee, W. (2010). The long war and parental combat deployment: Effects on military children and at-home spouses. *Journal of the American Academy of Child & Adolescent Psychiatry, 49*(4), 310–320. https://doi.org/10.1016/j.jaac.2010.01.003

Lieberman, A. F., & Van Horn, P. (2011). *Psychotherapy with infants and young children: Repairing the effects of stress and trauma on early attachment* (Reprint ed.). The Guilford Press.

Lipari, R., Palen, L., Ashley, O. S., Penne, M., Kan, M., & Pemberton, M. (2017). Examination of veteran fathers' parenting and their adolescent children's substance use in the United States. *Substance Use & Misuse., 52*(6), 698–708. https://doi.org/10.1080/10826084.2016.1253748

Mansfield, A. J., Kaufman, J. S., Marshall, S. W., Gaynes, B. N., Morrissey, J. P., & Engel, C. C. (2010). Deployment and the use of mental health services among U.S. army wives. *New England Journal of Medicine, 362*(2), 101–109. https://doi.org/10.1056/nejmoa0900177

Meadows, S. O., Tanielian, T. L., & Karney, B. R. (2016). *The deployment life study: Longitudinal analysis of military families across the deployment cycle*. RAND Corporation.

Military families resources for young children: sesame street. (n.d.). Retrieved July 26, 2020, from https://sesamestreetformilitaryfamilies.org/

Military OneSource. (2017). 2014 Demographics: Profile of the Military Community.

Millegan, J., Mclay, R., & Engel, C. (2014). The effect of geographic moves on mental healthcare utilization in children. *Journal of Adolescent Health, 55*(2), 276–280. https://doi.org/10.1016/j.jadohealth.2014.01.009

Monn, A. R., Zhang, N., & Gewirtz, A. H. (2018). Deficits in inhibitory control may place service members at risk for posttraumatic stress disorder and negative parenting behavior following deployment-related trauma. *Journal of Traumatic Stress, 31*, 866–875. https://doi.org/10.1002/jts.22351

Mustillo, S., Wadsworth, S. M., & Lester, P. (2015). Parental deployment and well-being in children. *Journal of Emotional and Behavioral Disorders, 24*(2), 82–91. https://doi.org/10.1177/1063426615598766

Nolan, J., Lindeman, S., & Varghese, F. P. (2019). Mobile app interventions for military and veteran families: Before, during, and after deployment. *American Psychological Association, 16*(2), 208–212. https://doi.org/10.1037/ser000027

O'Grady, A. E., Whiteman, S. D., Cardin, J., & Wadsworth, S. M. (2018). Changes in parenting and youth adjustment across the military deployment cycle. *Journal of Marriage and Family, 80*, 569–581. https://doi.org/10.1111/jomf.12457

O'Neal, C. W., Mallette, J. K., & Mancini, J. A. (2018). The importance of parents' community connections for adolescent well-being: An examination of military families. *American Journal of Community Psychology, 61*, 204–217.

Osofsky, J. D., & Chartrand, L. C. (2013). Military children from birth to five years. *The Future of Children, 23*(2), 61–77. https://doi.org/10.1353/foc.2013.0011

Padden, D., & Agazio, J. (2013). Caring for military families across the deployment cycle. *Journal of Emergency Nursing, 39*(6), 562–569. https://doi.org/10.1016/j.jen.2013.08.004

Paley, B., Lester, P., & Mogil, C. (2013). Family systems and ecological perspectives on the impact of deployment on military families. *Clinical Child and Family Psychology Review, 16*(3), 245–265. https://doi.org.ezproxy.libraries.wright.edu/10.1007/s10567-013-0138-y

Palmer, C. (2008). A theory of risk and resilience factors in military families. *Military Psychology, 20*, 205–217.

Rosenblum, K. L., & Muzik, M. (2014). STRoNG intervention for military families with young children. *Psychiatric Services, 65*(3), 399–399. https://doi.org/10.1176/appi.ps.650302

Services. (n.d.). Retrieved July 26, 2020, from https://focusproject.org/services-0

Sherman, M. D., Monn, A., Larsen, J. L., & Gewirtz, A. (2018). Evaluation of a Sesame Street multimedia intervention for families transitioning out of the military. *Journal of Child and Family Studies, 27*(8), 2533–2540. https://doi.org/10.1007/s10826-018-1083-7

Sories, F., Maier, C., Beer, A., & Thomas, V. (2015). Addressing the needs of military children through family-based play therapy. *Contemporary Family Therapy, 37*, 209–220. https://doi.org/10.1007/s10591-015-9342-x

Stepka, P., & Callahan, K. (2016). The impact of military life on young children and their parents. In A. H. In Gewirtz & A. M. Youssef (Eds.), *Risk and resilience in military and veteran families* (1st ed., pp. 11–26). Springer. https://doi.org/10.1007/978-3-319-12556-5

The military family advocacy program. (n.d.). Retrieved July 26, 2020, from https://www.militaryonesource.mil/family-relationships/family-life/preventing-abuse-neglect/the-family-advocacy-program

Transitioning to parents: The new parent support program. (n.d.). Retrieved July 26, 2020, from https://www.militaryonesource.mil/family-relationships/parenting-and-children/parenting-infants-and-toddlers/the-new-parent-support-program

Wadsworth, S. M., Cardin, J., Christ, S., Willerton, E., O'Grady, A. F., Topp, D., Coppola, E., Lester, P., & Mustillo, S. (2016). Accumulation of risk and promotive factors among young children in U.S. military families. *American Journal of Community Psychology, 57*, 190–101.

Walsh, T. B., Dayton, C. J., Erwin, M. S., Muzik, M., Busuito, A., & Rosenblum, K. L. (2014). Fathering after military deployment: Parenting challenges and goals of fathers of young children. *Health & Social Work, 39*(1), 35–44. https://doi.org/10.1093/hsw/hlu005

Wexler, H. K., & McGrath, E. (1991). Family member stress reactions to military involvement separation. *Psychotherapy: Theory, Research, Practice, Training, 28*(3), 515–519. https://doi.org/10.1037/0033-3204.28.3.515

Index

L. C. James et al. (eds.), *Clinical Health Psychology in Military and Veteran Settings*, https://doi.org/10.1007/978-3-031-12063-3

The manufacturer's authorised representative in the EU is Springer Nature Customer Service Centre GmbH, Europaplatz 3, 69115 Heidelberg, Germany. If you have any concerns regarding our products, please contact ProductSafety@springernature.com

Printed and bound by CPI Group (UK) Ltd, Croydon, CR0 4YY
30/09/2026
02225244-0007